Nursing Care: Concepts, Connections and Skills

Nursing Care: Concepts, Connections and Skills

Editor: Jim Carrey

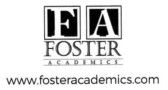

www.fosteracademics.com

www.fosteracademics.com

Cataloging-in-Publication Data

Nursing care : concepts, connections and skills / edited by Jim Carrey.
     p. cm.
Includes bibliographical references and index.
ISBN 978-1-64646-617-7
1. Nursing. 2. Nursing care plans. 3. Nursing--Practice. 4. Nursing services. 5. Medical care. I. Carrey, Jim.
RT41 .N87 2023
610.73--dc23

Foster Academics,
118-35 Queens Blvd., Suite 400,
Forest Hills, NY 11375, USA

ISBN 978-1-64646-617-7 (Hardback)

This book contains information obtained from authentic and highly regarded sources. Copyright for all individual chapters remain with the respective authors as indicated. All chapters are published with permission under the Creative Commons Attribution License or equivalent. A wide variety of references are listed. Permission and sources are indicated; for detailed attributions, please refer to the permissions page and list of contributors. Reasonable efforts have been made to publish reliable data and information, but the authors, editors and publisher cannot assume any responsibility for the validity of all materials or the consequences of their use.

Trademark Notice: Registered trademark of products or corporate names are used only for explanation and identification without intent to infringe.

Contents

Preface

This book aims to highlight the current researches and provides a platform to further the scope of innovations in this area. This book is a product of the combined efforts of many researchers and scientists, after going through thorough studies and analysis from different parts of the world. The objective of this book is to provide the readers with the latest information of the field.

Nursing care comprises collaborative and autonomous care of individuals of all ages, groups and communities in all settings. The primary objective of nursing care is to promote well-being and prevent illness. It is also responsible for providing emotional and psychological support to ill, disabled and dying people. There are various tasks performed by within nursing that includes the assessment of patients, conducting medical tests and creation of treatment plans. Some of the key skills which fall under the umbrella of this discipline are leadership, ability to stay calm, enthusiasm for learning, interpersonal skills and problem solving ability. This book unravels the concepts, connections and skills required for delivering nursing care. A number of latest researches have been included to keep the readers up-to-date with the global concepts in this area of study. The book is appropriate for students seeking detailed information in this area as well as for experts.

I would like to express my sincere thanks to the authors for their dedicated efforts in the completion of this book. I acknowledge the efforts of the publisher for providing constant support. Lastly, I would like to thank my family for their support in all academic endeavors.

Editor

The Nursing Performance Instrument: Exploratory and Confirmatory Factor Analyses in Registered Nurses

Knar Sagherian[1]* • Linsey M. Steege[2] • Jeanne Geiger-Brown[3] • Donna Harrington[4]

ABSTRACT

Background: The optimal performance of nurses in healthcare settings plays a critical role in care quality and patient safety. Despite this importance, few measures are provided in the literature that evaluate nursing performance as an independent construct from competencies. The nine-item Nursing Performance Instrument (NPI) was developed to fill this gap.

Purpose: The aim of this study was to examine and confirm the underlying factor structure of the NPI in registered nurses.

Method: The design was cross-sectional, using secondary data collected between February 2008 and April 2009 for the "Fatigue in Nursing Survey" ($N = 797$). The sample was predominantly dayshift female nurses working in acute care settings. Using Mplus software, exploratory and confirmatory factor analyses were applied to the NPI data, which were divided into two equal subsamples. Multiple fit indices were used to evaluate the fit of the alternative models.

Results: The three-factor model was determined to fit the data adequately. The factors that were labeled as "physical/mental decrements," "consistent practice," and "behavioral change" were moderately to strongly intercorrelated, indicating good convergent validity. The reliability coefficients for the subscales were acceptable.

Conclusions/Implications for Practice: The NPI consists of three latent constructs. This instrument has the potential to be used as a self-monitoring instrument that addresses nurses' perceptions of performance while providing patient care.

KEY WORDS:
nursing performance instrument (NPI), measures, validity, factor analysis.

Introduction

Nursing performance is an important measure of work productivity and patient safety. At the bedside, nurses are responsible for assessing and monitoring patients' changing conditions, coordinating their care, administering medications precisely, and communicating with the patients and their families (Battisto, Pak, Vander Wood, & Pilcher, 2009; Westbrook, Duffield, Li, & Creswick, 2011).

Thus, changes in their vigilance and performance may result in detrimental patient outcomes such as medical errors (Scott, Rogers, Hwang, & Zhang, 2006) and may deter the patients' recovery process and result in early discharge from the hospital (Zhan & Miller, 2003).

Highly stressful nursing work (Golubic, Milosevic, Knezevic, & Mustajbegovic, 2009) taxes the physical, mental, and perceptual abilities of the individual. Nurses who work long hours (Rogers, Hwang, Scott, Aiken, & Dinges, 2004), are fatigued or sleep deprived (Dorrian et al., 2008; Geiger-Brown et al., 2012), have high workloads (Aiken, Clarke, Sloane, Sochalski, & Silber, 2002; Montgomery, 2007), or encounter frequent interruptions (Hayes, Jackson, Davidson, & Power, 2015) are more likely to experience performance decrements during work hours that affect the timely provision and safe delivery of patient care.

Evaluating nursing work performance is a challenge because the construct is poorly defined in the literature and mostly operationalized in terms of competencies, nursing-sensitive quality indicators, and task-specific performance measures (DeLucia, Ott, & Palmieri, 2009). Competencies and task-specific measures that focus primarily on knowledge and skills (Zhang, Luk, Arthur, & Wong, 2001) are limited in terms of their ability to capture performance changes during work as they are either administered once when entering into the profession or periodically. Nursing-sensitive quality indicators are used to indicate the quality of nursing care or practices that patients receive through patient outcomes such as pressure ulcers, nosocomial infections, or falls (Idvall, Rooke, & Hamrin, 1997). However, these indicators are unit level measures that do not assess the individual performance of the nurse. Moreover, most of these indicators have a lag time between the provision of nursing care and the outcome.

There are few nursing performance instruments in the literature. The King's Nurse Performance scale is a competency checklist of observable nursing actions that is rated by an observer using 53 items in seven domains (e.g., physical,

[1]PhD, RN, Assistant Professor, College of Nursing, The University of Tennessee Knoxville, USA • [2]PhD, Assistant Professor, School of Nursing, University of Wisconsin-Madison, USA • [3]PhD, RN, Associate Dean for Research, School of Nursing, George Washington University, USA • [4]PhD, Professor, School of Social Work, University of Maryland, Baltimore, USA.

psychosocial, professional, teaching skills, and communication). However, this scale has been shown to have poor psychometric properties (Fitzpatrick, While, & Roberts, 1997). The Six Dimensional Scale of Nursing Performance by Schwirian (1978) is a reliable and valid instrument consisting of 52 items in six domains: leadership, critical care, planning and evaluation, interpersonal relations, and professional development. However, this scale includes 42 items that must be rated twice for the frequency and quality of the behaviors, which makes this a lengthy and time-consuming measure to complete. The Nurse Competence scale is another lengthy self-assessment tool consisting of 73 items divided into seven domains that measure nursing competence across the novice-to-expert continuum. It is considered reliable and valid, and the scale scores have been strongly correlated with Schwirian's nursing performance scale ($r = .83$, $p < .001$; Meretoja, Isoaho, & Leino-Kilpi, 2004). Thus, there is a need for short and psychometrically sound measures of nursing performance.

The Nursing Performance Instrument (NPI) is a self-rated, brief measure of work performance. The NPI consists of nine items that are not specific to any specialty area (e.g., intensive care, pediatrics) and represent behaviors or actions that are practiced by nurses when providing patient care. Nursing performance has been defined as a set of nursing activities or behaviors that are performed by nurses and directed toward the recovery and well-being of the patients assigned to their care. The main purpose is to meet the needs and expectations of the patients through this set of activities. The NPI was developed based on a conceptual framework of work performance that consists of task and contextual performance dimensions. In the occupational literature, task performance is job specific and prescriptive in nature and refers to a worker's ability to perform a set of tasks efficiently (Koopmans et al., 2011). For nurses, these tasks consist of direct patient care activities (e.g., intravenous access, medication administration, physical assessment, patient teaching), indirect patient care (e.g., documentation and communication, coordination of care, medication preparation), and tasks that are unrelated to nursing (e.g., waiting or searching for equipment; Battisto et al., 2009; DeLucia et al., 2009). Nursing task performance is focused on direct and indirect nursing tasks or activities that are geared toward or contribute the most to the care and recovery of the patients. These activities are either physical and/or mental in nature, with varying degrees of complexity. On the other hand, contextual performance is common across occupations. It is related to interpersonal relations, personality traits, and effective communication and is discretionary in nature. These are a set of proactive behaviors that provide psychosocial and organizational support to the work environment (Koopmans et al., 2011). In nursing, contextual performance includes a set of behaviors or practices that are common across nursing units and hospitals. Nurses perform these general practices (e.g., patient identification before administering

medications) to maintain nursing standards and support the safety and quality of patient care.

At the developmental stage of the NPI, Barker and her research team reviewed several existing performance measures: the Schwirian Six Dimension Scale of Nursing Performance (Schwirian, 1978), the Modified Scale of Nursing Performance (Battersby & Hemmings, 1991), the Self Report of Competence (Garland, 1996), and the Physician Mental Workload Measure (Bertram et al., 1992). In addition, the team reviewed the Work Limitations questionnaire, which is used to evaluate the abilities of workers in terms of mental and physical demands (Lerner et al., 2001). This scale was administered previously to investigate the relationship between low back pain and work performance in nurses (Denis, Shannon, Wessel, Stratford, & Weller, 2007). Twenty-nine items were adapted from the existing measures. Having in mind the dynamic nature of work performance, items that capture changes in behaviors or practices were created and included in the NPI as well. The initial NPI item list was sent for review to a panel of experts that consisted of nursing staff and members from the Board of Directors of the Virginia Nurses Association. The panel evaluated the NPI on content, readability, and clarity of both the items and the provided instructions. On the basis of their feedback, 20 items were removed or consolidated, and the final measure consisted of nine items on a 6-point Likert scale ranging from 1 = *strongly disagree* to 6 = *strongly agree*. At the final stage, two nurses reviewed the new NPI independently and approved the final version for use with registered nurses (Barker & Nussbaum, 2011). This process established the face and content validity of the NPI.

The factor structure of the NPI was hypothesized to consist of three domains: physical (Items 1, 4, and 8) and mental (Items 5 and 7) nursing tasks that are concept mapped to task performance and general performance tasks (Items 2, 3, 6, and 9) that are concept mapped to contextual performance. The purposes of this study were to (a) examine the underlying factor structure of the NPI and (b) confirm its factor structure in two samples of registered nurses.

Method

Design

The NPI data set for this secondary data analysis was from the Fatigue in Nursing Survey Set (Barker & Nussbaum, 2011). The original cross-sectional study aimed to explore perceived dimensions and states of fatigue and their relationship with perceived performance in a convenience sample of registered nurses in the United States.

Sample

One thousand nurses from different healthcare facilities (e.g., acute care hospitals, psychiatric facilities, educational settings, and long-term care) completed the online survey between February 2008 and April 2009. The details of the original study are presented elsewhere (Barker & Nussbaum, 2011). Two hundred three nurses had missing responses on the entire nine NPI items, resulting in a sample of 797 for the current study. There were no significant differences between the respondents and nonrespondents based on age, gender, marital status, education, hours of sleep, nursing experience, hours of work per week, and time spent on direct patient care. Details of these analyses are available from the author upon request.

Measure

Nursing performance instrument
The NPI consists of nine items on a 6-point Likert scale (1 = *strongly disagree* to 6 = *strongly agree*). These items address physical (1, 4, 8), mental (5, 7), and general (2, 3, 6, 9) tasks of performance during a work shift. Items 1, 2, 5, 7, and 9 are reverse coded, with higher item mean scores indicating higher nursing performance. The Cronbach's alpha in our sample (N = 797) for the total scale was .80.

Data Analysis

Descriptive statistics and exploratory data analyses were conducted using IBM SPSS Statistics Version 22.0 (IBM Inc., Armonk, NY, USA). The average missingness for the NPI items was 1.42% (range = 0.6%–2.8%). The average missingness for demographic and work-related variables was 1.34% (range = 0.3%–5.1%). Because missing data were less than the cutoff point of 5.0%, imputation was not necessary. The Little's missing completely at random (MCAR) test was not significant (χ^2 = 160.92, df = 138, p = .089), indicating that the missingness was randomly distributed across observations. In SPSS, the data set (N = 797) was randomly split into two equal subsamples. Independent samples t tests and chi-square statistics were examined to ensure that the two subsamples were comparable on sample characteristics and NPI items. There were no significant differences between the two subsamples (see Table 1 for the NPI items). The internal consistency reliability of the NPI subscales in the exploratory factor analysis (EFA) data was assessed using Cronbach's alpha. A value of ≥ .70 was considered acceptable (Nunnally, 1978) for a newly developed measure with subscales consisting of three items.

Using Mplus Version 7.31 (MPlus, Muthén & Muthén, Los Angeles, CA, USA), EFA and confirmatory factor analysis (CFA) were conducted. Because of the Likert-type scale, where response categories range from "*strongly disagree*" to "*strongly agree*," the data were treated as ordered categorical when the model parameters were estimated in Mplus. Missing data were handled with pairwise deletion when using the weighted least squares means and variance adjusted (WLSMV) estimator (Muthén & Muthén, 2010).

In the first random sample (n = 399), EFA using the oblique rotation (geomin) and the WLSMV estimator was conducted to identify the initial factor structure of the NPI scale. Oblique rotations allow for correlations between the hypothesized constructs (Costello & Osborne, 2005), and the WLSMV estimator is appropriate for the ordered categorical nature of the data in this study (Schmitt, 2011). Factor extraction was based on eigenvalues ≥ 1, the scree plot, multiple model fit indices (root mean square error of approximation [RMSEA] ≤ .06, comparative fit index [CFI] ≥ .95, and Tucker–Lewis Index [TLI] ≥ .95), and factor interpretability based on content (Costello & Osborne, 2005; Schmitt, 2011). Items with ≥ .40 factor loadings were included with their corresponding factor structures. Loadings less than .40 were considered weak, and loadings greater than .60 were considered strong (Costello & Osborne, 2005). If an item loaded on two factors, the item was assigned to the factor with the highest loading.

In the second random sample (n = 398), first-order (one, two, and three factors) and second-order CFA models were examined to confirm the structure of the NPI. Four fit indices (chi-square, RMSEA, CFI, and TLI) were evaluated to determine how well the models fit the ordinal categorical data.

Ethical Considerations

The institutional review board of the University of Maryland determined this secondary data analysis as nonhuman subjects research.

Results

The nurses in the total sample were mostly female (n = 745, 94.1%), White (n = 703, 88.9%), married (n = 531, 67.4%), and with a 4-year baccalaureate degree (n = 342, 43.7%). Nearly two thirds were 51–60 years old (n = 247, 31.1%), and slightly fewer were 41–50 years old (n = 216, 27.2%). Around 38.0% of the nurses (n = 295) reported sleeping 6–7 hours per day. However, more than one quarter of the sample (n = 231, 29.2%) reported sleeping less than 6 hours per day. More than three quarters worked in acute care settings (n = 651, 82.3%), and one quarter had more than 25 years of nursing experience (n = 215, 27.5%), followed by 1–5 years of nursing experience (n = 144, 18.4%). Day shifts were the most predominant work schedule (n = 402, 50.6%), and more than half of the sample worked 11–12 or more hours per shift (n = 474, 59.8%). Half of the sample (n = 391, 49.9%) reported spending 76%–100% of their time on direct patient care, and one fifth of the sample (n = 154, 19.7%) reported spending 51%–75% of their time on this activity. Over half reported working 21–40 hours during the week (n = 462, 58.3%), and two thirds reported working 41–60 hours during the week (n = 265, 33.5%).

TABLE 1.

Descriptive Statistics of NPI Items for Randomly Split Half-Samples of Online Survey Nurses (N = 797)

Variable	Subsample for EFA (n = 399)		Subsample for CFA (n = 398)		t	p
	M	SD	M	SD		
NPI 1: During a work shift, changes in my muscle strength, endurance, or physical energy affect my ability to perform physical tasks associated with my job (e.g., carry items, perform patient handling tasks, walk/drive from patient to patient, etc.).	3.64	1.51	3.63	1.48	0.083	.934
NPI 2: I sometimes find it necessary to take shortcuts in patient care.	4.00	1.50	4.03	1.41	−0.273	.785
NPI 3: I always apply the "5 rights" principle when administering medications to the patients.	5.06	1.12	5.00	1.12	0.834	.405
NPI 4: Throughout a work shift, I am able to perform fine motor tasks (e.g., inserting an IV, catheter insertion, medication preparation, etc.) with no difficulty.	4.99	0.98	4.97	0.96	0.295	.768
NPI 5: During a work shift, changes in my concentration or alertness affect my ability to perform patient monitoring, medication administration, and documentation tasks.	3.77	1.52	3.77	1.43	−0.048	.962
NPI 6: I am always able to carry out safe nursing practice.	4.69	1.18	4.62	1.15	0.784	.433
NPI 7: During a work shift, changes in my mood, mental energy, or attentiveness affect my ability to communicate clearly and effectively (e.g., express my opinions, understand what others are saying, etc.) with other nurses, physicians, clinicians, patients, or family members.	3.32	1.48	3.35	1.38	−0.281	.778
NPI 8: I always follow existing facility guidelines for safe patient handling (e.g., use of lift devices, two-person lifts, etc.).	4.35	1.34	4.38	1.25	−0.324	.746
NPI 9: I am sometimes forced to modify my standards to get the work done.	3.61	1.54	3.67	1.47	−0.614	.539

Note. Items 1, 2, 5, 7, and 9 are reverse coded. Higher scores indicate better or higher performance. EFA = exploratory factor analysis; CFA = confirmatory factor analysis; NPI = Nursing Performance Instrument.

Item Means

On average, the nurses' responses on eight of the nine NPI items were above the 3.5 midpoint of response scale. Overall, the sample perceived an absence of performance problems in areas that related to accomplishing physical tasks (NPI 1) and safe patient handling (NPI 8). There were possible ceiling effects on the NPI 3 ("always apply the '5 rights' when administering medications to the patients"; $M = 5.03$, $SD = 1.12$) and NPI 4 ("perform fine motor tasks with no difficulty"; $M = 4.98$, $SD = 0.97$) items. One item earned a mean score of 3.33 ($SD = 1.43$), with nurses reporting experiencing some communication problems with patients and healthcare team members because of changes in their mental energy, attentiveness, and mood during shift work.

Exploratory Factor Analysis

The scree plot indicated a three-factor structure. On the other hand, two factors were extracted based on eigen-values greater than 1 (4.0 and 1.3). The third factor had an eigenvalue of .96. Therefore, we examined the model fit indices of one-, two-, and three-factor structures, as shown in Table 2. The one-factor model did not fit the data based on a significant and high χ^2 of 376.31 and the low fit indices of CFI and TLI (below the cut point of .95). The RMSEA and standardized root mean square residual indicated areas of misfit in the residuals as well. The two-factor model had slightly improved fit indices, although the fit indices still did not reach the guidelines for adequate fit. The three-factor structure yielded an adequate fit to the data, with χ^2 remaining significant despite its decline to 60.07. The CFI and TLI fit indices increased to .979 and .936, respectively. The standardized root mean square residual was .029, indicating a good fit in standardized residuals, although the RMSEA of .100 indicated a mediocre fit in the errors.

The results in Table 3 indicate that the nine NPI items had significant factor loadings of greater than .40 in the

TABLE 2.
Model Fit Statistics Values in EFA and CFA

	χ^2	df	RMSEA	95% CI	CFI	TLI	SRMR
EFA (n = 399)							
One-factor	376.31**	27	.180	[0.164, 0.196]**	.845	.794	.098
Two-factor	223.21**	19	.164	[0.145, 0.184]**	.910	.829	.059
Three-factor	60.07**	12	.100	[0.076, 0.126]*	.979	.936	.029
CFA (n = 398)							
One-factor	527.35**	27	.213	[0.200, 0.232]**	.766	.687	-
Three-factor	96.62**	24	.087	[0.069, 0.106]**	.966	.949	-

Note. SRMR is not reported for CFA when data are treated as ordinal categorical and the WLSMV estimator is used. EFA = exploratory factor analysis; CFA = confirmatory factor analysis; df = degrees of freedom; CI = confidence interval; RMSEA = root mean square error of approximation; CFI = comparative fit index; TLI = Tucker–Lewis index; SRMR = standardized root mean square residual.
*p < .01. **p < .001.

one-, two-, and three-factor models. There was no cross-loading of items between the factors. In the one-factor model, item factor loadings were significant and ranged from .452 to .782. Similarly, in the two-factor model, the item factor loadings were significant and, in the expected direction, range from .42 to .86. However, neither of these models showed adequate fit, and they were not interpreted further.

On the basis of the adequate fit indices, we interpreted the model with the three factors and assigned labels based on the overall content they represented. In the three-factor structure, Factor 1, labeled "consistent practice," included NPI 3 ("5 rights principle"), NPI 4 ("perform motor tasks"), NPI 6 ("safe nursing practice"), and NPI 8 ("follow facility guidelines"). Factor 2, labeled "behavioral change," included NPI 2 ("take shortcuts") and NPI 9 ("modify standards"). Factor 3, labeled "physical/mental decrements," included NPI 1 ("perform physical tasks"), NPI 5 ("changes in concentration"), and NPI 7 ("changes in mental energy"). The three factors were found to have

moderate-to-strong correlations and significant intercorrelations. The correlations between steady performance with behavioral change and physical/mental decrements were moderate ($r_{1,2}$ = .463, $r_{1,3}$ = .435). Similarly, the correlation between behavioral change and physical/mental decrements was moderate to strong ($r_{2,3}$ = .585, p < .05). These relationships are in the expected direction.

Confirmatory Factor Analysis

The unidimensional structure of the NPI was examined as recommended by Kline (2011), and as expected, the model did not fit the data well. None of the fit indices were in the acceptable range (see Table 2). We interpreted the three-factor model (see Figure 1) based on the model fit indices that yielded adequate fit to the data. These findings were similar with the three-factor EFA. The χ^2 decreased to 96.62 but, however, remained significant. The CFI and TLI met the cutoff scores of ≥ .95, and the RMSEA of .087 suggested reasonable errors of approximation.

TABLE 3.
EFA Item Factor Standardized Loadings (N = 399)

NPI Item	One-Factor	Two-Factor Factor 1	Two-Factor Factor 2	Three-Factor Factor 1	Three-Factor Factor 2	Three-Factor Factor 3
NPI 1	.581*	.631*	−.001	−.011	.128	.553*
NPI 2	.666*	.436*	.343*	.054	.756*	−.011
NPI 3	.556*	−.072	.773*	.792*	.011	−.046
NPI 4	.452*	.134*	.416*	.484*	−.116	.223*
NPI 5	.782*	.783*	.062	.087	.117	.692*
NPI 6	.631*	.127*	.646*	.559*	.244*	.018
NPI 7	.753*	.861*	−.060	−.018	−.012	.895*
NPI 8	.533*	.002	.653*	.613*	.099	−.012
NPI 9	.694*	.481*	.326*	−.010	.805*	.035

Note. The bolded values indicate item factor loadings greater than .40. EFA = exploratory factor analysis.
*p < .05.

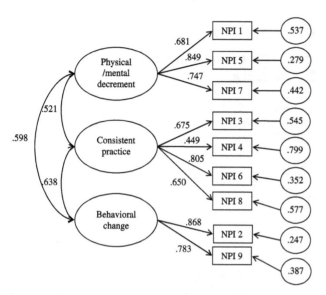

Figure 1. Confirmatory factor analysis of three-factor model standardized loadings (*N* = 398).

Eight of the NPI items had strong standardized factor loadings (> .60) with their corresponding latent constructs. Only one item, NPI 4 ("throughout a work shift I am able to perform fine motor tasks...without difficulty"), had a factor loading of < .60 but still > .40. The magnitude of the estimated correlations between the three latent constructs was considered moderate to strong (Cohen, 1988), and the directions were as expected. The relationships between physical/mental decrement and both consistent practice and behavioral change were .52 and .60, respectively. The relationship between consistent practice and behavioral change was .64. These correlations indicate good convergent validity, as they measure related aspects of nursing performance. Brown (2015) notes that factor correlations > .85 suggest "problematic discriminant validity" (p. 146). The factor correlations in this study were well below this criterion, suggesting adequate discriminant validity for the three factors.

Because the chi-square was significant and the RMSEA was slightly higher than desired, we examined the modification indices for the three-factor model. Having three modification indices suggested adding cross-loadings to improve model fit. However, in the absence of strong theoretical hypotheses and supportive literature, these changes were not made. Finally, we ran a second-order, three-factor model that showed statistically equivalent fit indices with the three-factor model. We adopted the three-factor model to avoid further model complexity and to be consistent with the literature on work performance.

Reliability

The Cronbach's alpha for the physical/mental decrement factor was .77. The Cronbach's alpha for the consistent practice factor was .69, almost at the cutoff point of .70.

These values are considered acceptable for newly developed scales (Nunnally, 1978).

Discussion

This is the first study to examine the underlying factor structure of the NPI in registered nurses. The findings from EFA and CFA support an NPI structure with three factors. These factors represent physical/mental decrements, consistent practice, and behavioral change constructs. Multiple goodness-of-fit indices were used to identify particular aspects of fit during the evaluation process of the one-, two-, and three-factor models. In EFA, the three-factor model indicated an adequate fit to the data. As shown in Table 2, these results were similar to the fit indices for the CFA three-factor model. The areas of misfit were related to the residuals where RMSEA indicated a mediocre fit to the data. The values for the χ^2 statistics showed a large decline, indicating an improvement of fit with subsequent models. It is possible that the remaining misfit may be related to the two underdeveloped constructs in the model that consist of two and three items only (Byrne, 2011).

The three factors with their corresponding items partially supported the factor structure that was hypothesized by the developers of the NPI. NPI 1 (physical performance) and NPIs 5 and 7 (mental performance) held together in the EFA. Conceptually, these items represent nursing tasks irrespective of their nature under the umbrella of nursing task performance in the study's adopted theoretical framework. NPIs 4 and 8 (physical performance) and NPIs 3 and 6 (general performance) also held together. These sets of items conceptually represent the contextual nursing performance in our theoretical framework. Interestingly, NPI 2 (take shortcuts) and NPI 9 (modify standards) represented a separate factor that indicated a form of behavioral change. In the literature, researchers such as Viswesvaran and Ones (2000) and Rotundo (2002) added the additional dimension of counterproductive work behavior to the conceptual framework of work performance that consists of task and contextual domains. This concept identifies certain employee behaviors that may cause harm to the organization. Examples of counterproductive behaviors include taking longer breaks, doing tasks incorrectly, disregarding safety, accidents, absenteeism, and presenteeism, among others (Koopmans et al., 2011). In healthcare, nurses may modify nursing standards or safety measures (e.g., patient identification, handwashing) to complete their work under workload-related time pressures (Gurses, Carayon, & Wall, 2009).

The directional relationships between the three latent constructs in nursing performance were in concordance with the relationships between the task, contextual, and counterproductive performance dimensions reported in the related literature (Koopmans et al., 2011). This provides confidence in the NPI's three subscales and its use in nursing performance studies.

In this study, the means for individual items were not interpreted in detail. However, there were possible ceiling effects in the items representing steady performance. A possible explanation relates to the 6-point response scale that may polarize nurses' responses. Conceptually, these items indicate that nurses, irrespective of being fatigued or being at the peak of their optimal performance, perceive their performances to be consistent and stable when implementing hospital policies and nursing standards. It is possible that these items are capturing social desirability in nurses that may be influenced by punitive or blaming environments when medical errors or undesirable events take place.

Limitations

One limitation of this study relates to the convenience sample that was used. The nurses in this sample were predominantly White and older in age. In addition, half worked regular day shifts, which is not the common work shift pattern in hospitals. A second limitation relates to the cross-sectional design that was used, which does not allow capturing within and between nursing performance variations throughout consecutive work shifts while providing patient care. A third limitation relates to mono-method bias, which limited our ability to test the construct validity of the NPI. In future research, these limitations may be addressed by (a) testing the factor structure in male nurses and those on night or rotating shifts, (b) administering an additional tool such as the Six Dimension Scale of Nursing Performance to establish convergent validity, and (c) testing the NPI in longitudinal studies to assess the sensitivity of the measures to change.

Conclusion/Implications for Practice

This study provides preliminary evidence for the factor structure of the NPI. The findings from the EFA and CFA provide indications of three forms of validity (factorial, convergent, and discriminant validity), and the subscales are considered reliable. Future plans include developing the latent constructs of "behavioral change" and "consistent practice" further, as the subscales consist of two and three items only, and conducting further validity testing. Additional work needs to be done to test for potential ceiling and social desirability effects. We are cautious in recommending

the use of the NPI at this developmental stage in hospital settings except for psychometric testing. This said, the findings suggest that the NPI is a promising performance measure in nursing, with the potential to be used as a self-monitoring

tool that assesses nurses' perceptions of performance while providing patient care.

References

Aiken, L. H., Clarke, S. P., Sloane, D. M., Sochalski, J., & Silber, J. H. (2002). Hospital nurse staffing and patient mortality, nurse burnout, and job dissatisfaction. *Journal of American Medical Association, 288*(16), 1987–1993. doi:10.1001/jama.288.16.1987

Barker, L. M., & Nussbaum, M. A. (2011). Fatigue, performance and the work environment: A survey of registered nurses. *Journal of Advanced Nursing, 67*(6), 1370–1382. doi:10.1111/j.1365-2648.2010.05597.x

Battersby, D., & Hemmings, L. (1991). Clinical performance of university nursing graduates. *The Australian Journal of Advanced Nursing, 9*(1), 30–34.

Battisto, D., Pak, R., Vander Wood, M. A., & Pilcher, J. J. (2009). Using a task analysis to describe nursing work in acute care patient environments. *The Journal of Nursing Administration, 39*(12), 537–547. doi:10.1097/NNA.0b013e3181c1806d

Bertram, D. A., Opila, D. A., Brown, J. L., Gallagher, S. J., Schifeling, R. W., Snow, I. S., & Hershey, C. O. (1992). Measuring physician mental workload: Reliability and validity assessment of a brief instrument. *Medical Care, 30*(2), 95–104.

Brown, T. A. (2015). *Confirmatory factor analysis for applied research* (2nd ed.). New York, NY: The Guilford Press.

Byrne, B. M. (2011). *Structural equation modeling with Mplus: Basic concepts, applications and programming.* New York, NY: Routledge.

Cohen, J. (1988). *Statistical power analysis for the behavioral sciences* (2nd ed.). Hillsdale, NJ: Lawrence Erlbaum Associates.

Costello, A. B., & Osborne, J. W. (2005). Best practices in exploratory factor analysis: Four recommendations for getting the most from your analysis. *Practical Assessment, Research & Evaluation, 10*(7), 1–9.

DeLucia, P. R., Ott, T. E., & Palmieri, P. A. (2009). Performance in nursing. *Reviews of Human Factors and Ergonomics, 5*(1), 1–40. doi:10.1518/155723409X448008

Denis, S., Shannon, H. S., Wessel, J., Stratford, P., & Weller I. (2007). Association of low back pain, impairment, disability & work limitations in nurses. *Journal of Occupational Rehabilitation, 17*(17), 213–226. doi:10.1007/s10926-007-9065-4

Dorrian, J., Tolley, C., Lamond, N., van den Heuvel, C., Pincombe, J., Rogers, A. E., & Drew, D. (2008). Sleep and errors in a group of Australian hospital nurses at work and during the commute. *Applied Ergonomics, 39*(5), 605–613. doi:10.1016/j.apergo.2008.01.012

Fitzpatrick, J. M., While, A. E., & Roberts, J. D. (1997). Measuring clinical nurse performance: Development of the King's Nurse Performance Scale. *International Journal of Nursing Studies, 34*(3), 222–230. doi:10.1016/S0020-7489(97)00009-6

Garland, G. A. (1996). Self report of competence. A tool for the staff development specialist. *Journal of Nursing Staff Development, 12*(4), 191–197.

Geiger-Brown, J., Rogers, V. E., Trinkoff, A. M., Kane, R. L., Bausell, R. B., & Scharf, S. M. (2012). Sleep, sleepiness, fatigue, and performance of 12-hour shift nurses. *Chronobiology International*, *29*(2), 211–219. doi:10.3109/07420528. 2011.645752

Golubic, R., Milosevic, M., Knezevic, B., & Mustajbegovic, J. (2009). Work-related stress, education and work ability among hospital nurses. *Journal of Advanced Nursing*, *65*(10), 2056–2066. doi:10.1111/j.1365-2648.2009.05057.x

Gurses, A. P., Carayon, P., & Wall, M. (2009). Impact of performance obstacles on intensive care nurses' workload, perceived quality and safety of care, and quality of working life. *Health Services Research*, *44*(2, Pt. 1), 422–443. doi:10. 1111/j.1475-6773.2008.00934.x

Hayes, C., Jackson, D., Davidson, P. M., & Power, T. (2015). Medication errors in hospitals: A literature review of disruptions to nursing practice during medication adminis-tration. *Journal of Clinical Nursing*, *24*(21–22), 3063–3076. doi:10.1111/jocn.12944

Idvall, E., Rooke, L., & Hamrin, E. (1997). Quality indicators in clinical nursing: A review of the literature. *Journal of Ad-vanced Nursing*, *25*(2), 6–17. doi:10.1046/j.1365-2648.1997. 1997025006.x

Kline, R. B. (2011). *Principles and practice of structural equation modeling* (3rd ed.). New York, NY: The Guilford Press.

Koopmans, L., Bernaards, C. M., Hildebrandt, V. H., Schaufeli, W. B., de Vet Henrica, C. W., & van der Beek, A. J. (2011). Conceptual frameworks of individual work performance: A systematic review. *Journal of Occupational and Environ-mental Medicine*, *53*(8), 856–866. doi:10.1097/JOM. 0b013e318226a763

Lerner, D., Amick, B. C. III., Rogers, W. H., Malspeis, S., Bungay, K., & Cynn, D. (2001). The work limitations questionnaire. *Medical Care*, *39*(1), 72–85.

Meretoja, R., Isoaho, H., & Leino-Kilpi, H. (2004). Nurse competence scale: Development and psychometric testing. *Journal of Advanced Nursing*, *47*(2), 124–133. doi:10.1111/ j.1365-2648.2004.03071.x

Montgomery, V. L. (2007). Effect of fatigue, workload, and environment on patient safety in the pediatric intensive care unit. *Pediatric Critical Care Medicine*, *8*(2, Suppl.), S11–S16. doi:10.1097/01.PCC.0000257735.49562.8F

Muthén, L. K., & Muthén, B. O. (2010). *Mplus user's guide* (6th ed.). Los Angeles, CA: Author.

Nunnally, J. (1978). *Psychometric theory* (2nd ed.). New York, NY: McGraw-Hill.

Rogers, A. E., Hwang, W. T., Scott, L. D., Aiken, L. H., & Dinges, D. F. (2004). The working hours of hospital staff nurses and patient safety. *Health Affairs*, *23*(4), 202–212. doi:10.1377/ hlthaff.23.4.202

Rotundo, M. (2002). The relative importance of task, citizen-ship, and counterproductive performance to global ratings of job performance: A policy-capturing approach. *Journal of Applied Psychology*, *87*(1), 66–80.

Schmitt, T. A. (2011). Current methodological considerations in exploratory and confirmatory factor analysis. *Journal of Psychoeducational Assessment*, *29*(4), 304–321.

Schwirian, P. M. (1978). Evaluating the performance of nurses: A multidimensional approach. *Nursing Research*, *27*(6), 347–351.

Scott, L. D., Rogers, A. E., Hwang, W. T., & Zhang, Y. (2006). Effects of critical care nurses' work hours on vigilance and patients' safety. *American Journal of Critical Care*, *15*(1), 30–37.

Visweswaran, C., & Ones, D. S. (2000). Perspectives on models of job performance. *International Journal of Selection and Assessment*, *8*(4), 216–226. doi:10.1111/1468-2389.00151

Westbrook, J. I., Duffield, C., Li, L., & Creswick, N. J. (2011). How much time do nurses have for patients? A longitudinal study quantifying hospital nurses' patterns of task time distribution and interactions with health professionals. *BMC Health Services Research*, *11*, 319. doi:10.1186/1472-6963-11-319

Zhan, C., & Miller, M. R. (2003). Excess length of stay, charges, and mortality attributable to medical injuries during hospi-talization. *Journal of the American Medical Association*, *290*(14), 1868–1874. doi:10.1001/jama.290.14.1868

Zhang, Z., Luk, W., Arthur, D., & Wong, T. (2001). Nursing competencies: Personal characteristics contributing to ef-fective nursing performance. *Journal of Advanced Nursing*, *33*(4), 467–474. doi:10.1046/j.1365-2648.2001.01688.x

2

The Development and Psychometric Testing on Psychiatric Nurses of a Nurse Case Management Competence Scale in Taiwan

Shing-Chia Chen[1] • Shih-Kai Lee[2] • Jiin-Ru Rong[3] • Chien-Chang Wu[4]
Wen-I Liu[5]*

ABSTRACT

Background: Case management is a complex process involving multiple activities. It is vital that nurses are competent in all related tasks for case management. A competence scale is a valuable tool for assessing task-related competency.

Purpose: The aims of this study were to examine the reliability and validity of an assessment scale for nurse case management competence and to use this scale to assess the current competency of nurses.

Methods: A nurse case management competence scale was developed in three stages: (a) selection of assessment items according to standards of practice for case management and literature review, (b) determination of content validity using the Delphi technique with a panel of experts, and (c) psychometric testing of the developed competence scale using a cross-sectional design. Convenience sampling was used to recruit psychiatric nurses at seven psychiatric centers in Taiwan to complete the scale anonymously. An exploratory factor analysis was performed to analyze construct validity. Discriminant validity, internal consistency, and 2-week test–retest reliability were also examined.

Results: Two hundred eighty-five psychiatric nurses completed an assessment scale comprising 18 items (originally 25 items). The content validity index reached 0.96 after the Delphi technique was applied twice in the expert panel. Seventy-eight percent of the total variance was explained by two dimension factors: coordination facilitation competence and direct care competence. Participants who had undertaken case management courses had superior case management ability compared with those who had not, indicating that the scale possesses excellent discriminant validity. Cronbach's α and the test–retest results showed excellent reliability. Of the two competence factors, direct care competence (3.03) was better than coordination facilitation competence (2.81).

Conclusions/Implications for Practice: There is a dearth of studies investigating the development and psychometric testing of case management competence scales. The results of this study provide evidence to support the reliability and validity of the developed case management competence scale among Taiwanese psychiatric nurses. It is a reliable and valid assessment instrument that may help identify educational needs and improve the case management competencies of nurses.

KEY WORDS:
case management, competence assessment instrument, reliability and validity, psychiatric nurses.

Introduction

Case management has become an important service delivery model in healthcare systems, and nurses typically serve as case managers (Dieterich et al., 2017). Case management is a complex process involving multiple activities. It is vital that nurse case managers are competent in all of the relevant tasks. A competence scale is a valuable assessment tool, with the results of assessment offering a baseline for improving the case management abilities of nurses. The purposes of this study were to examine the reliability and validity of an assessment scale for case management competency and to explore the current status of case management abilities among a group of nurses.

Defining ability and assessing core competence are crucial aspects of nursing education (Yanhua & Watson, 2011). Competence is generally defined as a person's capacity to integrate professional knowledge and skills and to play an effective, practical role (Cant, McKenna, & Cooper, 2013; Nursing and Midwifery Council, 2010). Core competencies of advanced practice nursing, standards of practice for case management, and case management roles and functions may be used as references for developing an advanced practice nursing competence scale (Henning & Cohen, 2008; Sastre-Fullana, De Pedro-Gómez, Bennasar-Veny, Serrano-Gallardo, & Morales-Asencio, 2014; Stanton, Swanson, & Baker, 2005; Tahan & Campagna, 2010). Although several case management competence scales have been developed, these previous works are characterized by a number of

[1]PhD, RN, Assistant Professor, School of Nursing, College of Medicine, National Taiwan University, and Supervisor, Department of Nursing, National Taiwan University Hospital • [2]MSN, RN, Director, Department of Nursing, Tsaotun Psychiatric Center, Ministry of Health and Welfare • [3]PhD, RN, Professor, School of Nursing, National Taipei University of Nursing and Health Sciences • [4]PhD, MD, Associate Professor, Department and Graduate Institute of Medical Education and Bioethics, College of Medicine, National Taiwan University • [5]PhD, RN, Professor, School of Nursing, National Taipei University of Nursing and Health Sciences.

methodological deficiencies, notably failure to show reliability and validity of the assessment instruments and small sample sizes (Hausdorf & Swanson, 2014; Henning & Cohen, 2008; Maijala, Tossavainen, & Turunen, 2015; Stanton et al., 2005; Yanhua & Watson, 2011).

Core Competencies for Case Management

The various currently available case management models may be categorized according to purpose, service content, and caseload. The four main categories are brokerage, managed care, full service, and strength models. Each has distinctive characteristics. The brokerage model focuses on referral rather than direct service provision, the managed care model emphasizes improved quality of care and equitable resource allocation, the full service model integrates the delivery of direct and/or indirect services, and the strength model focuses on developing clients' strengths to manage their own illness (Liu, 2011). All models identify the same crucial steps in the case management process: selecting cases, identifying and assessing needs, developing case management plans, providing needed services, and monitoring and evaluating provided services (Powell & Tahan, 2010; Tahan & Campagna, 2010). These steps are the core content of case management practice and are related to case management competence. In addition, these steps and practice standards play an essential role in the case management processes (Case Management Society of America [CMSA], 2016).

Case Management and Practice Standards

The CMSA (2016) established a set of case management practice standards. These include assessment, planning, facilitation, care coordination, evaluation, and advocacy for services to meet the comprehensive health needs of individuals and families. In all models and practice settings, requisite role activities for implementing case management include case management processes and services, resource utilization and management, sociopsychological and financial support, rehabilitation, effectiveness evaluation, and ethics and law (Tahan & Campagna, 2010). In Canada, the framework of case management competence emphasizes the importance of communication, collaboration, navigation, advocacy, management, and professional behavior (Frank, 2005). In addition, the CMSA (2016) developed methods for assessing, planning, promoting, and speaking for case management and related issues. The concrete content and practical activities related to practice standards for case management may provide a basis for measuring case management competence (CMSA, 2016; Powell & Tahan, 2010; Tahan & Campagna, 2010). To date, however, the suitability of case management content developed in the North American context for other countries with different healthcare systems and cultures has not been investigated.

Methods

Research Design and Subjects

The steps that have been established and widely used for developing competence scales are as follows: conduct a literature review, develop assessment content using the Delphi technique, and examine the reliability and validity of the resulting scale (Hwang, 2015; Lakanmaa et al., 2014; Maijala et al., 2015; Tahan & Campagna, 2010). The case management competence scale in this study was developed in line with these abovementioned three steps.

Stage 1: literature review

The literature was reviewed to identify appropriate case management processes, case management practice standards, case management planning, collaboration practices, professional roles, and practical activities related to evaluation, planning, facilitation, and advocacy. Essential practical activities for case management may be divided into six categories: case management processes and services, resource utilization and management, sociopsychological and financial support, rehabilitation activities, effectiveness evaluation, and ethics and law (Tahan & Campagna, 2010). Such practical activities constitute the foundation of a case management competence scale (CMSA, 2016; Henning & Cohen, 2008; Powell & Tahan, 2010; Tahan & Campagna, 2010). In this study, 31 items were initially included in the scale before implementing the next step (Delphi technique). Following Benner (Gardner, 2012), ability levels were divided into five categories: novice, advanced beginner, competent, proficient, and expert (scored from 1 to 5, with higher scores indicating better ability).

Stage 2: Delphi technique

The Delphi technique has been widely used to develop competence assessment scales that are designed to build consensus (Hwang, 2015; Lakanmaa et al., 2014; Maijala et al., 2015). Three iterations are sufficient to collect the needed information and to reach a consensus in most cases. If early group consensus is achieved, as few as two rounds may be needed (Hanafin, 2004). In this study, six experts in case management practice and education were invited to form an expert panel in an anonymous Delphi procedure. Four of the six were clinical practitioners (in oncology, long-term care, community chronic illness, and psychiatric case management), one was a case management supervisor with 5 years of experience supervising case managers in a long-term care management center, and one was a case management educator who taught a university course in case management.

In the first round, the experts independently evaluated the relevance and clarity of the 31 items in the initial version of the case management competence scale. A 4-point scale was used to assess the relevance and clarity of all the items (Polit & Beck, 2006). The experts could write comments, add additional items, and suggest rewordings. After the first round, the research assistant converted the collected information into a well-structured questionnaire. In the second round, all modifications were presented to the experts. Scale content validity index (CVI) was used to evaluate the extent of expert agreement on the relevance of the items (Polit & Beck, 2012; Su, Win, & Chung, 2013; Van Lancker et al., 2016). Polit and Beck (2006) recommended a scale CVI of 90.0%. The CVI was from .78 to .96 after the Delphi technique was applied twice. The content of the initial 31-item questionnaire was revised in line with feedback from the experts, and six similar questions were removed. Hence, the revised questionnaire contained 25 items.

Stage 3: psychometric testing

A cross-sectional research design was used to examine the validity and reliability of the scale. Two hundred fifty research subjects are required to assess a scale comprising 25 items (i.e., 10 research subjects are required for one item). Convenience sampling was employed to recruit psychiatric nurses (aged 20–64 years) who provided patient care in a psychiatric hospital. Nursing chiefs and supervisors were excluded.

Data Collection

After the study was approved by the ethics committee of National Taiwan University (IRB approval number 201203HS0002), research subjects were recruited from seven psychiatric teaching hospitals in northern, central, and southern Taiwan, each of which employed 100–250 psychiatric nurses. The data collection period was from April to August 2013. The principal investigator contacted the director of each hospital and requested that she or he invite staff to attend an information session about the project. At the meeting, the principal investigator explained the purpose of the research, obtained signed consent forms, and distributed envelopes containing the questionnaires to interested participants. The nurses were assured that there was no risk from participating in the study, that their responses would be treated in confidence (test–retest participants used a self-selected code), and that nonparticipation would not affect their present or future employment. To encourage participation, nurses who completed the questionnaire received a small gift as a token of thanks. After they had completed the questionnaires, which took approximately 10 minutes, the participants were asked to double-check their responses, seal their forms in the envelope, and return them to the research assistant.

Data Analysis

IBM SPSS 20.0 was used to perform the statistical analyses. An item–total correlation test and t test were performed to evaluate items for retention in the scale. The criterion for deleting items was an item–total correlation of less than .30

(Polit & Beck, 2012). An exploratory factor analysis (EFA) was performed to analyze construct validity. Discriminant validity, internal consistency (Cronbach's α), and 2-week test–retest reliability were also examined.

Results

Characteristics of Participants

Two hundred ninety-three psychiatric nurses met the inclusion criteria. Three of these did not wish to participate in the study and did not sign the consent form, and another four did not complete the questionnaire. One participant received a perfect score of 5 for all items. Therefore, 285 sets of data were available and submitted for statistical analysis.

The demographic characteristics of participants are shown in Table 1. Participants' average age was 35 (SD = 8.7) years, average length of employment as a nurse was 12 (SD = 8.8) years, and average length of time working in the department of psychiatry was 10 (SD = 7.7) years. Most participants (89.1 %) were female, and 210 participants (73.7%) had not undertaken a course related to case management. Slightly more than half of the study population (51.9%) held a bachelor's degree, and 36.8% held a college diploma.

Item Analysis

Item–total correlations for the initial 25-item competence scale ranged from .78 to .90. All of the items were retained, as the item–total correlation coefficients for these items were within the threshold of .30 (Chiou, 2010). In addition, the independent t test showed that the critical

TABLE 1.

Demographic Characteristics of Participants (N = 285)

Characteristic	Min	Max	Mean	SD
Age (years)	21	57	35	8.7
Length of nursing employment	1	35	12	8.8
Working years in the department of psychiatry	0	35	10	7.7

	n	%
Gender		
Male	31	10.9
Female	254	89.1
Educational level		
Vocational school	5	1.8
Junior college	105	36.8
Bachelor's degree	148	51.9
Master's degree	27	9.5
Had previously attended case management courses		
Yes	75	26.3
No	210	73.7

ratio of each item differed significantly between the higher-score group (upper 75%, score = 90) and the lower-score group (under 25%, score = 58). Hence, all of the initial 25 items had good title homogeneity and discrimination and were retained to test construct validity.

Construct Validity

An EFA was used to establish construct validity. We first performed the Kaiser–Meyer–Olkin (KMO) and sphericity tests. The KMO value reached .96, and the sphericity test was significant, indicating that factors were independent of one another and thus a factor analysis could be performed ($p < .001$). Factors were extracted using principal component analysis with the oblique rotation method (direct oblimin) using an eigenvalue greater than 1, a proportion of variance for each factor of at least 5%, and at least three items per dimension as the extraction criteria (Polit & Beck, 2012). Item factor loadings with an absolute value greater than .4 (Stevens, 2002) and difference of loading greater than .2 were retained. Hence, seven items were removed. One item was deleted at a time (Items 5, 14, 17, 9, 1, 4, and 24). For the remaining items, oblique rotations were performed in two dimensions. The results indicated that the KMO value reached .96 and that the sphericity test was significant. In addition, 78% of the total variance was explained (Table 2). The explained variance for Factor 1 was 71.90%, with initial eigenvalues of 12.94, comprising nine questions that were named collectively as "coordination facilitation competence" (12 items: 3, 6, 7, 8, 15, 16, 19, 20, 21, 22, 23, and 25). The explained variance for Factor 2 was 5.66%, with initial eigenvalues of 1.02, comprising six questions that were named collectively as "direct care competence" (six items: 2, 10, 11, 12, 13, and 24). The communality among the 18 items was between .62 and .88, and the factor loadings of the pattern matrix were between .53 and .98 (Table 3).

Discriminant Validity

We divided the participants into two groups to assess their case management abilities. Participants in the first group

TABLE 2.
Selected Analysis Results Using Oblique Rotation and Principal Component Extraction in the Case Management Competence Scale (18 Items)

Component	Initial Eigenvalue		
	Total	% of Variance	Cumulative %
1	12.94	71.90	71.90
2	1.02	5.66	77.56

Note. Components: 1, coordination facilitation competence; 2, direct care competence.

had attended case management courses for at least 4 hours, whereas those in the second group did not attend these courses. An independent sample t test was performed, and the average scores on the case management competence scale were analyzed. Overall, 75 participants had attended case management courses, and 210 participants had not. In two factor dimensions, the t values for direct care competence, coordination facilitation competence, and overall case management competence were 3.82, 4.89, and 4.69, respectively, and all p values were significant ($p < .001$). Therefore, in various dimensions, the case management ability of the participants who had attended case management courses was superior to that of those who had not attended, indicating that the scale possessed excellent discriminant validity.

Reliability

Regarding the 18 items and 2 factors, the Cronbach's α values that were associated with direct care competence and coordination facilitation competence were .94 and .97, respectively. The item–total correlations ranged from .75 to .88. The interitem correlations within the scale ranged from .60 to .88. The interitem correlations between the two dimensions ranged from .55 to .79 (see Table 3). The test–retest reliability with a 2-week interval for 30 participants was between .90 and .92, indicating that the case management competence scale had excellent reliability (Polit & Beck, 2012).

Case Management Ability

Case management competence was assessed using the 18-item scale. The average case management competence of the psychiatric nurses was 2.92 ($SD = 0.84$), which was below the score (3) that indicates competence in Benner's five-level typology (Gardner, 2012). Direct care competence earned the higher score (mean = 3.03, $SD = 0.88$), but coordination facilitation competence (mean = 2.81, $SD = 0.88$) did not reach the expected levels of competence (Table 4). In the scale, the items that were associated with the lowest competence level were as follows: (a) identifying usable personal and social resources (coordination facilitation competence), (b) determining whether targets are willing to receive case management services (direct care competence), (c) providing case management services according to related regulations (coordination facilitation competence), (d) helping cases and their family members to be independent (coordination facilitation competence), and (e) solving problems when case management services do not meet expectations (coordination facilitation competence).

Discussion

The demographic characteristics of nurse participants (age, length of employment as a nurse, and years of

TABLE 3.
Factor Loadings After Oblique Rotations for the Case Management Competence Scale

Item	Dimension 1	Dimension 2	ITC Coefficient	Critical Ratio t	Critical Ratio p	IIC Within Subscale	IIC Between Dimension
16	.98	−.20	.79	21.0	<.001	.63–.86	.57–.61
22	.96	−.06	.86	21.4	<.001	.69–.86	.60–.69
15	.92	−.08	.80	20.2	<.001	.63–.86	.58–.65
23	.87	.03	.86	25.2	<.001	.65–.86	.59–.75
19	.85	.07	.87	23.1	<.001	.69–.86	.65–.71
25	.82	.04	.81	18.5	<.001	.62–.76	.56–.72
20	.78	.15	.88	25.4	<.001	.69–.86	.63–.73
8	.79	.13	.85	25.0	<.001	.69–.82	.64–.70
3	.73	.09	.77	18.8	<.001	.63–.72	.55–.69
7	.71	.19	.84	23.3	<.001	.69–.80	.64–.71
6	.70	.22	.87	22.3	<.001	.70–.82	.67–.72
21	.67	.28	.88	24.7	<.001	.67–.86	.67–.74
11	−.06	.98	.81	23.1	<.001	.67–.88	.58–.70
10	−.00	.92	.81	22.7	<.001	.64–.88	.57–.73
12	.05	.89	.83	26.1	<.001	.68–.88	.60–.79
13	.09	.82	.81	22.0	<.001	.66–.88	.55–.74
24	.33	.56	.81	22.6	<.001	.60–.76	.61–.76
2	.30	.53	.75	19.3	<.001	.60–.68	.55–.69

Note. Extraction method: principal component analysis; rotation method: oblimin. ITC = item-to-total correlation; IIC = interitem correlation.

TABLE 4.
Eighteen Items, Two Factors, and Case Management Competence (N = 285)

Factor or Item	Mean	SD	Rank	Commonality
Dimension 1: coordination facilitation competence (12 items)	2.81	0.88		
3. Assessing cases' physical, mental, social, and financial conditions	2.84	0.99		.65
6. Developing care goals with cases and their family members	2.89	0.97		.79
7. Identifying usable personal and social resources	2.68	1.03	L1	.74
8. Developing care plans with cases, family members, and healthcare team members	2.78	1.00		.78
15. Communicating and coordinating with related divisions	2.88	1.04		.73
16. Establishing interdisciplinary cooperation with related healthcare systems	2.81	1.06		.75
19. Ability to solve problems when case management services do not meet expectations	2.75	1.00	L5	.82
20. Assessing the effect of case management services on cases' physical and mental health conditions and social situations	2.88	0.98		.82
21. Assessing the responses of cases and family members to services in order to ensure service quality	2.92	0.97		.81
22. Responding to environmental changes flexibly and in a timely manner	2.79	1.01		.83
23. Assisting cases and family members to be independent	2.74	1.00	L4	.80
25. Providing case management services according to relevant regulations	2.72	1.04	L3	.72
Dimension 2: direct care competence (six items)	3.03	0.88		
2. Determining whether cases are willing to receive case management services	2.68	1.00	L1	.62
10. Teaching cases to recognize and manage disease symptoms	3.23	0.98	H1	.85
11. Teaching cases to seek timely healthcare services or medical advice	3.18	1.02	H2	.88
12. Helping cases obtain medical or healthcare services	3.02	0.93	H4	.87
13. Providing cases and family members with service-related information	2.97	0.97	H5	.81
24. Protecting cases and family members' rights and interests according to ethical rules	3.07	1.04	H3	.72
Overall scale (18 items)	2.92	0.84		

employment in the department of psychiatry) were similar to those of other psychiatric nurses in Taiwan (Liu, 2014). Approximately 70% of psychiatric nurses had not attended courses related to case management (Liu, 2014; Liu, Rong, & Liu, 2014). The direct care and coordination facilitation competence that was investigated in this study is crucial for case management services, as described in previous studies. The roles of a case manager are to assess and provide required community services, to coordinate service processes, and to monitor service and evaluation (CMSA, 2016; Frank, 2005).

Studies investigating the development and psychometric testing of a case management competence scale are scant. Two relevant studies used a self-assessment checklist to evaluate the case management competence of nurse case managers (Henning & Cohen, 2008; Stanton et al., 2005). One of these identified a nonclinical competency model for case managers with five competencies (Hausdorf & Swanson, 2014), and another used the Delphi technique to identify the required case management competencies of nurse practitioners (Maijala et al., 2015). All of these studies failed to report the psychometric properties of their instruments. The results of this study provide evidence to support the reliability and validity of the developed case management competence scale among Taiwanese psychiatric nurses. Reliability was supported by high internal consistency and test–retest coefficients (> .90). Reliabilities above .90 are generally expected by clinicians and high-stakes decision-makers (Helms, Henze, Sass, & Mifsud, 2006). The closer a test–retest reliability score is to 1.00, the more stable an instrument is expected to be (Waltz, Strickland, & Lenz, 2010). Hence, the competence scale that was developed in this study may be deemed a consistent and stable instrument.

The overall validity of the developed scale was supported by its content validity, construct validity, and discriminant validity. The content validity reached 0.96 and showed good agreement among the six case manager experts in relation to the appropriateness of the competence instrument. Construct validity was examined using EFA, which showed that two dimensions explain 78% of the total variance in case management competencies (71.90% for Factor 1 and 5.66% for Factor 2). The total variance accounts for over 60%, and each factor over 5% met the criteria for EFA in social science research (Polit & Beck, 2012). Six items with fairly high loadings on two factors were deleted, and all the remaining 18 item loadings (which ranged from .53 to .98) were higher than .40, which was used as a cutoff value (Polit & Beck, 2012; Stevens, 2002). Hence, these items were clear in one dimension. Furthermore, the primary–secondary discrepancy was sufficiently large because the difference of loading was more than .2 (Matsunaga, 2015) among these items. The interitem correlation coefficients were .71 to .89, which is less than .9. According to the standard proposed by Field (2013), there was no multicollinearity in the data. However, the interitem correlations between two dimensions

were also over .70. This may support the use of the oblique rotation method in this study and suggests that some correlations between implementation and coordination may be present in the case management process. The case management process could represent most of the activities of nurse case managers, and these may occasionally overlap during the case management process.

The greatest differences that were identified between case management and nursing care were in the realms of multidisciplinary cooperation and resource coordination, which may explain why the coordination facilitation competence was relatively low. The abilities of participants in identifying usable personal and social resources and in determining whether clients were willing to receive services scored the lowest of all items. These abilities are crucial for providing care to clients who require multidisciplinary care, yet they receive little attention in nursing education. The importance of these two abilities is emphasized in the case management practice standards (CMSA, 2016), and both were included among the capabilities necessary for case management associates (social workers, coordinators, and specialists; Henning & Cohen, 2008).

The results showed that, even when senior psychiatric nurses used the case management method to provide continuous care, their case management ability did not reach the expected level of competence. The participants had an average of 10 years of working experience in the department of psychiatry. However, whereas their direct care competence reached the expected competence level (mean = 3.03, $SD = 0.88$), their coordination facilitation competence was low (mean = 2.81, $SD = 0.88$) and significantly lower than their direct care competence based on a paired sample t test ($p < .001$). Coordination facilitation competence is a therefore a priority area for improvement.

Conclusions

The case management competence scale with 18 items that was developed in this study may be replicated, used to assess the case management ability of nurses in other departments, and deployed as a tool in case management training. The scale may also be used to assess case management educational needs, the current status of the case management ability of nurses, and the effectiveness of continuing education in nursing. We recommend that priority be given to improving the coordination facilitation competence of psychiatric nurses. In this study, only psychiatric nurses served as research subjects. Thus, we recommend that nurses in other departments be recruited to further assess the reliability and validity of the case management competence scale. Future research may employ other instruments to examine the criterion-related validity of the scale.

Acknowledgments

The authors are grateful to the Taiwanese psychiatric nurses who participated in this study, which was funded by the National Science Council (NSC-101-2511-S-227-008). The views and opinions expressed in this manuscript are the authors' alone.

References

Cant, R., McKenna, L., & Cooper, S. (2013). Assessing preregistration nursing students' clinical competence: A systematic review of objective measures. *International Journal of Nursing Practice, 19*(2), 163–176. doi:10.1111/ijn.12053

Case Management Society of America. (2016). *Standards of practice for case management* (Rev. ed.). Little Rock, AR: Author.

Chiou, H. J. (2010). *Quantitative research and statistics: SPSS (PASW) data analysis examples*. Taipei City, Taiwan, ROC: Wunan. (Original work published in Chinese)

Dieterich, M., Irving, C. B., Bergm, H., Khokhar, M. A., Park, B., & Marshall, M. (2017). Intensive case management for severe mental illness. *Cochrane Database of Systematic Reviews*, CD007906. doi:10.1002/14651858.CD007906.pub3

Field, A. (2013). *Discovering statistics using IBM SPSS statistics* (4th ed.). London, England: Sage.

Frank, J. R. (Ed.). (2005). *The CanMEDS 2005 physician competency framework. Better standards. Better physicians. Better care*. Ottawa, Canada: The Royal College of Physicians and Surgeons of Canada.

Gardner, L. (2012). From novice to expert: Benner's legacy for nurse education. *Nurse Education Today, 32*(4), 339–340. doi:10.1016/j.nedt.2011.11.011

Hanafin, S. (2004). *Review of literature on the Delphi technique*. Dublin, Ireland: Office of the Minister for Children and Youth Affairs.

Hausdorf, P. A., & Swanson, S. (2014). A nonclinical competency model for case managers: Design and validation for home health care services. *Home Health Care Management and Practice, 26*(3), 154–162. doi:10.1177/1084822314521209

Helms, J. E., Henze, K. T., Sass, T. L., & Mifsud, V. A. (2006). Treating Cronbach's alpha reliability coefficients as data in counseling research. *The Counseling Psychologist, 34*(5), 630–660. doi:10.1177/0011000006288308

Henning, S. E., & Cohen, E. L. (2008). The competency continuum: Expanding the case manager's skill sets and capabilities. *Professional Case Management, 13*(3), 127–148. doi:10.1097/01.PCAMA.0000319966.30864.bf

Hwang, J. I. (2015). Development and testing of a patient-centred care competency scale for hospital nurses. *International Journal of Nursing Practice, 21*(1), 43–51. doi:10.1111/ijn.12220

Lakanmaa, R.-L., Suominen, T., Perttilä, J., Ritmala-Castrén, M., Vahlberg, T., & Leino-Kilpi, H. (2014). Basic competence in intensive and critical care nursing: Development and psychometric testing of a competence scale. *Journal of Clinical Nursing, 23*(5–6), 799–810. doi:10.1111/jocn.12057

Liu, W. I. (2011). *Nursing case management: Essential concepts and practices* (pp. 3–22). Taipei City, Taiwan, ROC: Farseeing. (Original work published in Chinese)

Liu, W. I. (2014). Examining Taiwanese psychiatric nurses' knowledge and confidence in case management. *The Journal of Continuing Education in Nursing, 45*(1), 43–48. doi:10.3928/00220124-20131015-07

Liu, W. I., Rong, J. R., & Liu, C. Y. (2014). Using evidence-integrated e-learning to enhance case management continuing education for psychiatric nurses: A randomized controlled trial with follow-up. *Nurse Education Today, 34*(11), 1361–1367. doi:10.1016/j.nedt.2014.03.004

Maijala, V., Tossavainen, K., & Turunen, H. (2015). Identifying nurse practitioners' required case management competencies in health promotion practice in municipal public primary health care. A two-stage modified Delphi study. *Journal of Clinical Nursing, 24*(17–18), 2554–2561. doi:10.1111/jocn.12855

Matsunaga, M. (2015). How to factor-analyze your data right: Do's, don'ts, and how-to's. *International Journal of Psychological Research, 3*(1), 97–110.

Nursing and Midwifery Council. (2010). *Standards for pre-registration nursing education*. London, England: Author.

Polit, D. F., & Beck, C. T. (2006). The content validity index: Are you sure you know what's being reported? Critique and recommendations. *Research in Nursing and Health, 29*(5), 489–497. doi:10.1002/nur.20147

Polit, D. F., & Beck, C. T. (2012). *Resource manual for nursing research: Generating and assessing evidence for nursing practice* (9th ed.). Philadelphia, PA: Wolters Kluwer Health/Lippincott Williams and Wilkins.

Powell, S. K., & Tahan, H. A. (2010). *Case management: A practical guide for education and practice* (3rd ed.). Philadelphia, PA: Wolters Kluwer Health/Lippincott Williams and Wilkins.

Sastre-Fullana, P., De Pedro-Gómez, J. E., Bennasar-Veny, M., Serrano-Gallardo, P., & Morales-Asencio, J. M. (2014). Competency frameworks for advanced practice nursing: A literature review. *International Nursing Review, 61*(4), 534–542. doi:10.1111/inr.12132

Stanton, M. P., Swanson, C., & Baker, R. D. (2005). Development of a military competency checklist for case management. *Lippincott's Case Management, 10*(3), 128–135. doi:10.1097/00129234-200505000-00003

Stevens, J. P. (2002). *Applied multivariate statistics for the social science*. Mahwah, NJ: Lawrence Erlbaum Associates.

Su, Y.-Y., Win, K. T., & Chung, T.-C. (2013). Identifying the Taiwanese electronic health record systems evaluation framework and instrument by implementing the modified Delphi method. In R. Bali, I. Troshani, S. Goldberg, & N. Wickramasinghe (Eds.), *Pervasive health knowledge management* (pp. 351–371). New York, NY: Springer. doi:10.1007/978-1-4614-4514-2_25

Tahan, H. A., & Campagna, V. (2010). Case management roles and functions across various settings and professional disciplines. *Professional Case Management, 15*(5), 245–277. doi:210.1097/NCM.1090b1013e3181e94452

Van Lancker, A., Beeckman, D., Verhaeghe, S., Van Den Noortgate, N., Grypdonck, M., & Van Hecke, A. (2016). An instrument to collect data on frequency and intensity of symptoms in older palliative cancer patients: A develop-ment and validation study. *European Journal of Oncology Nursing, 21,* 38–47. doi:10.1016/j.ejon.2015.11.003

Waltz, C. F., Strickland, O. L., & Lenz, E. R. (2010). *Measurement in nursing and health research* (4th ed.). New York, NY: Springer.

Yanhua, C., & Watson, R. (2011). A review of clinical compe-tence assessment in nursing. *Nurse Education Today, 31*(8), 832–836. doi:10.1016/j.nedt.2011.05.003

3

The Effectiveness of Function-Focused Care Interventions in Nursing Homes

Su Jung LEE[1] • Mi So KIM[2] • You Jin JUNG[3] • Sung Ok CHANG[4]*

ABSTRACT

Background: Since the Omnibus Budget and Reconciliation Act was passed in South Korea in 1987, function-focused care (FFC) has been used in long-term care to achieve the highest possible levels of self-care and independence for older adults. However, many perceive nursing home residents with cognitive function impairments as having little restorative potential.

Purpose: The purpose of this review is to report on evidence and strategies relating to FFC interventions in nursing home settings and to summarize the effects of FFC on the functional abilities of resident subgroups.

Methods: A literature review using EMBASE, MEDLINE, and Cumulative Index to Nursing and Allied Health Literature was conducted for articles published between January 1, 2000, and February 20, 2016. Twenty-two eligible studies were identified. Relevant data were extracted, and the results were synthesized into an integrated literature review. Study quality was appraised using the Cochrane Risk of Bias tool and the Risk of Bias Assessment tool for Non-randomized Studies.

Results: This review included 22 trials that were of moderate to high quality. Our systematic review confirmed the FFC interventions as integrated and dedicated processes; the five key strategies underpinning effective FFC interventions; and the effectiveness of FFC interventions on physical, psychosocial, and cognitive functions. The five key strategies underpinning FFC interventions included interactive learning for caregivers, the content of learning programs for caregivers, residents' preferences and interests, optimizing approaches according to residents' functional status, and the conceptual frameworks of FFC interventions. Most of the studies (n = 15) evaluated psychosocial functions and found significant improvements in aspects such as mood, affect, and behavioral problems. Likewise, the 13 studies assessing physical function found significant improvements in effectiveness in aspects such as movement, balance, and activities of daily living. Only four studies looked at cognitive function effectiveness, using measures such as place finding, verbal use, and memory.

Conclusions/Implications for Practice: Our review found scientific evidence that FFC interventions improve functional abilities across various levels of cognitive function in nursing homes. Nursing homes may employ effective strategies to maximize the effects of FFC interventions and use educational materials to teach caregivers to implement FFC interventions competently.

KEY WORDS:
aged care, caring intervention, daily activities of living, integrated care, nursing homes.

Introduction

Restorative care is an innovative nursing care philosophy that emphasizes evaluating residents' underlying functional capabilities and helping them to optimize a variety of functional abilities and increase physical activity (Resnick, Galik, Gruber-Baldini, & Zimmerman, 2011). Research on restorative care with respect to nursing homes (NHs) and home care elderly populations (Baker, Gottschalk, Eng, Weber, & Tinetti, 2001) has been increasing. More recently, function-focused care (FFC) has begun to be used interchangeably with restorative care (Resnick, Galik, & Boltz, 2013). FFC interventions have centered on different function areas (e.g., self-care, mobility, psychosocial, cognitive, and incontinence) and included several elements (individualized assessment, staff education, teamwork, goal setting, and documenting outcomes) to break residents' cycles of dependency and optimize individual functioning (Shanti et al., 2005). As mandated by the Omnibus Budget and Reconciliation Act, NHs have attempted to implement FFC programs to provide care that allows residents to attain and maintain their highest functional ability across a variety of activities (Resnick et al., 2013). Older adults in NHs are categorized as one of the most

[1]PhD, RN, Research Professor, Korea University College of Nursing, Seoul, Republic of Korea • [2]PhD, RN, Research Professor, Korea University College of Nursing, Seoul, Republic of Korea • [3]MSN, RN, Doctoral Student and Associate Research Fellow, National Evidence-Based Healthcare Collaborating Agency, Seoul, Republic of Korea • [4]PhD, RN, Professor, Korea University College of Nursing, Seoul, Republic of Korea.

functionally disabled groups and are typically in need of extensive assistance related to dressing, transfers, toileting, eating, personal hygiene, mobility, and locomotion (Carpenter, Hastie, Morris, Fries, & Ankri, 2006). In addition, it has been estimated that 41% of older NH residents in the United States have moderate to severe cognitive impairment (Zimmerman, Sloane, & Reed, 2014). Rapidly decreasing functional abilities have serious implications for the severity of health risks related to decreased mobility, the amount of functional care required, rising care costs, and, ultimately, residents' quality of life (Resnick et al., 2004, 2006; Taylor & Sloan, 2000). Moreover, the most disabled groups, that is, NH residents with cognitive impairments such as aphasia, motor apraxia, and memory loss, create a particular challenge for FFC interventions (Rabins, Lyketsos, & Steele, 2006). In short, FFC interventions that promote the optimization of functional abilities and maintain the dignity of frail residents in NHs remain a significant priority for research and clinical practice.

An analysis of FFC interventions is needed to stimulate future increases in the functional abilities of disabled older adults in NHs, to competently perform FFC, and to employ appropriate care strategies for improving residents' functioning and increasing their activity time. A recent review of the FFC approach identified studies addressing the overall effect of FFC on residents in a variety of settings (Resnick et al., 2013). This integrative review is intended to contribute to a wider project by specifically analyzing and building on the existing published work of Resnick et al. (2013). We summarize the results of the current key components of FFC interventions and analyze these components using recent trial studies. In particular, we focus on a variety of resident cognitive conditions because intervention with residents with moderate to severe cognitive impairment confers the most critical health benefits. We examine the effectiveness of FFC interventions in different functional areas, including physical, psychosocial, and cognitive, and summarize findings related to the various cognitive function subgroups. We focus on NH settings for older adults rather than on other community living facilities because a meaningful examination and comparison of FFC intervention outcomes requires data from homogeneous care environments. The object of the current study is a comprehensive evaluation of the effects of FFC interventions on a variety of functional abilities with regard to specific strategies and their efficacy and a review of the overall evidence for FFC interventions in NH settings.

Methods

Search Strategy

The following search terms were used: FFC, restorative care, dedicated and care or intervention or program, integrated and care or intervention or program, combination and care or intervention or program, abilities-focused care, skills training,

nursing home, and long-term care facility. The initial search was conducted using two key databases for nursing and allied health literature: MEDLINE and the Cumulative Index to Nursing and Allied Health Literature. The initial search of these two databases identified a large number of articles (approximately 2,000). Because of the large-scale nature of the literature review, the search database was limited to three major nursing-related databases: Ovid MEDLINE (1946 to present), Embase (1974 to 2016 Week 07), and Cumulative Index to Nursing and Allied Health Literature.

Inclusion Criteria

The inclusion criteria were studies that (1) focused on populations of older adults in NHs; (2) addressed the FFC (or restorative care) intervention focused on physical, psychosocial, or cognitive function care programs with components such as individualized assessment, staff education, teamwork, goal setting, or documented outcomes; (3) included physical, psychosocial, or cognitive functions as outcomes; (4) used nonrandomized controlled trials (non-RCTs) or RCTs; (5) were written in the English language; and (6) were published between 2000 and February 20, 2016.

Exclusion Criteria

Studies were excluded if they (1) included only caregiver outcomes for the FFC intervention, (2) tested a medical intervention, or (3) were qualitative or review articles.

Search Outcome

The Preferred Reporting Items for Systematic Reviews and Meta-Analyses flow chart in Figure 1 shows how the articles used in this review were selected. The initial electronic database searches identified 3,310 studies, which were imported into Endnote software (Clarivate Analytics, Philadelphia, PA, USA). After duplicates were deleted, 2,056 studies remained. Two independent investigators considered all of the titles and abstracts. Where there was disagreement or uncertainty about inclusion, the two reviewers were required to work out a consensus opinion. Thus, the pool of studies was reduced to 96 articles. A full-text screening process using the criteria discussed previously excluded a further 75 studies; an additional eligible study found through a reference was included. The two researchers analyzed the remaining 22 studies.

Quality Appraisal

The methodological quality of the studies was evaluated using the following tools: Cochrane Risk of Bias (RoB) tool for RCTs (Higgins & Green, 2011) and the Risk of Bias Assessment tool for Non-randomized Studies (RoBANS; Park et al., 2011). The RoB tool considers seven criteria, including random sequence generation, allocation concealment, blinding of participants and personnel, blinding

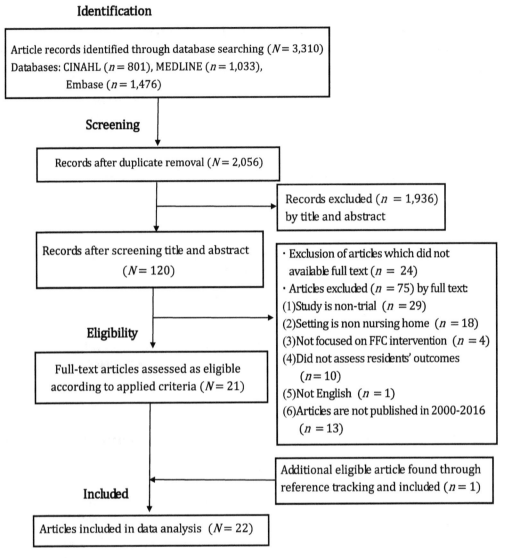

Identification

Article records identified through database searching ($N = 3,310$)
Databases: CINAHL ($n = 801$), MEDLINE ($n = 1,033$),
Embase ($n = 1,476$)

Screening

Records after duplicate removal ($N = 2,056$)

Records excluded ($n = 1,936$)
by title and abstract

Records after screening title and abstract
($N = 120$)

· Exclusion of articles which did not
  available full text ($n = 24$)
· Articles excluded ($n = 75$) by full text:
(1) Study is non-trial ($n = 29$)
(2) Setting is non nursing home ($n = 18$)
(3) Not focused on FFC intervention ($n = 4$)
(4) Did not assess residents' outcomes
     ($n = 10$)
(5) Not English ($n = 1$)
(6) Articles are not published in 2000-2016
     ($n = 13$)

Eligibility

Full-text articles assessed as eligible
according to applied criteria ($N = 21$)

Additional eligible article found through
reference tracking and included ($n = 1$)

Included

Articles included in data analysis ($N = 22$)

Figure 1. Systematic review: PRISMA (Preferred Reporting Items for Systematic Reviews and Meta-Analyses) flow chart.

of outcome assessment, incomplete outcome data, selective reporting, and other sources of bias, and rates quality as low, high, or uncertain. The RoBANS instrument considers six criteria, including selection of participants, confounding variables, intervention measurement, blinding of outcome assessment, incomplete outcome data, and selective outcome reporting, and likewise rates quality as low, high, or uncertain. After two independent reviewers had assessed the quality of each study, the evidence used for evaluation was recorded on the sheet and utilized for discussion and reevaluation when resolving differing appraisals of a particular study's quality. This study used the RoB tool to assess the quality of all nine RCTs and determined that five studies were of high quality and four were of moderate quality. The RoBANS tool was used to assess the quality of all 13 non-RCTs; 10 studies were of high quality, and three were of moderate quality. Table 1 describes the characteristics of these studies and key information on their FFC intervention components.

Data Extraction

Data were extracted from the set of 22 selected studies for this review using a tool that incorporated the following information: author, year, country, population sample, study design, quality assessment, residents' cognitive function level, intervention method, outcome measures, and relevant findings. A data extraction sheet was displayed in tabular summaries, and an integrated review of findings from 22 key studies was constructed from narrative descriptions, complemented by tabular summaries.

Results

Trial Characteristics

Of the 22 selected studies that reported residents' functional outcomes, 13 used quasi-experimental designs (59%) and nine were RCTs (41%). The sample sizes of these 22 studies

TABLE 1.

Articles Reviewed on FFC Intervention in Nursing Homes

Author, Year (Country)	Study Design/Quality Assessment (Theoretical Bases)	Sample Size (Mean Age [Years])	Inclusion Criteria in Terms of Resident Cognitive Function
Beck et al., 2002 (United States)	Randomized controlled trial (RCT)/ High (basic psychosocial needs)	N = 127 (83.64)	Residents with dementia; moderate or severe cognitive impairment (MMSE ≤ 20)
Blair, Glaister, Brown, & Phillips, 2007 (United States)	Quasi-experimental design (QED)/ High (none)	N = 84 (79.25)	Residents had mild to moderate cognitive impairment (MMSE > 18)
Bonanni et al., 2009 (United States)	Single-group repeated-measure design/ Moderate (none)	N = 50 (50% were aged 85+)	Residents with a probability of functional decline
Bossers et al., 2015 (Netherlands)	RCT/ High (none)	N = 109 (85.5)	Residents with mild to moderate cognitive impairment (23 ≥ MMSE ≥ 9)
Chan & Pang, 2010 (China)	QED/ High (none)	N = 121 (83.54)	Residents without cognitive problems
Dechamps et al., 2010 (France)	RCT/ High (none)	N = 49 (83.2)	Residents with dementia; moderate or severe cognitive impairment (MMSE ≤ 20)
Finnema et al., 2005 (Netherlands)	RCT with matched groups/ Moderate (adaptation–coping model)	N = 146 (83.7)	Residents with dementia; mild to severe cognitive impairment
E. M. Galik et al., 2008 (United States)	Single-group repeated-measure design/ High (self-efficacy theory)	N = 46 (82.61)	Residents with dementia; moderate or severe cognitive impairment
E. Galik, Resnick, Hammersla, & Brightwater, 2014 (United States)	A cluster RCT/ Moderate (social ecological model)	N = 103 (83.7)	Residents with dementia; moderate or severe cognitive impairment (MMSE ≤ 15)
Huang, Chung, Chen, Chin, & Wang, 2016 (Taiwan)	RCT/ High (none)	N = 75 (79.43)	Residents with mild to moderate cognitive impairment (MMSE ≥ 13)

Intervention	Measure of Resident Outcome	Principal Resident Outcome
Three types of treatment: psychosocial activity, activities of daily living (ADLs), and a combination of the two	Disruptive Behavior Scale, Observable Displays of Affect Scale, Apparent Affect Rating Scale, Positive Visual Analogue Scale, and Negative Visual Analogue Scale	Findings indicated that treatment groups were positively affected but disruptive behaviors were not reduced.
Nursing staff training of "Orem's Systems of Nursing Care (OSNC)" and Skinner's "Applied Behavioral Analysis" and morning ADL intervention for residents	ADLs (Barthel self-care ratings), Worry Questionnaire for Continuing Care Residents, Rosenberg Self-Esteem Scale, and Geriatric Depression Scale (GDS)	There was no difference in worry or depression, ADLs, or self-esteem among the treatment groups, but the OSNC program was more independent regarding ADLs than other programs.
Training nursing staff and dedicated restorative intervention included ambulation, passive range of motion, active range of motion, balance and strength training, transfer and mobility training, splint use, and ADL intervention	ADL, locomotion and walking score, bladder continence, and depression	There was a significant improvement in ADL scores and walking and locomotion.
Combined aerobic and strength training versus aerobic-only training on cognitive and motor function	Assessment of motor functions: walking endurance, leg strength, knee extension, mobility, and balance assessment of cognitive functions: verbal memory, visual memory, face recognition, and executive functions	The combined treatment group was more positively affected than the aerobic-only group in motor decline and slowing cognitive function.
The storytelling approach	Quality of life, end-of-life care preferences	Significant improvements in functioning based on treatment preference stability and communication of treatment preferences were noted.
Cognition–action intervention using standardized exercises to enhance social interactions and communication.	Neuropsychiatric inventory (NPI), GDS, Berg Balance Scale, quality-of-life activity measure for postacute care, and muscle strength	There was a significant reduction in NPI scores and an improvement in Berg total scores. GDS scores were reduced, and muscle strength and quality of life were improved.
Integrated emotion-oriented care and usual care	Dutch Behavior Observation Scale for Psychogeriatric Inpatients, Cornell Scale for Depression in Dementia (CSDD), Cohen-Mansfield Agitation Inventory (CMAI), Geriatric Resident Goal Scale, and the Philadelphia Geriatric Center Morale Scale	Positive effects found in maintaining an emotional balance and preserving a positive self-image.
Nursing staff training and Res-Care intervention for residents	The Barthel Index, Physical Activity Survey in Long-Term Care (PASLTC), ActiGraph, CSDD, and CMAI	There was significant improvement in behavioral symptoms and mood with a decrease in physical activity but no significant change in overall physical activity or physical function.
Nursing staff training and function-focused care for the cognitively impaired intervention	Tinetti scale, Barthel Index, ActiGraph, PASLTC, CMAI-Short Form, CSDD, and Apathy Inventory	There were significant improvements in physical functioning and physical activity and a decrease in the number of fall events in the treatment group compared with the control group.
Cognitive–behavioral strategies and an exercise program	Fear of falling, depression (Taiwanese Depression Questionnaire), mobility (Tinetti Mobility Scale), and muscle strength using a MicroFET 2 device.	There was significant improvement in fear of falling, incidences of falls, mobility, depressive inclination, and muscle strength.

(continues)

TABLE 1.
Articles Reviewed on FFC Intervention in Nursing Homes, Continued

Author, Year (Country)	Study Design/Quality Assessment (Theoretical Bases)	Sample Size (Mean Age [Years])	Inclusion Criteria in Terms of Resident Cognitive Function
Kolanowski, Litaker, & Buettner, 2005 (United States)	Crossover experimental design with repeated-measures/ High (needs-driven dementia-compromised behavior [NDB] model)	$N = 30$ (82.3)	Residents with dementia; mild to severe cognitive impairment (MMSE $\leq$ 24)
Landi, Russo, & Bernabei, 2004 (Italy)	Case–control study/ High (none)	$N = 30$ (80.9)	Residents with moderate to severe cognitive impairment
Nolan, Mathews, & Harrison, 2001 (United States)	A multiple-baseline experimental design/ High (none)	$N = 3$ (86.33)	Residents with dementia with severe Alzheimer's disease (residents' respective MMSE scores were 7, 4, and 6.)
Mezey et al., 2000 (Canada)	QED/ High (none)	$N = 40$ (88.63)	Residents with dementia; moderate or severe cognitive impairment (MMSE < 19)
Resnick et al., 2006 (United States)	Single-group repeated-measure design/ Moderate (self-efficacy theory)	$N = 21$ (88.3)	Residents with mild to moderate dementia cognitive impairment (MMSE $\geq$ 15)
Resnick et al., 2009 (United States)	Randomized controlled repeated-measure design/ Moderate (self-efficacy theory)	$N = 487$ (83.8)	Residents with mild to moderate cognitive impairment (MMSE $\geq$ 11)
Schnelle et al., 2002 (United States)	RCT/ High (none)	$N = 190$ (87.5)	Residents were able to obey a one-step instruction
Shanti et al., 2005 (Canada)	QED/ High (none)	$N = 84$ (82.6)	Residents who are likely to benefit from care
Talley et al., 2015 (United States)	A longitudinal analysis of nursing home MDS data/ Moderate (none)	$N = 7,735$ (85.8)	None (excluded residents who had an end-stage disease)
Tappen, Williams, Barry, & Disesa, 2002 (United States)	Randomized trial/ Moderate (none)	$N = 55$ (87)	Residents with Alzheimer's disease; mild to severe cognitive impairment (MMSE $\leq$ 23)
van Weert, van Dulmen, Spreeuwenberg, Ribbe, & Bensing, 2005a (Netherlands)	QED/ High (none)	$N = 120$ (83.2)	Residents with dementia; moderate or severe cognitive impairment
van Weert et al., 2005b (Netherlands)	QED/ High (none)	$N = 125$ (83.3)	Residents with dementia; moderate or severe cognitive impairment

Note. FFC = function-focused care; MMSE = Mini-Mental State Examination.

Intervention	Measure of Resident Outcome	Principal Resident Outcome
Recreational activities derived from the NDB model	Affect Rating Scale, Dementia Mood Picture Test, activity engagement time, and CMAI	Agitation and negative affect were significantly improved in all treatment groups, but there was no significant change in mood.
Moderate-intensity exercise program (a combination of aerobic/endurance activities, flexibility training, strength training, and balance training)	Behavioral problems: physical and verbal abuse, wandering, and sleep disorders	There was a statistically significant reduction in behavioral problems and the use of hypnotic and antipsychotic medications.
Two external memory aids (photographs and signs) were placed outside residents' bedrooms	Room finding	Displaying large-print signs and photographs increased the probability of room finding.
Educational programs for caregivers on how to provide abilities-focused morning care	Interaction behaviors, level of agitation, level of function (mental disorientation/confusion, physical disability, disengagement, and socially inappropriate behavior)	The program enhanced residents' personal attendance, functional behaviors, levels of overall function, and decreased levels of agitation.
Training for nursing staff and restorative care intervention for residents	The Barthel Index, Dementia Quality of Life Instrument, self-efficacy for functional ability, outcome expectations for functional ability, and resident participation index, muscle contractures and strength	There was no difference in Res-Care Intervention; however, positive trends were shown in quality of life, outcome expectations, self-efficacy, and participation in restorative care activities, and there was decreased pain.
A two-tiered self-efficacy-based intervention focused on motivating nursing assistants and residents to engage in functional and physical activities	Barthel Index, Tinetti Gait and Balance, grip strength (muscle contractures and strength), Dementia Quality-of-Life Scale, self-efficacy, and Outcome Expectations Scales for Function	There was significant improvement in the Tinetti gait and balance subscores as well as stair climbing, walking, and bathing.
Functional incidental training (FIT) intervention that was integrated with incontinence care and exercise	Fecal and urinary incontinence frequency, maximum pounds lifted with upper body, level of assistance required to stand, average and maximum distance walked	The FIT intervention improved or prevented a decline in continence, upper-body strength, and mobility.
The "restorative care education and training program" consisting of a 5-week workshop and resource manual for both supervisory and direct care staff	Goal Attainment Scaling (GAS), Timed Up and Go, Functional Independence Measure (FIM), Multidimensional Observation Scale for Elderly Subjects (MOSES), and hierarchical assessment of balance and mobility (HABAM)	Residents who received restorative care improved significantly in GAS, FIM, MOSES self-care, and HABAM.
Restorative care programs	ADL dependency score	There was no significant improvement in ADL dependency scores.
Three types of treatment: conversation, walking, and a combination of the two	Communicative ability: total words, conciseness, and information units	The conversation-only intervention significantly improved communication performance in conciseness and the number of nonredundant units.
Training for caregivers and individual 24-hour Snoezelen program for residents	Indicators of nonverbal communication, indicators of verbal communication	Regarding residents, significant treatment effects were found for smiling, certified-nursing-assistant-directed gazing, negative verbal behaviors (less disapproval and anger), and verbally expressed autonomy.
Training for caregivers and individual 24-hour Snoezelen program for residents	Dutch Behavior Observation Scale for Psychogeriatric In-patients, CMAI-Dutch version, CSDD (Dutch version), observer assessed behavior (INTERACT) and mood (FACE)	There were significant treatment effects on levels of apathetic behavior, loss of decorum, rebellious behavior, aggressive behavior, and depression.

ranged from 3 to 7,735, comprising 9,830 participants with a mean age of 85 years.

Function-Focused Care Interventions as an Integrated and Dedicated Process

In 11 of the selected studies, the FFC intervention used an integrated process that generally addressed complex situations such as morning care. Mezey et al. (2000) and Blair et al. (2007) conducted abilities-focused programs where caregivers were engaged in activities related to dressing, bathing, toileting, and grooming residents. Shanti et al. (2005) implemented an FFC workshop program for NH staff and incorporated FFC care into daily routines. In another study, 99 NH staff members participated in a training course and incorporated emotion-oriented care into their normal, 24-hour care procedures (Finnema et al., 2005). Van Weert, van Dulmen, Spreeuwenberg, Ribbe, and Bensing (2005a, 2005b) examined the effectiveness of the Snoezelen method, a method of multisensory stimulation using light, sound, smell, and feel, implemented by certified nursing assistants who were involved in the FFC intervention during 24-hour care. Five studies suggested implementing FFC intervention components, including evaluating residents' functioning; evaluating environment and policy, education, and care goal setting; and motivating and monitoring staff for residents' participation in functional activities and exercises in daily activities (E. Galik et al., 2014; E. M. Galik et al., 2008; Resnick et al., 2006, 2009; Talley et al., 2015).

The other 11 studies used an FFC-exclusive process in which designated research or NH staff provided a scheduled program at an appointed time. One functional incidental training study applied dedicated FFC processes after research staff had assessed residents' baseline functional abilities (Schnelle et al., 2002). Schnelle et al. (2002) designed FFC processes that were scheduled every 2 hours, at which times residents received care from research staff that was designed to increase functional ability. Another four studies, completed within a predetermined time, tested dedicated FFC processes that were designed to utilize therapeutic techniques (conversational, occupational, and recreational) that were applied by trained interveners and therapists (Kolanowski et al., 2005; Tappen et al., 2002). The remaining eight studies used hired staff who were trained in FFC interventions to implement various programs (activities, room finding, exercise, and conversation) that were related to functional abilities (Beck et al., 2002; Bonanni et al., 2009; Bossers et al., 2015; Chan & Pang, 2010; Dechamps et al., 2010; Huang et al., 2016; Landi et al., 2004; Nolan et al., 2001).

Key Strategies Underpinning Effective Function-Focused Care Interventions

Interactive learning for caregivers

(Mezey et al. 2000) provided an educational program on abilities-focused morning care to caregivers who provide functional care services. This program employed role-playing and simulations and incorporated exercises that required caregiver participation and stimulated discussions to share applied learning experiences. Another study provided a restorative care education and training program to NH staff in the form of an interactive workshop conducted by a multidisciplinary team, which included an educator. This program used teaching methods such as role-playing, group strategizing, case studies, and practice exercises (Shanti et al., 2005). In another study, NH staff members participated in a training course, received supervision through nursing consultations, were given feedback via multidisciplinary consultations and emotion-oriented groups, and exchanged experiences and information to receive support (Finnema et al., 2005).

Content of the learning programs for caregivers

Several studies conducted educational sessions that were designed to teach caregivers intervention skills and knowledge to improve the functional abilities of residents (Table 2). Mezey et al. (2000) provided detailed information on the construction of their FFC intervention. The content was intended to enhance residents' social and self-care abilities through improving their skills in the realms of attention and conversation by the use of memory books, verbal cues, motor cues, and verbal prompts and the creation of relaxing environments. In another study (Shanti et al., 2005), NH staff participated in a five-module workshop designed to build skills and promote confidence; physical activity; communication; feeding and eating; positioning, mobility, and transfers; and assessment and evaluation. In a study of emotion-oriented approaches (Finnema et al., 2005), NH staff were trained in emphatic skills so that they could apply an emotion-oriented approach to daily care. Two studies (van Weert et al., 2005a, 2005b) trained certified nursing assistants to improve their practical skills and knowledge with regard to communication and Snoezelen, which involves reviewing specific behavior problems, identifying residents' sensory preferences, and applying sensory stimulation in daily care. In other studies (E. M. Galik et al., 2008; Resnick et al., 2009; Talley et al., 2015), an FFC intervention began with an in-service educational component for caregivers that included verbal encouragement or physiological feedback to foster resident self-efficacy while performing personal care activities.

Residents' preferences and interests

Schnelle et al. (2002) implemented FFC interventions after conducting repeated interviews to assess residents' preferences. Beck et al. (2002) carried out an assessment of residents' interests, which resulted in FFC interventions that were significantly more interesting to the residents ($p = .028$). In a study of theory-based recreational activities (Kolanowski et al., 2005), FFC interventions were classified according to residents' types of interest so that the program matched

TABLE 2.
The Contents of the Function-Focused Care Learning Program

Educational Module	Content
Communication	• Skills of attention, conversation, use of memory books, verbal cues, motor cues, verbal prompts, verbal encouragement, cueing with self-modeling
	• Social conversation, jokes, greetings, showing agreement/affection/partnership, conversations about sensory stimuli, supporting demented residents in responsiveness, avoiding correcting residents' subjective perceptions, cueing with self-modeling
Focusing on residents' emotions	• Being alert to the effects of residents' past experiences and acknowledging residents' experiences
	• (Non)verbal emphatic skills, showing affection and empathy with eye contact, instrumental touch, affective touch, smiling
	• A relaxing environment
Physical activity	• Specific exercises for bed- or wheelchair-bound residents and those with urinary incontinence, arthritis, and osteoporosis
	• Exercise training activities, range-of-motion exercises, brace and splint training, and amputation-prosthesis care
Positioning, mobility, and transfers	• Correct use of gait aids, transfer techniques for resident positioning (in bed and chairs), and other strategies for safe, independent ambulation
Activities of daily living	• Feeding/eating: hydration and aspiration problems; strategies to promote safe, independent eating practices; bathing; dressing; grooming; bowel and bladder training
Physiological feedback	• Pain management: medications, complementary techniques
	• Fear management: building confidence
	• Fatigue management: schedule rest times and reinforce their benefits
	• Management of shortness of breath: encourage breathing skills or use oxygen
Assessment and evaluation	• Setting individualized goals, awareness of residents' needs

residents' preferences for novelty (openness) and social stimulation (extraversion). This interest-matching strategy improved residents' behavioral function much more than treatment alone. Two studies of Snoezelen-integrated care focused on the discovery of which stimuli residents liked most and the integration of those stimuli into daily care (van Weert et al., 2005a, 2005b).

Individualized approach for each functional status
A notable study by Beck et al. (2002) applied an activities of daily living (ADL) intervention that used different behavioral methods that were designed to address residents' individual cognitive deficits. For example, residents with ideomotor apraxia required strategies such as physical guidance and touch to begin movement, whereas residents with dementia received single-step recommendations to guide ADL performance using behavior and communication techniques. In another study, the FFC intervention used a needs-driven dementia-compromised behavior (NDB) model that was intended to meet individual need and skill (physical and cognitive function) levels (Kolanowski et al., 2005). For example, passive residents became more functional and joined activities that were designed to provide social stimulation and novelty because the intervention reduced their with-

drawn behavior. One study addressed FFC intervention strategies for residents with functional impairments (Shanti et al., 2005). It examined residents with communication impairments (speech, voice, language, hearing, cognition, and/or vision) resulting from conditions such as dementia, stroke, and other neurological or medical conditions. Because of the potential diversity of functional status of older adults with complex diseases, Shanti et al. (2005) and E. Galik et al. (2014) focused on developing an individualized goal-setting strategy and then documenting outcomes. Two studies of Snoezelen-integrated care incorporated an underlying philosophy of person-centered care, which intends to maintain personhood even in cases of failing mental powers by grasping knowledge of the individual and showing affective involvement (van Weert et al., 2005a, 2005b).

Conceptual frameworks of function-focused care interventions
The theoretical basis of the FFC intervention study by Beck et al. (2002) was that the basic psychosocial needs of residents include territoriality, autonomy, communication, personal identity, self-esteem, cognitive understanding, safety, and security and that meeting these needs reduces disruptive behavior. The recreational activities efficacy study

of Kolanowski et al. (2005) hypothesized that residents would realize improved psychosocial outcomes when the NDB model was implemented. The NDB model changes negative behavioral symptoms into appropriate ones by meeting residents' needs. Finnema et al. (2005) reported designing an emotion-oriented FFC intervention specifically for residents with dementia, using an adaptation–coping model based on the crisis and stress–appraisal–coping models. Resnick et al. (2006, 2009) and E. M. Galik et al. (2008) applied self-efficacy and outcome expectations according to the self-efficacy theory and showed that efficacy expectations are enhanced by mastery experiences, verbal encouragement, vicarious experiences, and the management of affective and physiological states. Finally, E. Galik et al. (2014) used the Social Ecological Model, which addresses the effect of intrapersonal, interpersonal, policy, and environmental factors on behavior, as an FFC intervention framework.

Effectiveness of Function-Focused Care Interventions on Physical, Psychosocial, and Cognitive Functions

Most studies ($n = 19$, 86%) reported significant effects associated with FFC interventions as principal outcomes. These studies will be discussed according to NH residents' levels of cognitive function.

Of the nine studies of FFC interventions for residents with moderate to severe cognitive impairment, seven reported improvements and two reported mixed effects (no change or improvement). One experimental study (Nolan et al., 2001) revealed a 50% greater probability of residents with severe cognitive impairments finding their rooms using external memory aids. One RCT (E. Galik et al., 2014) found significant improvements in physical function at 3 months ($p = .01$) and physical activity (according to actigraphies and surveys) at 6 months ($p = .05$, $p = .01$) and a decrease in the number of fall events in the treatment group compared with the control group (28% vs. 50%, respectively; $p = .02$). The two RCTs for residents with moderate to severe dementia who received behavioral interventions reported the following effects—positive facial expressions ($p < .001$), contentment ($p = .037$), interest ($p = .028$), positive body posture/movements ($p < .001$), improved neuropsychiatric inventory scores ($p < .01$), improved Berg balance scores ($p = .01$), improved depressive symptoms ($p < .001$), improved quality of life ($p < .01$), and improved strength ($p < .01$; Beck et al., 2002; Dechamps et al., 2010)—but found also that disruptive behaviors were not significantly reduced (Beck et al., 2002). One quasi-experimental study (Mezey et al., 2000) that was conducted on participants with moderate to severe dementia showed that an abilities-focused program led to postintervention improvements in residents' psychosocial functions on the three subscales of personal attending, calm-functional behaviors, and agitation ($p = .046$) and in their level of overall function ($p = .023$). Two quasi-experimental studies of residents with moderate to severe dementia (van Weert et al.,

2005a, 2005b) found significant Snoezelen-integrated care effects for verbal expressed autonomy ($p < .01$), negative verbal behaviors ($p < .05$), nursing staff-directed gaze ($p < .05$), smiling ($p < .01$), apathetic behavior ($p < .05$), aggressive behavior ($p < .05$), loss of decorum ($p < .05$), rebellious behavior ($p < .05$), depression ($p < .05$), well-being (e.g., mood, enjoyment, happiness, sadness), and adaptive behavior (e.g., responding to speaking, normal-length sentences). One case–control study that incorporated physical activity with a psychosocial and behavior management training program (Landi et al., 2004) found a significant reduction in behavioral problems, such as physical and verbal abuse, wandering, and sleep disorders; as a consequence, the use of hypnotic and antipsychotic medications was reduced. Another study of 46 subjects (E. M. Galik et al., 2008) that employed a Res-Care intervention found an improvement in behavioral symptoms ($p = .04$) and mood ($p < .02$) and a decrease in physical activity, as measured by actigraphy ($p = .005$), but no significant change in overall physical activity or physical function.

Of the six studies of FFC interventions that were conducted on residents with mild to moderate cognitive impairment, four reported improvement and two reported no significant effects. One RCT study of restorative care (Resnick et al., 2009) found that physical performance such as gait and balance, stair climbing, walking, and bathing improved significantly ($p < .05$). Specifically, there was a significant improvement in overall balance and mobility from baseline to 4 months and a reduced decline in gait function at 12 months. Two RCTs for residents with mild to moderate dementia (Bossers et al., 2015; Huang et al., 2016) that was composed of behavioral and exercise interventions reported improvements in cognitive function ($p < .001$), visual memory ($p < .001$), verbal memory ($p = .003$), executive function ($p < .001$), walking endurance ($p = .004$), leg muscle strength ($p < .001$), balance ($p = .002$), fear of falling ($p < .001$), mobility ($p < .001$), depressive symptoms ($p < .001$), and muscle strength in the extremities ($p < .001$ or .01). One quasi-experimental study (Chan & Pang, 2010) that addressed residents with mild to moderate dementia found significant effects for the Let-Me-Talk advanced care planning program on treatment preference stability ($p \leq .001$) and communication treatment preferences ($p = .012$) as well as positive effects on existential distress ($p = .038$). However, two studies of residents with mild to moderate dementia (Blair et al., 2007; Resnick et al., 2006), which did not find significant results using an FFC intervention, did show some positive trends in terms of quality of life, outcome expectations, self-efficacy, participation in care activities, decline in pain, and independence during ADLs.

Of the seven studies that used an FFC intervention on residents with various cognitive conditions, six reported improvements and one found no significant effects. One RCT study (Tappen et al., 2002) on residents with mild to severe levels of cognitive impairment that implemented conversation and exercise interventions found significant improvement in the conciseness ($p = .0101$) and number of information units ($p = .0433$) in the conversation-only treatment group compared with the control group. Another RCT on residents who were able to obey instructions found that functional incidental training exercise improved continence, upper-body strength, and mobility significantly ($p = .0001–.05$; Schnelle et al., 2002). In addition, another RCT study on residents with mild to severe levels of cognitive impairment that implemented integrated emotion-oriented care found positive effects for the care approach in terms of maintaining emotional balance ($p = .04$) and preserving a positive self-image ($p = .04$; Finnema et al., 2005). A quasi-experimental study (Shanti et al., 2005) on residents who were able to benefit from an FFC intervention found that physical function in Goal Attainment Scaling ($p = .05$), Functional Independence Measure ($p < .001$), the Multidimensional Observation Scale for Elderly Subjects self-care ($p = .04$), and a hierarchical assessment of balance and mobility ($p = .03$) were improved significantly by the Restorative Care Education and Training Program. A trial of a dedicated restorative care program that was conducted on residents with a probability of functional decline found that ADL scores (33% of the residents), walking (30% of the residents), and locomotion (20% of the residents) had improved at 6 months (Bonanni et al., 2009). Another experimental study (Kolanowski et al., 2005) that was conducted on residents with mild to severe levels of cognitive impairment found that agitation ($p < .001$) and negative affect ($p = .056$) had significantly improved in the treatment groups. However, a longitudinal study (Talley et al., 2015) that analyzed data from a national NH survey found no increase in the ADL dependency score.

Discussion

The findings of this systematic review offer several recommendations for making FFC interventions more effective. This review revealed that both integrated and dedicated FFC intervention processes were accompanied by training and that dedicated-process caregivers, usually external staff, were trained in advance. This review covered an equal number of integrated-process ($n = 11$) and dedicated-process ($n = 11$) studies of FFC interventions. Because of the variety of measures of residents' functional abilities and types of study designs, this review was unable to determine which FFC intervention programs were most effective or whether integrated or dedicated processes are better. The decision to choose either an integrated or dedicated FFC intervention process may be made based on the preferences of the specific NH nursing work force (Schnelle et al., 2002).

Caregiver education about FFC interventions is an effective approach to optimizing the functioning of residents. A summary of the potential educational content for FFC interventions is provided in Table 2. An example of FFC interventions during ADLs is encouraging residents to walk to the bathroom rather than using a commode in their beds.

Regarding education method, interactive teaching is suggested to provide the knowledge and skills related to the FFC intervention because this method provides feedback from simulations (Shanti et al., 2005). Another suggestion is that education alone is insufficient and that supervisory support is crucial for successful implementation (Blair et al., 2007). These educational strategies may enhance the positive care behavior of caregivers and their communications related to the delivery of FFC interventions to residents.

Some studies used several conceptual frameworks. Self-efficacy theory was the most frequently used. Evidence is accumulating regarding the importance of theory-based FFC interventions. Thus, various educational materials are used in FFC interventions to train caregivers to encourage residents' self-efficacy and outcome expectations. In addition, the findings emphasized that FFC interventions should focus on individual resident-centered care by considering individual needs and preferences. The NDB model states that individuals have basic psychosocial needs and that negative behaviors may relate to these needs (Kolanowski et al., 2005). Even in studies that did not directly refer to this theory, the FFC intervention was conducted in a similar way because it was based on the social cognitive theory, which focuses on perceived self-efficacy and beliefs (Liu, Galik, Nahm, Boltz, & Resnick, 2015). Overall consideration of these conceptual frameworks suggests that functional interventions based on FFC philosophy will be more effective when they focus on the self-motivation and empowerment of the individual.

In terms of the effects of FFC, the effects on physical function, as reported in 13 studies, belonged to three outcome types: motor function, self-care ability, and incontinence. Motor function was presented as muscle strength or balance and mobility, and self-care ability was presented as independence measurements using ADL items. Of these 13 studies, 10 trials showed that the FFC interventions not only delay declines in physical function but also may improve physical function significantly.

Regarding the effects on psychosocial function, 12 of the 15 studies reported the positive effects of FFC on disruptive behavior or mood-specific outcomes. Because of the prevalence of behavioral problems in NH residents with dementia, FFC testing was often performed using psychosocial measurements. In particular, Harwood, Barker, Ownby, and Duara (2000) noted that behavioral symptoms (agitation and passivity) accounted for poor health outcomes, including social isolation and weakened physical functioning. In addition, FFC interventions stimulated more positive care interactions and emotional balance. The present review indicated that the resident-centered FFC approach made the relationship between caregivers and residents more satisfying and cooperative.

From an analysis of the three studies that focused directly on the effects on cognitive functions, we found that finding place and communication performance using words and information, memory, and Mini-Mental State Examination/Geriatric Depression Scale points was better. Although no shift in cognitive functioning level from moderate to mild or from severe to moderate was reported because of the progressive nature of dementia, the results did confirm additional benefits. Several studies indirectly confirmed improvements in psychosocial functioning that were related to behavioral symptoms associated with dementia.

Most of the studies included in this review used multiple positive measures of functional ability outcomes. Therefore, it was impossible to accurately determine which functional ability had improved the most. These findings support a previous research review (Resnick et al., 2013) on FFC interventions in multiple care settings that showed that FFC interventions with older adults showed positive results, either of less functional decline or of functional maintenance. Overall, this review further confirmed that implementing FFC interventions, regardless of the cognitive status of residents, is beneficial for optimizing their physical, psychosocial, and cognitive functional abilities.

There were some limitations of this review. Although several search strategies were employed to identify published FFC intervention studies, it is possible that some relevant published studies may have been missed because of the search terms used. In addition, because this review included only 22 studies, the combined sample is not large enough to generalize the findings widely beyond the surveyed populations. However, on the basis of currently published articles, these results provide evidence to support the efficacy of FFC interventions in NHs and an overview of various aspects of implementation for FFC interventions.

On the basis of this review, caregivers working in NH practice should accept FFC interventions as effective for residents who are more active and should consider the multidimensional benefits of FFC interventions on their residents' physical, psychological, and cognitive functions. Expanding this work to cover interventions that were designed to address residents with differing functional statuses across a larger population of residents will be critical, so as to optimize all of the functions necessary to develop a comprehensive FFC intervention.

Conclusions

The studies that were included in this review describe different FFC intervention programs and the numerous ways in which these programs were implemented. Most of the studies on the integrated FFC intervention process educated caregivers on related communication skills and on how to focus properly on residents' emotions, physical activity, physiological feedback, positioning, mobility and transfers, ADL, and assessment and evaluation. These FFC interventions used social cognitive theory as a framework to motivate residents. Most FFC interventions relate to physical and psychosocial functions. However, the lack of studies on cognitive and spiritual functions in the literature means that relational interventions have been developed in various ways.

Therefore, future studies should focus on these functional areas to identify effective FFC interventions that optimize comprehensive functional abilities.

Acknowledgments

This research was supported by the Basic Science Research Program under the National Research Foundation of Korea (NRF) and funded by the Ministry of Education, Science and Technology (NRF-2015R1D1A1A01057258).

References

Baker, D. I., Gottschalk, M., Eng, C., Weber, S., & Tinetti, M. E. (2001). The design and implementation of a restorative care model for home care. *The Gerontologist, 41*(2), 257–263. https://doi.org/10.1093/geront/41.2.257

Beck, C. K., Vogelpohl, T. S., Rasin, J. H., Uriri, J. T., O'Sullivan, P., Walls, R., … Baldwin, B. (2002). Effects of behavioral interventions on disruptive behavior and affect in demented nursing home residents. *Nursing Research, 51*(4), 219–228. https://doi.org/10.1097/00006199-200207000-00002

Blair, C. E., Glaister, J., Brown, A., & Phillips, C. (2007). Fostering activities of daily living by intact nursing home residents. *Educational Gerontology, 33*(8), 679–699. https://doi.org/10.1080/03601270701364149

Bonanni, D. R., Devers, G., Dezzi, K., Duerr, C., Durkin, M., Hernan, J., & Joyce, C. (2009). A dedicated approach to restorative nursing. *Journal of Gerontological Nursing, 35*(1), 37–44. https://doi.org/10.3928/00989134-20090101-02

Bossers, W. J., van der Woude, L. H., Boersma, F., Hortobágyi, T., Scherder, E. J., & van Heuvelen, M. J. (2015). A 9-week aerobic and strength training program improves cognitive and motor function in patients with dementia: A randomized, controlled trial. *The American Journal of Geriatric Psychiatry, 23*(11), 1106–1116. https://doi.org/10.1016/j.jagp.2014.12.191

Carpenter, G. I., Hastie, C. L., Morris, J. N., Fries, B. E., & Ankri, J. (2006). Measuring change in activities of daily living in nursing home residents with moderate to severe cognitive impairment. *BMC Geriatrics, 6*, 7. https://doi.org/10.1186/1471-2318-6-7

Chan, H. Y., & Pang, S. M. (2010). Let me talk—An advance care planning programme for frail nursing home residents. *Journal of Clinical Nursing, 19*(21–22), 3073–3084. https://doi.org/10.1111/j.1365-2702.2010.03353.x

Dechamps, A., Alban, R., Jen, J., Decamps, A., Traissac, T., & Dehail, P. (2010). Individualized cognition-action intervention to prevent behavioral disturbances and functional decline in institutionalized older adults: A randomized pilot trial. *International Journal of Geriatric Psychiatry, 25*(8), 850–860. https://doi.org/10.1002/gps.2427

Finnema, E., Dröes, R. M., Ettema, T., Ooms, M., Adèr, H., Ribbe, M., & van Tilburg, W. (2005). The effect of integrated emotion-oriented care versus usual care on elderly persons with dementia in the nursing home and on nursing assistants: A randomized clinical trial. *International Journal of Geriatric Psychiatry*, 20(4), 330–343. https://doi.org/10.1002/gps.1286

Galik, E., Resnick, B., Hammersla, M., & Brightwater, J. (2014). Optimizing function and physical activity among nursing home residents with dementia: Testing the impact of function-focused care. *The Gerontologist*, 54(6), 930–943. https://doi.org/10.1093/geront/gnt108

Galik, E. M., Resnick, B., Gruber-Baldini, A., Nahm, E. S., Pearson, K., & Pretzer-Aboff, I. (2008). Pilot testing of the restorative care intervention for the cognitively impaired. *Journal of the American Medical Directors Association*, 9(7), 516–522. https://doi.org/10.1016/j.jamda.2008.04.013

Harwood, D. G., Barker, W. W., Ownby, R. L., & Duara, R. (2000). Relationship of behavioral and psychological symptoms to cognitive impairment and functional status in Alzheimer's disease. *International Journal of Geriatric Psychiatry*, 15(5), 393–400. https://doi.org/10.1002/(SICI)1099-1166(200005)15:5<393::AID-GPS120>3.0.CO;2-O

Higgins, J. P. T., & Green, S. (Ed.). (2011). *Cochrane handbook for systematic reviews of interventions* (version 5.1.0). London, England: The Cochrane Collaboration. Retrieved from http://handbook-5-1.cochrane.org/

Huang, T. T., Chung, M. L., Chen, F. R., Chin, Y. F., & Wang, B. H. (2016). Evaluation of a combined cognitive–behavioural and exercise intervention to manage fear of falling among elderly residents in nursing homes. *Aging & Mental Health*, 20(1), 2–12. https://doi.org/10.1080/13607863.2015.1020411

Kolanowski, A. M., Litaker, M., & Buettner, L. (2005). Efficacy of theory-based activities for behavioral symptoms of dementia. *Nursing Research*, 54(4), 219–228. https://doi.org/10.1097/00006199-200507000-00003

Landi, F., Russo, A., & Bernabei, R. (2004). Physical activity and behavior in the elderly: A pilot study. *Archives of Gerontology and Geriatrics*, (9), 235–241. https://doi.org/10.1016/j.archger.2004.04.033

Liu, W., Galik, E., Nahm, E. S., Boltz, M., & Resnick, B. (2015). Optimizing eating performance for long-term care residents with dementia: Testing the impact of function-focused care for cognitively impaired. *Journal of American Medical Directors Association*, 16(12), 1062–1068. https://doi.org/10.1016/j.jamda.2015.06.023

Mezey, M., Fulmer, T., Wells, D. L., Dawson, P., Sidani, S., Craig, D., & Pringle, D. (2000). Effects of an abilities focused program of morning care residents who have dementia and on caregivers. *Journal of the American Geriatrics Society*, 48(4), 442–449. https://doi.org/10.1111/j.1532-5415.2000.tb04704.x

Nolan, B. A., Mathews, R. M., & Harrison, M. (2001). Using external memory aids to increase room finding by older adults with dementia. *American Journal of Alzheimer's Disease & Other Dementias*, 16(4), 251–254. https://doi.org/10.1177/153331750101600413

Park, J., Lee, Y., Seo, H., Jang, B., Son, H., Kim, S., ... Hahn, S. (2011). *Risk of bias assessment tool for non-randomized studies (RoBANS): Development and validation of a new instrument.* Retrieved from https://abstracts.cochrane.org/2011-madrid/risk-bias-assessment-tool-non-randomized-studies-robans-development-and-validation-new

Rabins, P. V., Lyketsos, C. G., & Steele, C. D. (2006). *Practical dementia care* (2nd ed.). New York, NY: Oxford University Press.

Resnick, B., Galik, E., & Boltz, M. (2013). Function focused care approaches: Literature review of progress and future possibilities. *Journal the American Medical Directors Association*, 14(5), 313–318. https://doi.org/10.1016/j.jamda.2012.10.019

Resnick, B., Galik, E., Gruber-Baldini, A., & Zimmerman, S. (2011). Testing the effect of function-focused care in assisted living. *Journal of the American Geriatrics Society*, 59(12), 2233–2240. https://doi.org/10.1111/j.1532-5415.2011.03699.x

Resnick, B., Gruber-Baldini, A. L., Zimmerman, S., Galik, E., Pretzer-Aboff, I., Russ, K., & Hebel, J. R. (2009). Nursing home resident outcomes from the Res-Care intervention. *Journal of the American Geriatrics Society*, 57(7), 1156–1165. https://doi.org/10.1111/j.1532-5415.2009.02327.x

Resnick, B., Simpson, M., Bercovitz, A., Galik, E., Gruber-Baldini, A., Zimmerman, S., & Magaziner, J. (2004). Testing of the Res-Care pilot intervention: Impact on nursing assistants. *Geriatric Nursing*, 25(5), 292–297. https://doi.org/10.1016/j.gerinurse.2004.08.002

Resnick, B., Simpson, M., Bercovitz, A., Galik, E., Gruber-Baldini, A., Zimmerman, S., & Magaziner, J. (2006). Pilot testing of the restorative care intervention: Impact on residents. *Journal of Gerontological Nursing*, 32(3), 39–47.

Schnelle, J. F., Alessi, C. A., Simmons, S. F., Al-Samarrai, N. R., Beck, J. C., & Ouslander, J. G. (2002). Translating clinical research into practice: A randomized controlled trial of exercise and incontinence care with nursing home residents. *Journal of the American Geriatrics Society*, 50(9), 1476–1483. https://doi.org/10.1046/j.1532-5415.2002.50401.x

Shanti, C., Johnson, J., Meyers, A. M., Jones, G. R., Fitzgerald, C., Lazowski, D. A., ... Ecclestone, N. A. (2005). Evaluation of the restorative care education and training program for nursing homes. *Canadian Journal on Aging*, 24(2), 115–126. https://doi.org/10.1353/cja.2005.0065

Talley, K. M., Wyman, J. F., Savik, K., Kane, R. L., Mueller, C., & Zhao, H. (2015). Restorative care's effect on activities of daily living dependency in long-stay nursing home residents. *The Gerontologist*, 55(1, Suppl.), S88–S98. https://doi.org/10.1093/geront/gnv011

Tappen, R. M., Williams, C. L., Barry, C., & Disesa, D. (2002). Conversation intervention with Alzheimer's patients: Increasing the relevance of communication. *Clinical Gerontologist*, 24(3–4), 63–75. https://doi.org/10.1300/J018v24n03_06

Taylor, D. H., Jr., & Sloan, F. A. (2000). How much do persons with Alzheimer's disease cost Medicare? *Journal of the American Geriatrics Society*, 48(6), 639–646. https://doi.org/10.1111/j.1532-5415.2000.tb04721.x

van Weert, J. C., van Dulmen, A. M., Spreeuwenberg, P. M., Ribbe, M. W., & Bensing, J. M. (2005a). Effects of Snoezelen, integrated in 24 h dementia care, on nurse–patient communication during morning care. *Patient Education & Counseling*, 58(3), 312–326. https://doi.org/10.1016/j.pec.2004.07.013

van Weert, J. C., van Dulmen, A. M., Spreeuwenberg, P. M., Ribbe, M. W., & Bensing, J. M. (2005b). Behavioral and mood effects of Snoezelen integrated into 24-hour dementia care. *Journal of the American Geriatrics Society*, 53(1), 24–33. https://doi.org/10.1111/j.1532-5415.2005.53006.x

Zimmerman, S., Sloane, P. D., & Reed, D. (2014). Dementia prevalence and care in assisted living. *Health Affairs*, 33(4), 658–666. https://doi.org/10.1377/hlthaff.2013.1255

4

Palliative Nursing for Cancer Patients as an Abstract Concept: A Hermeneutic Study

Leili BORIMNEJAD[1] • Marjan MARDANI-HAMOOLEH[2]* • Naimeh SEYEDFATEMI[3] • Mamak TAHMASEBI[4]

ABSTRACT

Background: Understanding the outcomes of palliative care (PC) that is provided to patients with cancer is necessary.

Purpose: The aim of this study was to explore the lived experiences of Iranian nurses with regard to PC outcomes in cancer patients.

Methods: This hermeneutic study interviewed 14 nurses to understand their lived experiences with regard to PC outcomes in cancer patients. A seven-stage process of data analysis was employed.

Results: One constitutive pattern "palliative nursing for cancer patients is an abstractive concept" and the two associated themes of "providing excellent PC" and "PC as an alarm" were identified. Providing excellent PC had two subthemes: being a unique nurse and experiencing the humanistic approach to caring. PC as an alarm also had two subthemes: caring-related concerns and challenging issues caused by caring.

Conclusions: The findings provide a deeper understanding of the nursing experience with regard to PC outcomes in cancer patients.

KEY WORDS:
cancer, hermeneutic phenomenology, nurse, palliative care, patient.

Introduction

Cancer remains one of the main causes of human death worldwide, although the mortality rate for cancer has been in continual decline for the past two decades (Siegel, Miller, & Jemal, 2015). Cancer is a growing concern in Middle Eastern countries (Daher, 2011). In Iran, cancer is the third most common cause of death after heart disease and road accidents (Heidari & Mardani-Hamooleh, 2016). The incidence of cancer in Iran is estimated to be around 48–112 and 51–144 persons per year per million for women and men, respectively (Seyedfatemi, Borimnejad, Mardani Hamooleh, & Tahmasebi, 2014). Sadly, nonscientifically based cultural attitudes regarding cancer still widely persist, indicating that cancer-related taboos have not yet been broken (Borimnejad, Mardani Hamooleh, Seyedfatemi, & Tahmasebi, 2014).

Cancer negatively affects the lives of patients, with many requiring palliative care (PC), which is a holistic, humanistic, and cooperative mode of care that promotes the quality of life of patients and their families and helps them deal with the physical, psychological, spiritual, religious, cultural, and social aspects of their cancer experience (Negarandeh, Mardani Hamooleh, & Rezaee, 2015). There is a worldwide need for PC in the care of cancer patients (Human Rights Watch, 2011). Despite the emphasis on comprehensive and humanitarian care, providing PC is stressful for nursing personnel. Moreover, the physical and psychological fatigue of nurses negatively affects their effectiveness in providing PC (Hamooleh, Borimnejad, Seyedfatemi, & Tahmasebi, 2013).

In Iran, the main barrier faced by nursing discipline in offering PC to patients with cancer is the lack of a clear structure for nursing personnel, as PC does not receive sufficient consideration in the education curriculum (Iranmanesh, Axelsson, Häggström, & Sävenstedt, 2010). In fact, the 4-year nursing curriculum that is required to receive a bachelor's degree in nursing in Iran provides no PC-related academic credits or clinical training (Rassouli & Sajjadi, 2014). Given the rising incidence of cancer in Iran and the importance of increasing the level of quality of life in cancer patients, PC is of fundamental importance for these patients. In Iran, PC services are provided to patients with incurable diseases, particularly those with end-phase diseases. PC is client centered, which implies that a holistic approach is required to meet patient needs. Contrary to the development of the fundamental healthcare program in Iran, a progressive program for giving professional PC services does not exist yet, as healthcare services do not give planned end-of-life PC to patients. The PC plan for cancer includes promoting the establishment of palliative and supportive medical units across the country. In the past few years, attention to PC has increased in Iran. However, coverage is irregular, with PC provided at a few centers only. Thus, many cancer patients are deprived of appropriate PC. Only one referral public hospital currently provides PC services to cancer patients in Iran (Tahmasebi, 2013), and improving PC-related services is being actively discussed for the Iranian oncology setting (Seyedfatemi et al., 2014). As understanding the outcomes of PC is an essential part of caring for cancer patients effectively, it is important for nurses

[1]PhD, Associate Professor, Center for Nursing Care Research, Iran University of Medical Sciences, Tehran, Iran • [2]PhD, Assistant Professor, Iran University of Medical Sciences, Tehran, Iran • [3]PhD, Professor, Center for Nursing Care Research, Iran University of Medical Sciences, Tehran, Iran • [4]MD, Consultant in Palliative Medicine, and Associate Professor, Cancer Institute, Tehran University of Medical Sciences, Tehran, Iran.

to address these outcomes. Therefore, studying these nurses and their perceptions related to the outcomes of PC in cancer patients is essential. In addition, understanding the perspectives and experiences of other nurses regarding the outcomes of PC may offer oncology nurses a chance to develop their own modes of care.

A review of the literature indicates that few qualitative research studies have assessed PC outcomes in cancer patients in Iran. This study was thus designed to explore the lived experiences of nurses in Iran regarding the PC outcomes of cancer patients.

Methods

Design

This qualitative research was accomplished using a hermeneutic phenomenological method, a method that elicits the perspective of respondents on the meaning of "being in the world" (Heidegger, 1962). Using the hermeneutic phenomenological method in the present research was intended to permit the participant nurses to focus on their lived experiences through explaining their experiences caring for PC for cancer patients.

Participants

This study was performed in the oncology wards of two teaching hospitals in Tehran, Iran, specializing in the treatment of patients with cancer. The wards in these hospitals have 15–32 beds and offer PC to cancer patients. Nurses with full-time work experience of at least 1 year in oncology nursing were included in the study. We employed a purposeful maximum variation sampling of 14 baccalaureate degree nurses (eight women and six men). Nine were married, and the remainder were single. The participants ranged from 28 to 46 years old, had been working in oncology wards from 3 to 15 years, and had 4–18 years of nursing work experience. To ensure that all of the qualified nurses at the target teaching hospitals were offered a chance to participate, the wards were frequently visited by the second author, covering all three nursing shifts. The key criterion for inclusion was the experience of providing PC to cancer patients.

Data Collection

The data were collected during the spring and summer of 2015. Face-to-face, semistructured individual interviews lasting around 35–50 minutes were held in the oncology wards. Fourteen participants were selected before reaching data saturation, that is, the point at which no new themes appeared in the ongoing data analysis. Each participant was interviewed once, with 14 interviews conducted. Over a 3-month period, the participants were interviewed by the second author in their wards. An interview guide was used, and the interviews were audiotaped. The interviews were done in Persian by the second

author. The segments of the interviews that were relevant to the present article were translated into English by a specialist translator and then back translated into Persian for verification by the first author. The key question asked in the interviews was "What is your lived experience with regard to the PC outcomes in cancer patients?" After the participants responded to the above question, more questions were asked to enrich the data such as "Would you clarify this further?", "What do you mean by that?", and "Could you please provide me an example in order to assist us to better comprehend your point of view?"

Data Analysis

Data gathering and analysis occurred simultaneously. Teamwork was used to analyze the data, and a seven-stage data analysis procedure (Diekelmann, Allen, & Tanner, 1989) was employed to gain a better understanding of the lived experiences of the nurses.

Stage 1: Each interview text was read through completely to gain a general understanding.

Stages 2 and 3: Probable common meaning units were recognized using extracts to support the interpretation. The authors repeatedly listened to the tape recordings to extract the real meaning from the data.

Stage 4: The research group evaluated their interpretations for similarities and dissimilarities, gaining more insight and agreement by revisiting the primary text.

Stage 5: All of the texts were revised to verify the emergent themes and subthemes. Next, these themes and subthemes were then classified by the research team.

Stage 6: A constitutive pattern was recognized that presented the connection between these themes and subthemes across all of the texts.

Stage 7: The research team created a final report, including quotes that were provided to each participant for their review and confirmation of the accuracy of the contents.

Rigor

The trustworthiness of this study is supported by four criteria: credibility, dependability, conformability, and transferability (Lincoln & Guba, 1985). To achieve credibility, interview texts, extracted meaning units, and themes and subthemes were discussed by several of the participants and two persons with doctoral degrees in nursing. To establish data dependability, the views of an external viewer who is a well-known phenomenological researcher were adopted. To attain conformability, all of the actions were recorded, and a report was arranged on the progression of the study. To ensure data transferability, data were collected and analyzed from two nurses who were outside this study and who had circumstances similar to the participants.

Ethical Consideration

The study proposal was confirmed by the ethics committee of Tehran University of Medical Sciences (Proposal code: 194-1195-1353, Ethical code: 952133), and legal permissions were obtained before conducting the interviews. The data gathering process was accomplished after confirming oral consent and obtaining signed informed consent from all of the participating nurses. The participants were guaranteed that all of the data would remain confidential and that they had the right to withdraw at any time during or after the interviews. If participants wished, they could obtain the audio files. The interview setting was a quiet place within the participant's cancer ward, and interviews were held at the convenience of each participant. There were no dependency relationships or conflicts of interests between the interviewer and interviewees.

Results

The findings were organized under two main themes: providing excellent PC and PC as an alarm. Providing excellent PC had two subthemes: being a unique nurse and experiencing the humanistic approach to caring. PC as an alarm also had two subthemes: caring-related concerns and challenging issues caused by caring. These themes and subthemes reflected the meaning for the participants of PC outcomes in cancer patients. The constitutive pattern of this study was "palliative nursing for cancer patients is an abstractive concept." The study themes and the participants' quotations are explained below.

Providing Excellent Palliative Care

Participants reported that being a unique nurse and adopting a humanistic approach to caring were important to providing excellent PC to cancer patients.

Being a unique nurse

Nurses perceived that thanking God during difficult situations and being more grateful in their personal life were outcomes that they received from their PC work in the cancer ward: "*Facing patients' difficulties caused me to say that my difficulties are very small in comparison with them and I have become more thankful to God for what I have.*" (Participant [P] 4)

Stronger spiritual beliefs and self-confidence represent another aspect of being a unique nurse in the cancer ward, reducing fear of death and increasing kindness to others: "*My spiritual beliefs have increased and are influencing my personal life. Working in this ward has reduced my fear of death.*" (P6)

Understanding that I had the greatest blessings in this ward but had been unaware of them is like a mountain whose reflection has returned to me and increased my self-confidence. (P3)

I feel that providing PC to cancer patients has made me kinder and that that it has influenced my care of patients. (P8)

I always PC to cancer patients is a way to heaven. (P12)

Moreover, nurses expressed feeling blessed by their work in the cancer ward: "*My father believes that the blessings of this work return to my own life and I think he is right because I had some successes in my work that I know are rooted in working in this ward.*" (P2)

Experiencing the humanistic approach to caring

PC strengthened the ability of cancer patients to fight against cancer or helped him or her to have a peaceful death: "*We help patients to fight death or have a peaceful death to increase their life quality.*" (P5)

The participants expressed the belief that providing PC to cancer patients helped preserve human dignity, reduce pain, and support patients: "*In my opinion, one outcome of PC is preserving the human dignity of the patients in an appropriate way. Respect for the patient is considered in PC.*" (P11)

I have noticed that when I do PC, narcotics reduce patients' pain and they seem satisfied. (P10)

When PC is done for a patient in a good way, he actually receives multilateral support, which results in a better life. (P14)

Palliative Care as an Alarm

Nurses mentioned a range of caring-related concerns and challenging issues.

Caring-related concerns

Repeated vein puncture in cancer patients and fatigue in the ward made nurses averse to PC: "*Vein puncture in most cancer patients is difficult and bothers them but I have to do it, which is aversive to me.*" (P13)

Patients' inability to express their sexual needs made nurses worried:

One of my distresses with regard to cancer patient PC is that they cannot not talk about their sexual needs or are so ashamed while doing it. (P7)

Most cancer patients have some problems in their sexual relationship with their spouse but hide it because of cultural boundaries. This issue makes nurses worried. (P1)

This point, that nurses did not observe the positive results of PC in the cancer ward, was an alarm that made nurses depressed: "*If I knew that PC could result in having a normal life, I would not get depressed. My personal life may be influenced by this depression.*" (P9)

In addition, nurses mentioned the stressful identity of cancer patient PC, which was aversive to them: "*Working with terminal patients is really hard and stressful...most of them know they have short lives and their stress is transmitted to us.*" (P8)

> *Seeing a patient that knows death is near bothers me.* (P2)

In fact, dealing with patients in the final stages of life and their deaths was an alarm of PC that may increase the concerns of nurses: "*I feel sad while confronting the patient's family who are mourning for the patient that is still alive.*" (P5)

> *Once I was responsible for calling discharged patients. I called 6 families, all of whom said the patient died! I felt bad, did not call any more families and I was even so sad at home.* (P10)

Challenging issues caused by caring

Nurses believed that cancer patient PC would result in occupational burnout, a motivation to work, and reduction of job satisfaction: "*Once a goldsmith asked me where I work? When I replied in a cancer ward he said selling flowers in a stall is better than working in the cancer ward! Run away! My family and friends tell me 'quit your job!' Hearing such words causes occupational burnout in nurses in the long term.*" (P6)

> *High mortality rate in this ward motivates us to offer PC and causes challenges in the nursing system.* (P12)

> *No one could believe that once we had 5 deaths in a night shift! It is easy to say but really reduces nurses' job satisfaction.* (P7)

> *In my opinion, nurses who provide PC should be moved to another ward occasionally with the aim of increasing their job satisfaction.* (P11)

However, offering PC to cancer patients is frequently stigmatized. Furthermore, working in the cancer ward for long periods may cause nurse burnout and result in nurses leaving their jobs: "*Fewer nurses accept working here, they think cancer patient PC is a disgrace! Nurses who work in this ward for a long time will become exhausted and finally quit nursing.*" (P13)

The Constitutive Pattern: Palliative Nursing for Cancer Patients as an Abstract Concept

According to the lived experiences of the participants, providing palliative nursing to cancer patients is an abstract concept.

They claimed that, on the one hand, these impacts exalted their personal and occupational life and, on the other hand, were a threat to them. Nevertheless, their perceptions showed that their negative points about PC had not yet resulted in negative absolutism. Real obstacles could not prevent nurses from providing PC to their patients but caused them to find deeper layers of PC that give continuity to the care provided.

Discussion

The participants in this study perceived distinct outcomes of cancer patient PC that may have varied effects on their personal and occupational life. In addition, PC fluctuated between different contradictions. According to Roach (1987), caring is the unique manifestation of a person's being in the world. It may be shown through love or compassion, sorrow or joy, and sadness or despair. It is humankind fired with zeal, concern, or solicitude or humanity bruised to the very core of its being.

In this study, providing excellent PC included being a unique nurse and experiencing a humanistic approach to caring. Generally, being thankful to God in difficult times and having the strength to cope with them, reinforcement of spiritual beliefs, increased self-confidence, becoming kinder, finding a way to heaven, being more grateful in life, lessening the fear of death, and success in personal affairs represent the perceptions of the participants regarding providing excellent PC. In Iran, nurses have a spiritual outlook toward their job, believe in spiritual rewards for their profession, and, because of their spiritual outlook, do their work to satisfy God. In addition, providing PC to terminal patients changed their points of view about life and death. Watson (1985) explains nursing as a human science, with the main focus being the process of human care. Roach also discussed that caring is the human mode of being, with nursing as the profession-alization of human caring.

Findings of this study are consistent with the result of a study that showed that oncology nurses use some coping strategies with stresses at work to empower them to solve personal and occupational problems (Zander, Hutton, & King, 2013). In general, participants claimed that reducing pain, preserving human dignity, and receiving multilateral support are positive reactions of PC. Eriksson (1992) perceives suffering and pain as normal human phenomena. She claimed that nurses should try to alleviate pain in all caring functions. In addition, Watson reported that caring in nursing is expressed in the context of not only caring for patients' basic needs but also caring for patient values. She highlighted the nursing act of helping individuals while preserving the dignity and worth of the patient regardless of his or her condition. Other studies have confirmed these findings (Borimnejad et al., 2014; Fernandes et al., 2013; Hamooleh et al., 2013).

In this study, the participants helped patients to experience a peaceful death, which, in the participants' opinions, had positive results for the patients. Prior research has shown that nurses make death more peaceful for terminal patients in accordance with those patients' requests (Neergaard et al., 2009). In fact, nursing personnel have an exclusive role to bolster the right of patients to improve their quality of life and to experience a dignified and undisturbed death (Elcigil, 2011).

On the other hand, this study investigated whether the participants perceived PC in terms of a range of alarms covering caring-related concerns and challenging issues. The participants reported that PC was upsetting and stressful. They believed that care-related alarms affected their personal life. Likewise, prior research has shown that caregivers of cancer patients experience negative feelings that change their personal life and ultimately affect the patient care process (de Duarte, Zanini, & Nedel, 2012). In addition, our results revealed that the high mortality rate and even being informed about the death of a patient affected the nurses considerably. In other words, nurses perceived the death of patients as a significant emotional challenge. Findings of a study indicated that nurses experienced acute emotional suffering because of facing the death of their patients (Huang, Chen, & Chiang, 2016).

Another concern of nurses that was associated with alarms of care for cancer patients was their sexual needs. The participants expressed that they felt that their patients were typically unable or ashamed to express these needs. Similarly, other research has indicated that cancer patients are ashamed to express their sexual needs (Abdollahzadeh et al., 2014; Heidari & Mardani-Hamooleh, 2016). These cultural findings reveal that talking about sexual needs is difficult for patients in Iran. These results support the need to further expand and enhance cultural-related intervention and to address the concept of cultural care in palliative nursing. Leininger (2002) found humans as inseparable from their cultural environment. She said that caring is a worldwide phenomenon and proposed that views of caring may vary with cultural context. In the culture-based perspective, healthcare providers may be able to provide better care based on the cultural attitudes that support cancer patients in improving, maintaining, and regaining health in the contexts of their life conditions (Surbone & Baider, 2013). In addition, as the findings of this study showed that participants encounter cultural barriers related to their sexual needs, we may reduce these barriers through education.

The participants perceived challenging issues that included occupational burnout, reduced job satisfaction, and motivation to work or to quit due to PC alarms. The participants further mentioned that working in the cancer ward reduced job satisfaction. They believed that PC may result in professional burnout and their quitting in the longer term. The participants linked their provision of PC with a loss of job motivation. In their opinion, this situation challenges the nursing system. These findings are consistent with the results of a study that showed care for cancer patients to be challenging (Kovács, Szabó, & Fülöp, 2013). Moreover, nurses stated that friends, associates, and society prohibited them from and reproached them for working in cancer wards. In

fact, the participants noted that working with cancer patients increased the already negative public perception of oncology nurses. From their point of view, this may lead to occupational burnout. In addition, some of the participants perceived providing PC to patients as a stigma, leaving them disinclined to work in cancer wards. However, considering the PC as a stigma endangers the continuum of patient care (Ramchandran & Von Roenn, 2013). On the basis of the experiences of the authors, all of whom work in cancer wards in Iran, the stigmatization of cancer is associated with severe and negative effects on nurses. Thus, their perspectives on cancer care are influenced by culture. Caring for cancer patients faces nurses with myriad challenges. PC services are especially challenging for nurses. These services may lead to many disagreeable and risky outcomes such as stress, depression, burnout, and low job satisfaction. Recognition of these nursing challenges has implications for clinical improvements in supporting nurses during this challenging situation. Continued effort is necessary to overcome these and other challenges to the successful provision of PC.

This is the first qualitative study in Iran to generate information on the perspectives of nurses on providing PC to cancer patients. Thus, we believe that the findings are uniquely important. We suggest that additional qualitative studies be conducted widely on this subject to provide richer data and to expand understanding of related issues. Furthermore, research into the lived experiences of members of other healthcare groups may enhance our understanding of related outcomes.

Conclusions

The findings of the present research highlight certain aspects of the outcomes of patients with cancer in Iran. The lived experiences of the nurses in this study revealed that the negative effects of PC did not prevent them from providing PC to patients. Consequently, considering social and cultural situations in Iran, it seems that Iranians prefer rational outcomes to nonrational outcomes in light of the inclination that participants expressed toward the positive effects of PC in cancer wards despite their perceived negative feedback. Our results show that palliative nursing for cancer patients is influenced by a variety of conditions. Thus, a deep understanding of these circumstances is critical to help nursing managers design effective strategies for managing cancer care.

Limitations

The present research did not limit its focus to a specific type or stage of cancer. Thus, the nurse participants worked in wards that included a broad range of patients with different types and stages of cancer.

Acknowledgments

The authors wish to express their appreciation and special thanks to all of the nurses who kindly participated in this study.

References

Abdollahzadeh, F., Moradi, N., Pakpour, V., Rahmani, A., Zamanzadeh, V., Mohammadpoorasl, A., & Howard, F. (2014). Un-met supportive care needs of Iranian breast cancer patients. *Asian Pacific Journal of Cancer Prevention, 15*(9), 3933–3938. https://doi.org/10.7314/APJCP.2014.15.9.3933

Borimnejad, L., Mardani Hamooleh, M., Seyedfatemi, N., and Tahmasebi, M. (2014). Human relationships in palliative care of cancer patient: Lived experiences of Iranian nurses. *Materia Socio-Medica, 26*(1), 35–38. https://doi.org/10.5455/msm.2014.26.35-38

Daher, M. (2011). Opioids for cancer pain in the Middle Eastern countries: A physician point of view. *Journal of Pediatric Hematology/Oncology, 33*(1, Suppl.), S23–S28. https://doi.org/10.1097/MPH.0b013e3182121a0f

de Duarte, M. L., Zanini, L. N., & Nedel, M. N. (2012). The daily routine of parents of children hospitalized with cancer: Nursing challenges. *Revista Gaucha de Enfermagem, 33*, 111–118.

Diekelmann, N., Allen, D., & Tanner, C. (1989). *The NLN criteria for appraisal for baccalaureate programs: A critical hermeneutic analysis*. New York, NY: National League for Nursing.

Elcigil, A. (2011). The current status of palliative care in Turkey: A nurse's perspective. *Journal of Pediatric Hematology/ Oncology, 33*(1, Suppl.), S70–S72. https://doi.org/10.1097/MPH.0b013e318212244a

Eriksson, K. (1992). The alleviation of suffering—The idea of caring. *Scandinavian Journal of Caring Science, 6*(2), 119–123. https://doi.org/10.1111/j.1471-6712.1992.tb00134.x

Fernandes, M. A., Evangelista, C. B., Platel, I. C., Agra, G., Lopes Mde, S., & Rodrigues Fde, A. (2013). The perception by nurses of the significance of palliative care in patients with terminal cancer. *Ciencia and Saude Coletiva, 18*(9), 2589–2596. https://doi.org/10.1590/S1413-81232013000900013

Hamooleh, M. M., Borimnejad, L., Seyedfatemi, N., & Tahmasebi, M. (2013). Perception of Iranian nurses regarding ethics-based palliative care in cancer patients. *Journal of Medical Ethics and History Medicine, 6*, 12.

Heidari, H., & Mardani-Hamooleh, M. (2016). Cancer patients' informational needs: Qualitative content analysis. *Journal of Cancer Education, 31*(4), 715–720. https://doi.org/10.1007/s13187-015-0887-z

Heidegger, M. (1962). *Being and time* (Macquarie, J., & Robenson, E., Trans., 1st ed.). Oxford, UK: Basil Blackwell.

Huang, C. C., Chen, J. Y., & Chiang, H. H. (2016). The transformation process in nurses caring for dying patients. *The Journal of Nursing Research, 24*(2), 109–117. https://doi.org/10.1097/jnr.0000000000000160

Human Rights Watch. (2011). *Global state of pain treatment. Palliative care as a human right*. Retrieved from www.hrw.org/reports/2011/06/02/global-state-pain-treatment-0

Iranmanesh, S., Axelsson, K., Häggström, T., & Sävenstedt, S. (2010). Caring for dying people: Attitudes among Iranian and Swedish nursing students. *Indian Journal of Palliative Care, 16*(3), 147–153. https://doi.org/10.4103/0973-1075.73643

Kovács, Z., Szabó, C., & Fülöp, E. (2013).Therapy helps—Psychosocial support for patients diagnosed with breast cancer, reducing anxiety and depression. *Psychiatria Hungarica, 28*(4), 454–463.

Leininger, M. (2002). Culture care theory: A major contribution to advance transcultural nursing knowledge and practices. *Journal of Transcultural Nursing, 13*(3), 189–192.

Lincoln, Y. S., & Guba, E. G. (1985). *Naturalistic inquiry*. London, England: Sage Publications.

Neergaard, M. A., Vedsted, P., Olesen, F., Sokolowski, I., Jensen, A. B., & Søndergaard, J. (2009). Associations between home death and GP involvement in palliative cancer care. *The British Journal of General Practice, 59*(566), 671–677. https://doi.org/10.3399/bjgp09X454133

Negarandeh, R., Mardani Hamooleh, M., & Rezaee N. (2015). Concept analysis of palliative care in nursing: Introducing a hybrid model. *Journal of Mazandaran University of Medical Sciences, 25*(130), 40–51.

Ramchandran, K., & Von Roenn, J. H. (2013). Palliative care always. *Oncology (Williston Park), 27*(1), 13–16.

Rassouli, M., & Sajjadi, M. (2014). Palliative care in Iran: Moving toward the development of palliative care for cancer. *American Journal of Hospice and Palliative Care, 33*(3), 240–244. Retrieved from http://journals.sagepub.com/doi/abs/10.1177/1049909114561856. https://doi.org/10.1177/1049909114561856

Roach, M. S. (1987). *The human act of caring: A blueprint for health professions*. Toronto, Canada: Canadian Hospital Association.

Seyedfatemi, N., Borimnejad, L., Mardani Hamooleh, M., & Tahmasebi, M. (2014). Iranian nurses' perceptions of palliative care for patients with cancer pain. *International Journal of Palliative Nursing, 20*(2), 69–74. https://doi.org/10.12968/ijpn.2014.20.2.69

Siegel, R. L., Miller, K. D., & Jemal, A. (2015). Cancer statistics, 2015. *CA Cancer Journal for Clinicians, 65*(1), 5–29. https://doi.org/10.3322/caac.21254

Surbone, A., & Baider, L. (2013). Personal values and cultural diversity. *Journal of Medicine and the Person, 11*(1), 11–18. https://doi.org/10.1007/s12682-013-0143-4

Tahmasebi, M. (2013). Palliative care for the end-of-Life cancer patients in the emergency department in Iran. *Iranian Journal of Cancer Prevention, 6*(4), 231–232.

Watson, J. (1985). *Nursing: Human science and human care—A theory of nursing*. New York, NY: National League of Nursing Press.

Zander, M., Hutton, A., & King, L. (2013). Exploring resilience in paediatric oncology nursing staff. *Collegian, 20*(1), 17–25. https://doi.org/10.1016/j.colegn.2012.02.002

5

The Shared Subjective Frames of Interdisciplinary Practitioners Involved in Function-Focused Care in a Nursing Home: Q-Methodology

Mi So KIM[1] • Gyu-Tae KIM[2] • Su Jung LEE[1] • Min Sun PARK[1] • Eun-hye JEONG[3] • Sung Ok CHANG[4]*

ABSTRACT

Background: An interdisciplinary team-based approach in nursing homes has been suggested in the literature as a strategy for delaying functional decline in residents. Function-focused care is a philosophy-based approach in which interdisciplinary practitioners assess functional capacity and help older adults to optimize and maintain their remaining abilities.

Purpose: This study explored and described the shared subjective frames of interdisciplinary practitioners as regards function-focused care for nursing home residents.

Methods: Q-methodology was used to analyze the subjectivity of each factor of function-focused care for nursing home residents. Data were collected from August to September 2016. Thirty-four Q-statements were selected and scored by the 30 interdisciplinary practitioners on a 9-point scale with a normal distribution. Data were analyzed using the PQ Method 2.33 program.

Results: The results revealed four factors of function-focused care, including (a) using a wait-and-see approach to encourage self-care, (b) maintaining interactive communications to identify and respond to changes, (c) reinforcing residents' inner and outer strengths for homeostasis, and (d) using a tailored approach based on comparisons between the past and the present. Shared subjectivity may provide an important collaborative framework to identify and solve complex problems related to the functional needs of nursing home residents.

Conclusions: The results of this study elucidate the subjectivities of interdisciplinary practitioners and better enable their provision of effective care in support of the remaining functional abilities of older adults living in nursing homes. The findings may be used as a reference to establish communication methods and shared documentation for interdisciplinary practitioners in nursing homes and construct interdisciplinary function-focused care practice guidelines.

KEY WORDS:
function-focused care, interdisciplinary, nursing homes, Q-methodology, subjective frames.

Introduction

The world population is aging rapidly, with the percentage of those over the age of 65 years expected to increase from 8.5% in 2015 to 16.7% in 2050 (He, Goodkind, Kowal, & U.S. Census Bureau, 2016). The older adult populationin Asia, which is growing at a much faster rate than in Europe or North America, is an increasing social burden. To ameliorate this problem, Japan in 2000 became the first country in Asia to introduce a long-term care insurance system. South Korea introduced its long-term care system in 2008; as a result, the number of nursing homes (NHs) has risen by 135.4%, from 1,332 in 2008 to 3,136 in 2016 (Statistics Korea, 2017).

In general, older adults residing in NHs are frail and have chronic illnesses and complex health statuses (Congressional Budget Office, 2013). Several studies have recommended an interdisciplinary team-based approach to prevent or slow functional decline, with teams including nursing staff (advanced nurse practitioners, registered nurses, and nursing assistants), geriatricians, pharmacists, psychologists, dietitians, physical therapists, occupational therapists, and social workers (Aniemeke et al., 2017; de Mazières et al., 2017; Eckstrom et al., 2016). Function-focused care (FFC) is a philosophy that focuses on assessment of the underlying function-related capabilities of older adults to assist these individuals optimize and maintain their remaining abilities through continual increases in the time spent performing physical activities (Resnick & Galik, 2013). Many long-term care settings such as NHs attempt to implement FFC programs to help residents optimize performance across a broad range of functional abilities

[1]PhD, RN, Research Professor, College of Nursing, Korea University, Seoul, ROK • [2]PhD, Professor, School of Electrical Engineering, Korea University, Seoul, ROK • [3]RN, Doctoral Student, College of Nursing, Korea University, Seoul, ROK • [4]PhD, RN, Professor, College of Nursing, Korea University, Seoul, ROK.

(Lee, Kim, Jung, & Chang, 2019). The core members of the interdisciplinary team working in NHs include physical therapists, who restore, maintain, and promote physical function of NH residents; occupational therapists, who develop, recover, and improve skills necessary for daily living; social workers, who provide psychosocial assessments and interventions to maintain and enhance physical and mental health; and nursing staff, who help maximize residents' remaining functional abilities through systematic assessment and individualized interventions (American Physical Therapy Association, 2019; Lim et al., 2014; Vongxaiburana, Thomas, Frahm, & Hyer, 2011).

Interdisciplinary practitioners use their subjectivities to provide care for residents and to promote functioning. The subjectivities of a practitioner reflect philosophical viewpoints, values, attitudes, and experiences (Akhtar-Danesh, Dehghan, Morrison, & Fonseka, 2011; Simons, 2013) and have the characteristics of a self-directory (Doo & Lee, 2016). Thus, the FFC provided by interdisciplinary practitioners in NH settings reflects both individual and shared subjectivity among interdisciplinary practitioners. Shared cognition in realms such as knowledge, information, beliefs, and attitudes shapes explanations and expectations of tasks, which may in turn coordinate behaviors and ultimately help shape an effective interdisciplinary team approach (Razzouk & Johnson, 2012; Washington et al., 2017). No prior study has examined the shared FFC-related subjectivities of interdisciplinary practitioners working in NHs. Therefore, the purpose of this study was to explore the shared FFC-related subjectivity of these practitioners.

Methods

Research Design

This study used a Q-methodological approach to explore and describe the FFC-related subjectivities of interdisciplinary practitioners working in an NH setting. The Q-methodology, developed by Stephenson (1935) to explore individual subjectivity, combines the strengths of qualitative and quantitative research to enable individuals to express their subjectivities and perspectives on an issue (as cited in Simons, 2013). The Q-methodology has been broadly applied in healthcare-related research (Spurgeon, Humphreys, James, & Sackley, 2012).

Procedure

Data were collected from August to September 2016. Figure 1 depicts the steps that were used in the Q-methodology for this study.

Concourse and Q-Sample

The concourse, that is, the sum of thoughts from the participants, was developed using interviews with 30 interdisciplinary practitioners (nurses, physical therapists, occupational therapists, and social workers) working in NHs. In-depth interviews were conducted with NH interdisciplinary practitioners on FFC-related assessments and interventions until theoretical saturation was achieved. The statements of the participants were recorded and analyzed to construct a Q-population, and their identified subjectivities were reconfirmed. The questions used to develop the Q-population included the following:

1. What considerations affect your assessment of resident function in NH settings?
2. What subjective framework do you use to select and implement interventions for the remaining functional abilities of the residents in NHs?

Eighty-one statements comprising the concourse used in this study were obtained, and two research nurses assessed the content validity of these statements. To select the self-referencing statements (Q-samples), the 81 Q-samples were

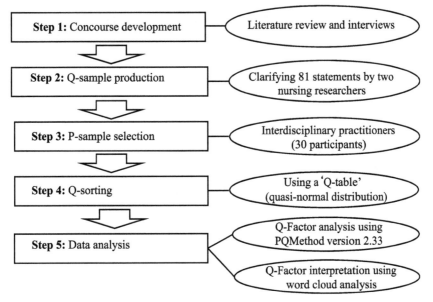

Figure 1. The practical steps in Q-methodology.

read repeatedly until the researchers confirmed and categorized the viewpoints regarding interdisciplinary FFC in NHs into 34 Q-statements. Six practitioners were recruited for a pilot study to test the validity and reliability of the items. Vague or ambiguous statements were eliminated or modified to ensure the clarity of each Q-statement.

P-sample

Q-methodology does not require large or representative samples ($N = 20/40$ is normal) because the intent is to select participants with various subjectivities and key viewpoints (Spurgeon et al., 2012; Watts, 2015). As shown in Spurgeon et al. (2012), 23 participants responding to as few as 39 statements are sufficient to provide valid results. Therefore, a purposive sample of 30 interdisciplinary practitioners from five NHs was recruited for the Q-population and Q-sorting procedures. As interdisciplinary practitioners have been identified in literature reviews as critical providers of FFC to residents of NHs (American Physical Therapy Association, 2019; Bureau of Labor Statistics, U.S. Department of Labor, 2019; Vongxaiburana et al., 2011), they were presumed capable of providing sufficient data on the research topic addressed in this study. The P-sample in this study consisted of 10 nurses, 10 social workers, nine physical therapists, and one occupational therapist, with 1–15 years (mean = 5.5 years) of experience providing FFC to older adult residents of NHs.

Q-sort

Thirty interdisciplinary practitioners produced 34 Q-statements, each of which was rated on a scale of 1–9. Practitioners of Q-sorting read the cards with the Q-statements and classified them into agree (+), disagree (–), or neutral feelings (0). Simultaneously, each Q-statement was placed in a sorting grid with nine tiers, shown in Figure 2. Follow-up interviews were conducted to discern the reason and meaning of the practitioner's choices for the Q-statements that were extreme (–4, +4). Each practitioner spent approximately 30 minutes completing the Q-sorting procedure.

Data Analysis

Q-factor analysis

A proprietary software package (PQMethod Version 2.33; Peter Schmolck, formerly of Military University Munich, Germany) was used to establish a shared subjective framework for FFC interdisciplinary practitioners who care for NH residents. Each practitioner's score was entered into the software by recording the number of the card allocated to each of the 34 Q-statements. Thus, 30 Q-sets of data were entered, and the PQMethod was used to analyze the sort. The analysis was conducted to identify groups of Q sorts with similar configurations. In the factor analysis phase, the software automatically creates a factor array, consensus statements, and the significantly distinguishing statements to represent that factor (Watts, 2015).

Q-factor interpretation

The factor arrays formed the basis of the different Q-factor interpretations. The purpose of factor interpretation is to understand and explain the shared subjectivity of the participants who were captured in one factor. The significant statements form the basis of the interpretation but do not explain the factors completely. Therefore, when interpreting the results, statements showing strong agreement or strong disagreement for each factor presented in the Q-factor analysis, consensus statements, statements with more agreement or less agreement than other factors, supporting reasons for the most strongly agree or disagree statements of the P-samples in a Q-sort, and existing literature and general characteristics data were used (Kim, 2008; Watts, 2015).

The participants were asked to provide more information regarding Q-statements that they had placed at the extreme ends of the sorting grid (Simons, 2013). Follow-up interviews may significantly improve the ability of researchers to interpret emergent viewpoints, identify shared viewpoints, and gain deeper insights (Watts, 2015). In this study, in addition to interpreting the reasons why participants assigned most agree/disagree judgments to the Q-statements, the Q-factor was analyzed using a word cloud analysis on follow-up interview

Strongly Disagree		Disagree		Neutral		Agree		Strongly Agree
-4	-3	-2	-1	0	1	2	3	4

Figure 2. Q-sort grid with array position value.

texts that reflected their decisions. A word cloud is a combination of words that appear in different colors and sizes that depict the frequency of occurrence of each word. The size of a word correlates with how frequently it is used. The validity of the factor interpretation was validated using visualization that focused on extracting repeated and meaningful keywords.

Ethical Considerations

This study was approved by the institutional review board of the university (1040548-KU-IRB-16-201-A-1), and each participant provided permission for their involvement. The purpose and process of this study were explained to the participants. All of the participants volunteered to participate. Participants were assured that the information they provided would be kept confidential.

Results

A Q-factor analysis of the subjectivity related to FFC for residents of NHs using the PQ-Method 2.11 program resulted in four frame-of-reference factors, including (a) using a wait-and-see approach to encourage self-care, (b) maintaining interactive communications to identify and respond to changes, (c) reinforcing residents' inner and outer strengths for homeostasis, and (d) using a tailored approach based on comparisons between the past and the present. These four factors explained 48% of the total variance among the 30 participants (10 nurses, 10 social workers, nine physical therapists, and one occupational therapist), with 17% of the total variance explained by Factor 1, 14% by Factor 2, 9% by Factor 3, and 8% by Factor 4. Of the participants, 10 were classified under Factor 1, six were classified under Factor 2, seven were classified under Factor 3, and three were classified under Factor 4. The remaining four participants were not included under any factor.

Table 1 presents the list of Q-statements with factor arrays. Of the 34 statements, 26 showed significant differences between the factors ($p < .05$). Next, these 26 statements were analyzed qualitatively in a three-step process to interpret the factors. In the first step, the transcripts of the interviews were repeatedly read and summarized to obtain an overview of the subjectivity of the participants related to providing FFC to NH residents. In the second step, the factors were interpreted using the 26 distinguishing statements and statements showing strong agreement or strong disagreement for each factor presented in Table 1. In the third step, the factors were further interpreted using the reasons for the "most strongly agree" and "most strongly disagree" statements of the P-samples in the Q-sort.

Consensus Q-statements were found for three statements (Q6, Q11, and Q26), of which Q6 showed the strongest level of agreement across all factors. "*It is important to remember the common answers and attitudes of the residents. This is because they can be used as criteria to identify changes in*

cognitive functions of older adults" (Q6). Although the focus of providing FFC to NH residents differed from factor to factor, the importance of comparing the past and present responses of the recipients of care and of identifying changes in their remaining functional abilities was reflected in all of the factors.

Factor 1: Using a Wait-and-See Approach to Encourage Self-Care

The four social workers, three nurses, and three physical therapists grouped under Factor 1 were between 27 and 58 years old and had between 1 year 5 months and 10 years 4 months of experience providing FFC in NHs. In terms of providing FFC, Factor 1 focuses on using the various perspectives of interdisciplinary practitioners to assess the remaining functional abilities of NH residents when these residents have diverse problems (Q3, Q25; numbers in brackets refer to the Q-sort statements in Table 1). Furthermore, to help residents maintain or improve remaining function independently, practitioners should monitor the status of remaining functional abilities and allow self-care, providing instruction, demonstration, and assistance as necessary rather than proactively (Q21, Q20). Participant P-3 had the highest factor weight in Factor 1. P-3 noted, "*I think that waiting for the residents to finish their meal or move around regardless of how long it takes is most important when providing FFC. It helps the residents utilize their remaining functional abilities (Q20). They are capable of doing a lot of things if we assist them. We need to wait while supporting and observing their activities, and give verbal/nonverbal cues and demonstrations when they make a mistake (Q25).*"

As shown in Figure 3, the word cloud analysis for Factor 1 identified "remaining function" as the most frequently used term, followed by "independently," "multiple problems," "depend on condition," "combining view," "see," and "wait." Thus, synthesizing the perspectives of multiple interdisciplinary practitioners to closely monitor the remaining functional abilities of residents with multiple problems and then waiting and observing to ensure that these residents practice self-care as much as possible constitute key elements of Factor 1.

Factor 2: Maintaining Interactive Communications to Identify and Respond to Changes

The three social workers and three physical therapists grouped under Factor 2 were between 27 and 36 years old and had between 1 year 9 months and 12 years of experience providing FFC in NHs. In terms of providing FFC, Factor 2 focuses on identifying the various needs related to the functional status of the residents through verbal and nonverbal communication with residents and their families (Q21, Q2) and on identifying changes in functional abilities through talking with residents and constantly comparing residents' reactions with their

TABLE 1.
List of Q-Statements and Factor Arrays

Q-Statement	Factor Array (N = 26)			
	Factor 1 (n = 10)	Factor 2 (n = 6)	Factor 3 (n = 7)	Factor 4 (n = 3)
1. I think the basic function-focused care approach is administering different function-focused care based on the nursing home resident's disposition and his or her rehabilitation needs, rather than the individual administering general care.	3	4	−1**	4
2. I think that, when assessing nursing home residents for admission, the family's subjective evaluation should only be a reference and that the function status assessment should be based on the data confirmed through a direct encounter with the patient.	0**	−3**	2*	4*
3. Nursing home residents usually have multiple problems, so the function status assessment of a resident should be judged by combining views from interdisciplinary experts working in the facility who co-manage the residents.	4	3	4	2
4. Assessing nursing home residents' spiritual desire to find meaning in life is important. The identification of their meaning in life can work as a driving force for them to utilize their remaining function for the rest of their lives.	0	0	−2*	−3*
5. Identifying nursing home residents' MMSE confirms not only dementia but also the subject's communication function, program participation function, and ability to build social relations. Therefore, it should be the primary assessment factor.	2	1*	2	−2**
6. It is important to remember the content and attitudes of the resident's responses to questions in everyday communication. This recollection can be a criterion for identifying cognitive function change.	2	3	1	2
7. Because pain most affects daily life, ROM and pain assessment of a resident should take place constantly.	−2*	2	1*	3
8. When a resident with normal physical function and mild dementia suddenly cannot feed herself, this is a clinical indicator of cognitive decline.	−2	0	3**	−4**
9. When a resident with normal physical function and mild dementia begins to have incontinence of urine and stool, this is a clinical indicator of cognitive decline.	0	−1	3**	1*
10. When a resident with normal physical function and mild dementia shows a decline in the ability to maintain his or her balance, this is a clinical indicator of physical function decline.	−1	−2	3**	−1
11. For a resident with normal physical function but who has severe dementia, a fall risk assessment should be paired with a walking function assessment.	1	0	0	2
12. For a resident with normal physical function but who has severe dementia, a wandering assessment can be a clinical indicator of an anxious mental state.	−3*	1**	−1	−1
13. In the case of a resident in a bedridden state without severe cognitive function damage, caregiver should focus on the psychosocial factor assessment.	0**	−3	−2	−2
14. In the case of a resident in a bedridden state without severe cognitive function damage, caregiver should focus on the remaining muscle assessment.	−2	−1	−1	1**
15. In the case of a resident in a bedridden state without severe cognitive function damage, a decline in communication ability is a clinical indicator of depression.	−3	−3	1*	−1*
16. In the case of a resident in a bedridden state with severe dementia, the occurrence of pressure sores is an important clinical indicator of overall function failure.	−4**	0**	2**	−2**
17. In case of a resident in a bedridden state with severe dementia, their eye expression, facial expression, and complexion are the main clinical indicators for pain assessment.	0	2	2	0
18. I think that cognitive function intervention with residents should start from having conversations and that these conversations should focus on recalling memories to improve cognitive function.	1*	−2	0	0

(continues)

TABLE 1.
List of Q-Statements and Factor Arrays

Q-Statement	Factor Array (N = 26)			
	Factor 1 (n = 10)	Factor 2 (n = 6)	Factor 3 (n = 7)	Factor 4 (n = 3)
19. I think that spiritual function intervention with residents should make the continued religious life possible according to their religious preferences.	−1**	3**	−4	−4
20. I think that residents should work independently when training or doing daily activities to enhance their remaining functional abilities, even if it takes a long time.	4**	−2**	1	0
21. Because the caregiver's actions or language affects the nursing home resident's emotional status, they play a critical factor in psychosocial function assessment.	3**	4**	−2	−2
22. When elderly residents refuse daily activities or training, it is important to invest time and effort to entertain and encourage them.	1	2	0*	1
23. In order to prevent (joint) contracture, it is important to train residents to get out of their rooms regularly, with the assistance of wheelchairs if necessary, regardless of their condition.	−4	−4	−3**	1**
24. Environmental intervention such as providing as relaxing an atmosphere as their home is the primary consideration for improving their functions.	2	1	1	−1*
25. For a resident with normal physical function and minor dementia, considering their remaining functional abilities for sustentation is a common intervention practice.	3	−2	0	3
26. For a resident with normal physical function but who has severe dementia, it is most important to intervene by focusing on the individual's remaining sociopsychological function.	−1	1	0	0
27. For a resident with normal physical function but who has severe dementia, providing satisfaction and pleasure through the simplest program possible is suggested.	0**	−1	−2	−3
28. For a resident with normal physical function but who has severe dementia, it is necessary to show them daily activities step-by-step in detail and have them imitate the steps.	−2**	1	−1**	2
29. For a resident in a bedridden state without severe damage to their cognitive function, spiritual and emotional intervention are the most important because their cognitive function still remains.	2**	−4	−1**	−3
30. For a resident in a bedridden state without severe cognitive function damage, communication intervention for improving social function is the most important.	1*	−1	−3**	−1
31. For a resident in a bedridden state without severe cognitive function damage, sensory stimuli intervention such as watching TV are important for improving their remaining sense functions.	−1	−1	−4**	1**
32. In the case of a resident in a bedridden state with severe dementia, designing a suitable ingestion method should be considered the priority to prevent nutritional problems caused by cognitive malfunctions or swallowing disorders.	−1	0	4**	0
33. In the case of a resident in a bedridden state with severe dementia, because the resident has difficulty in expressing his or her opinions, abnormalities in the skin or joints need to be checked for to prevent accidents.	1	2	0	3
34. In the case of a resident in a bedridden state with severe dementia, sensory stimuli intervention such as a body massage are the most important for improving remaining sensory functions.	−3	0	−3	0

Note. Factor Q-sort values were identified by a Q-sort factor analysis and indicated the statements ranked from +4 = *most agree* to −4 = *most disagree.*
*p < .05; **p < .01.

normal state (Q6). Because problems may not be attributable to a single change in functional status (Q15), interdisciplinary practitioners should communicate and share perspectives on the physical, cognitive, social, and spiritual functional changes of NH residents and provide FFC (Q3).

Participant P-14 had the highest factor weight in Factor 2. P-14 noted, "*I think that the actions and words of the caregiver, the care environment, and the mood have greater positive impacts on the elderly than providing one-sided FFC (Q21).*"

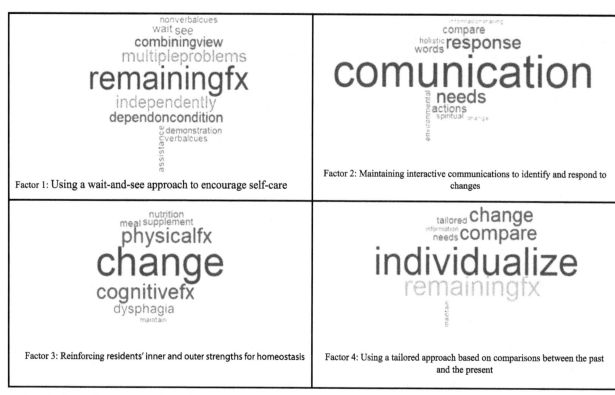

Factor 1: Using a wait-and-see approach to encourage self-care

Factor 2: Maintaining interactive communications to identify and respond to changes

Factor 3: Reinforcing residents' inner and outer strengths for homeostasis

Factor 4: Using a tailored approach based on comparisons between the past and the present

Figure 3. Word cloud representation of the subjective frames of interdisciplinary practitioners in the function-focused care of nursing home residents. The size and prominence of a word depend on the number of times that it appears.

The word cloud analysis for Factor 2 identified "communication" as the most frequently used term, followed by "needs," "response," "compare," "words," "actions," "information sharing," and "change." Thus, Factor 2 uses continuous interaction to compare the current and past responses of residents to detect changes over time and better understand resident care needs through information sharing.

Factor 3: Reinforcing Residents' Inner and Outer Strengths for Homeostasis

The six nurses and one occupational therapist grouped under Factor 3 were between 31 and 58 years old and had 6 months to 7 years of experience providing FFC in NHs. In terms of providing FCC, Factor 3 focuses on using various methods of ingestion to prevent decreased nutrition intake because of dementia or dysphagia, which may affect physical and cognitive functioning adversely (Q8, Q32). The participants grouped according to this factor expressed the opinion that cues that indicate changes in physical and cognitive functions such as inability to self-feed, inability to control feces, and inability to maintain balance should be taken into consideration when providing FFC (Q9, Q10). Participant P-21 had the highest factor weight in Factor 3. She noted, *"There are times when an elderly resident does not eat well or refuses to eat. I chose the No. 32 card as the 'most agree' card because malnutrition weakens the bodily functions and eventually inhibits daily life. If residents have dysphagia, I give muscle training by encouraging them to swallow repeatedly.*

I also provide nutrition by adjusting portions or altering food shapes for those who struggle to eat although they want to eat. I try to sympathize with their emotional struggles (Q32)."

The word cloud analysis for Factor 3 identified "change" as the most frequently used term, followed by "cognitive function," "physical function," "dysphagia," "supplement," "nutrition," "meal," and "maintain." Thus, monitoring dietary and nutritional status to help assess physical–cognitive functional status and increase both inner and outer strength for homeostasis is stressed in Factor 3.

Factor 4: Using a Tailored Approach Based on Comparisons Between the Past and the Present

The one nurse and two physical therapists grouped under Factor 4 were between 29 and 45 years old and had between 2 years 2 months and 15 years of experience providing FFC in NHs. In terms of providing FCC, Factor 4 focuses on comparing the functional status of NH residents at the time of admission with current functional status and on regularly observing changes in physical status such as pain or range of movement problems (Q2, Q7, Q33). Moreover, personalized functional care should be provided based on the remaining functions and needs of the resident (Q1, Q25). Participant P-16 had the highest factor weight in Factor 4. She noted, *"I only take the family's comments as a reference. I assess the resident's functioning status based on the data acquired from an actual consultation with the resident and an accurate assessment. Remembering the initial state and the normal state is a good basis for being aware of any changes (Q2)."*

The word cloud analysis for Factor 4 identified "individualization" as the most frequently used term, followed by "remaining function," "compare," "change," "needs," and "tailored." Thus, identifying the remaining functional abilities and needs of the residents through comparisons of current and past functional status and the status of other residents is stressed in Factor 4.

Discussion

This study focused on determining the subjectivity of interdisciplinary practitioners with regard to providing FFC to residents of NH facilities. On the basis of the findings, a shared subjective framework for the management of remaining function of residents in NH facilities should incorporate a wait-and-see approach to encourage residents to self-care. In addition, this framework should provide encouragement; maintain communications with residents to monitor changes; create a therapeutic environment that strengthens physical, cognitive, and psychological functioning from a homeostatic standpoint; and regularly compare residents' current and previous functional abilities to provide personalized care. Because this study used subjectivity to identify four types of practitioners, this framework may be referenced and adopted by practitioners of different disciplines. Shared cognition is a collective activity that affects overall group goals and activities. In complex settings, higher levels of shared cognition are associated with similar problem conceptualizations and solution approaches (Razzouk & Johnson, 2012). Therefore, shared subjectivity may be presented as a collaborative framework to identify and solve complex and diverse problems related to the functional abilities of NH residents.

Talley et al. (2015) and Galik, Resnick, Hammersla, and Brightwater (2014) suggested that verbal encouragement or physiological feedback that improves self-efficacy should be provided to promote independent living in residents of NHs. This approach will likely be more effective than direct interventions in optimizing FFC. Improving the ability of older adults to live independently is critical to the improvement of remaining functional ability and underpins the practical care philosophies of the practitioner. The related characteristics are incorporated into Factor 1, which focuses on observing the remaining functional abilities of residents with multiple problems for an appropriate period to determine the best approach to providing assistance.

The important role of communication in acquiring and assessing the medical and functional histories and individual needs of recipients of care has been addressed in the literature (Gentleman, 2014; McGilton et al., 2009). Practitioners may assess changes in the health status of older adults with dementia who lack verbal communication skills by observing nonverbal communications such as facial expressions and behaviors (Broughton et al., 2011; Lee & Chang, 2010). The focus of Factor 2 is on the role of verbal and nonverbal communication

with NH residents as a shortcut to the identification of their expressed and unexpressed functional needs and on sharing this information among interdisciplinary practitioners to detect unrecognized needs. The findings of this study regarding Factor 2 are unique in that the communications of practitioners were regularly compared to accurately identify changes in the remaining functional abilities of the NH residents over time.

Promoting nutritional balance and physical activity has been noted in several studies as an effective intervention to maintain homeostasis, which becomes difficult as older adults lose remaining functional abilities and grow increasingly frail (Garatachea, Santos-Lozano, Hughes, Gómez-Cabello, & Ara, 2017; Mañas & Sinclair, 2017). Because NHs are residential rather than medical care facilities, promoting stability and improving quality of life are the focus of Factor 3. To achieve this goal, interdisciplinary practitioners must share indicators of changes in physical–cognitive functioning to reinforce the inner and outer strengths of NH residents.

Numerous studies have addressed the need for and effectiveness of the tailored care reflected in Factor 4 (de Mazières et al., 2017; Liebel, Powers, Friedman, & Watson, 2012; Muntinga et al., 2012). Factor 4 recognizes that the needs and remaining functional abilities of each resident are unique and that providing customized care is another focus of FFC. In addition, Factor 4 is unique in recognizing the status of NHs as residential spaces and the embedded nature of practitioners in the daily lives of residents. Thus, the past and present status of residents' remaining functional abilities and levels of desire may be regularly compared with other residents and addressed.

This study supports the subjective framework of providers as practical in the following ways: First, the findings may be used as a resource to establish communication methods or documentation for sharing among interdisciplinary practitioners in NHs. Second, the findings may be used as an educational component that guides interdisciplinary practitioners to provide FFC to older adult residents of NHs. Finally, the findings may be used to construct a practical conceptual framework that may be shared among interdisciplinary practitioners and used in practice.

Limitations

Thirty participants were included in this study. However, small sample sizes are considered to be significant in Q-methodology because of the focus on intraindividual differences rather than interindividual differences. Increasing the number of participants in future studies will permit more subjective frameworks to be identified and more robust knowledge shared. A second limitation is that interpreting Q-factors is as important as the Q-factors themselves in Q-studies. In addition to the traditional interpretation of Q-methodology, the word cloud method was used in this study to visualize the subjectivity of the words that were expressed by the participants. This helped avoid hermeneutical errors and improved the credibility, trustworthiness, and validity of this study. Third, the participants did not include sufficient numbers for each occupational group because four occupational groups were included. Therefore, the focus of this study focused was on the ideas that were shared among the various subjective frameworks. Thus, the subjective framework from each discipline for FFC for NH residents may exist independently and deserves further study.

Conclusions

This study described the FFC-related subjectivities of interdisciplinary practitioners with regard to NH residents and how these were shared in an interdisciplinary setting. The results may help interdisciplinary practitioners better understand shared subjectivity and enable them to provide FFC more effectively to residents of NHs. Finally, the findings of this study may be used as a resource for developing interdisciplinary FFC practice guidelines.

Acknowledgments

This research was supported by the Basic Science Research Program through the National Research Foundation of Korea, funded by the Ministry of Education, Science and Technology (2015R1D1A1A01057258), and by a Korea University Grant.

Author Contributions

Study conception and design: SOC, MSK
Data collection: MSK, SJL, MSP, EJ
Data analysis and interpretation: SOC, MSK, GTK
Drafting of the article: MSK, SOC
Critical revision of the article: SOC, MSK

References

Akhtar-Danesh, N., Dehghan, M., Morrison, K. M., & Fonseka, S. (2011). Parents' perceptions and attitudes on childhood obesity: A Q-methodology study. *Journal of the American Academy of Nurse Practitioners, 23*, 67–75. https://doi.org/10.1111/j.1745-7599.2010.00584.x

Aniemeke, C., Finley, M. R., Harnetiaux, K. M., Macias, G., Patel, N. K., Prince, R., & Ye, Y. (2017). An interdisciplinary team-developed nursing home orientation as a quality improvement tool in improving community perceptions of post acute and long term care services. *JAMDA: The Journal of Post-Acute and Long-Term Care Medicine, 18*(3), B12. https://doi.org/10.1016/j.jamda.2016.12.031

American Physical Therapy Association. (2019). *Who are physical therapists?* Retrieved from http://www.apta.org/AboutPTs/

Broughton, M., Smith, E. R., Baker, R., Angwin, A. J., Pachana, N. A., Copland, D. A., … Chenery, H. J. (2011). Evaluation of a caregiver education program to support memory and communication in dementia: A controlled pretest-posttest study with nursing home staff. *International Journal of Nursing Studies, 48*(11), 1436–1444. https://doi.org/10.1016/j.ijnurstu.2011.05.007

Bureau of Labor Statistics, U.S. Department of Labor. (2019). *Occupational outlook handbook, occupational therapists.* Retrieved from https://www.bls.gov/ooh/healthcare/occupational-therapists.htm

Congressional Budget Office. (2013). *Rising demand for long-term services and supports for elderly people.* Retrieved from https://www.cbo.gov/sites/default/files/113th-congress-2013-2014/reports/44363-ltc.pdf

de Mazières, C. L., Morley, J. E., Levy, C., Agenes, F., Barbagallo, M., Cesari, M., … Rolland, Y. (2017). Prevention of functional decline by reframing the role of nursing homes? *JAMDA: The Journal of Post-Acute and Long-Term Care Medicine, 18*(2), 105–110. https://doi.org/10.1016/j.jamda.2016.11.019

Doo, H. J., & Lee, Y. J. (2016). Perception of nursing students' experience of simulation based learning: An application of q-methodology. *International Journal of Bio-Science and Bio-Technology, 8*, 313–328. https://doi.org/10.14257/ijbsbt.2016.8.1.28

Eckstrom, E., Neal, M. B., Cotrell, V., Casey, C. M., McKenzie, G., Morgove, M. W., … Lasater, K. (2016). An interprofessional approach to reducing the risk of falls through enhanced collaborative practice. *Journal of the American Geriatrics Society, 64*(8), 1701–1707. https://doi.org/10.1111/jgs.14178

Galik, E., Resnick, B., Hammersla, M., & Brightwater, J. (2014). Optimizing function and physical activity among nursing home residents with dementia: Testing the impact of function-focused care. *The Gerontologist, 54*, 930–943. https://doi.org/10.1093/geront/gnt108

Garatachea, N., Santos-Lozano, A., Hughes, D. C., Gómez-Cabello, A., & Ara, I. (2017). Physical exercise as an effective antiaging intervention. *BioMed Research International, 2017*, 7317609. https://doi.org/10.1155/2017/7317609

Gentleman, B. (2014). Focused assessment in the care of the older adult. *Critical Care Nursing Clinics of North America, 26*, 15–20. https://doi.org/10.1016/j.ccell.2013.09.006

He, W., Goodkind, D., Kowal, P., & U.S. Census Bureau. (2016). *An aging world: 2015—International population reports.* Washington, DC: U.S. Government Publishing Office.

Kim, H. K. (2008). *Q methodology: Philosophy of science, theories, analysis, and application.* Seoul, Korea: Communication Books. (Original work published in Korean)

Lee, S. J., & Chang, S. O. (2010). A study on the types of pain identification by nurses for nursing home patients with dementia. *Journal of the Korean Academy of Fundamentals of Nursing, 17*(4), 508–519. (Original work published in Korean)

Lee, S. J., Kim, M. S., Jung, Y. J., & Chang, S. O. (2019). The effectiveness of function-focused care interventions in nursing homes: A systematic review. *The Journal of Nursing Research, 27*(1), e9. https://doi.org/https://doi.org/10.1097/jnr.0000000000000268

Liebel, D. V., Powers, B. A., Friedman, B., & Watson, N. M. (2012). Barriers and facilitators to optimize function and prevent disability worsening: A content analysis of a nurse home visit intervention. *Journal of Advanced Nursing, 68*, 80–93. https://doi.org/10.1111/j.1365-2648.2011.05717.x

Lim, S. Y., Chang, S. O., Kim, S. J., Kim, H. J., Choi, J. E., & Park, M. S. (2014). Nurses' management of nursing home residents' remaining functional ability: Concept development. *Journal of the Korean Academy of Fundamentals of Nursing, 21*, 57–68. (Original work published in Korean)

Mañas, L. R., & Sinclair, A. J. (2017). Diabetes and functional limitation: The emergence of frailty and disability. In A. J. Sinclair, T. Dunning, L. R. Mañas, & M. Munshi (Eds.), *Diabetes in old age* (4th ed., pp. 213–224). Hoboken, NJ: Wiley. https://doi.org/10.1002/9781118954621

McGilton, K. S., Boscart, V., Fox, M., Sidani, S., Rochon, E., & Sorin-Peters, R. (2009). A systematic review of the effectiveness of communication interventions for health care providers caring for patients in residential care settings. *Worldviews on Evidence-Based Nursing, 6*, 149–159. https://doi.org/10.1111/j.1741-6787.2009.00155.x

Muntinga, M. E., Hoogendijk, E. O., van Leeuwen, K. M., van Hout, H. P., Twisk, J. W., van der Horst, H. E., ... Jansen, A. P. (2012). Implementing the chronic care model for frail older adults in the Netherlands: Study protocol of ACT (frail older adults: care in transition). *BMC Geriatrics, 12*, 19. https://doi.org/10.1186/1471-2318-12-19

Razzouk, R., & Johnson, T. (2012). Shared cognition. In N. M. Seel (Ed.), *Encyclopedia of the sciences of learning* (1st ed., pp. 3056–3058). Boston, MA: Springer.

Resnick, B., & Galik, E. (2013). Using function-focused care to increase physical activity among older adults. *Annual Review of Nursing Research, 31*, 175–208. https://doi.org/10.1891/0739-6686.31.175

Simons, J. (2013). An introduction to Q methodology. *Nurse Researcher, 20*, 28–32. https://doi.org/10.7748/nr2013.01.20.3.28.c9494

Spurgeon, L., Humphreys, G., James, G., & Sackley, C. (2012). A Q-methodology study of patients' subjective experiences of TIA. *Stroke Research and Treatment, 2012*, 486261. https://doi.org/10.1155/2012/486261

Statistics Korea. (2017). *Welfare facilities for the elderly*. Retrieved from http://www.index.go.kr/potal/main/EachDtlPageDetail.do?idx_cd=2766 (Original work published in Korean)

Stephenson, W. (1935). Technique of factor analysis. *Nature, 136* (3434), 297.

Talley, K. M., Wyman, J. F., Savik, K., Kane, R. L., Mueller, C., & Zhao, H. (2015). Restorative care's effect on activities of daily living dependency in long-stay nursing home residents. *The Gerontologist, 55*(1, Suppl.), S88–S98. https://doi.org/10.1093/geront/gnv011

Vongxaiburana, E., Thomas, K. S., Frahm, K. A., & Hyer, K. (2011). The social worker in interdisciplinary care planning. *Clinical Gerontologist, 34*, 367–378.

Washington, K. T., Demiris, G., Parker Oliver, D., Swarz, J. A., Lewis, A. M., & Backonja, U. (2017). A qualitative analysis of information sharing in hospice interdisciplinary group meetings. *American Journal of Hospice and Palliative Care, 34*, 901–906. https://doi.org/10.1177/1049909117693577

Watts, S. (2015). Develop a Q methodological study. *Education for Primary Care, 26*, 435–437. https://doi.org/10.1080/14739879.2015.1101855

6

The Conceptual Structure of the Management by Nurses of the Ego Integrity of Residents of Nursing Homes

Sun-Young LIM[1] • Sung Ok CHANG[2]*

ABSTRACT

Background: The number of older people admitted to nursing homes has continued to rise with the recent expansion of the Republic of Korea's long-term care system. Maintaining ego integrity is a major task for older people approaching the end of life. As efforts to maintain ego integrity include the final stages of life, this concept is critically important for older people in nursing homes. This study was designed to assess issues related to ego integrity in the nursing home environment to determine how nurses should play a key role in managing this important life task.

Purpose: The management by nurses of the ego integrity of residents of nursing homes is a new phenomenon that is central to promoting long-term, quality care. This study was designed to clarify and conceptualize this management phenomenon in the context of nursing homes.

Methods: A hybrid model of concept development was used to analyze the ways in which nurses manage the ego integrity of residents of nursing homes. In the theoretical phase, a working definition of the management by nurses of residents' ego integrity is developed using a literature review. In the fieldwork phase, in-depth interviews are conducted with eight nurses from six nursing homes in Seoul and three other provinces. Finally, in the final analytical phase, the theoretical and fieldwork findings are interpreted and compared.

Results: Two components, assessment and intervention, of the approach by nurses to managing the ego integrity of residents of nursing homes were identified. Assessment incorporates 10 attributes in the following three dimensions: "identifying the extent to which residents' basic needs are being fulfilled," "determining how residents achieve friendly relationships with others," and "determining how each resident creates a harmonious view of his or her life." Intervention incorporates nine attributes in the following two dimensions: "helping residents develop a positive view of life" and "helping residents make the best use of their remaining functional abilities."

Conclusions/Implications for Practice: By managing the ego integrity of residents, nurses have a significant influence on residents' sociopsychological adaptation, especially in the challenging environment of a nursing home. This study supports that managing the ego integrity of residents of nursing homes is an important and practical component of the role played by nurses and of the aid and care they provide. Furthermore, the findings verify the effectiveness of intervention studies in examining assessment tools and developing guidelines for ego-integrity management.

KEY WORDS:
ego integrity, hybrid model, nursing home.

Introduction

Population aging introduces new healthcare challenges such as adding complexity to the medical environment and transferring social care for diversely functional older adults from home and medical facility settings to nursing homes (Kojima, 2015). As more older adults are living longer with geriatric illnesses, nursing homecare is becoming more prevalent (Paek et al., 2016).

The proportion of the population in South Korea aged 65 years or older is expected to increase from 14.3% in 2018 to 41% in 2060 (Korean Statistical Information Service, 2018). To accommodate this aging society, the number of nursing homes has increased significantly since Korea implemented long-term care insurance in July 2008.

As life expectancy continues to increase, efforts have been made to highlight the positive aspects of an aging society, including concepts related to successful aging, gerotranscendence, and ego integrity (Martineau & Plard, 2018; Westerhof et al., 2017; Wong & Yap, 2016). Successful aging suggests sociopsychological completeness in healthy older adults who are able to maintain relatively healthy physical and cognitive functions in the community setting (Chodzko-Zajko et al., 2009), gerotranscendence implies a positive and continually evolving change in the worldview of older people (Wong & Yap, 2016), and ego integrity refers to positive sociopsychological adaptation in older adults.

[1]PhD, RN, *Visiting Professor, College of Nursing, Baekseok Culture University, ROK* • [2]*PhD, RN, Professor, College of Nursing, Korea University, ROK.*

As nursing homes require that residents engage in sociopsychological adaptation, practitioners have used ego integrity to induce positive adaptation in nursing home settings (Erikson, 1963; Lim & Chang, 2018a; Torges et al., 2008). Nursing home practitioners manage the ego integrity of residents by helping them establish a more harmonious and positive relationship with their caregivers (Torges et al., 2008). The management by nurses of residents' ego integrity relies on nursing-specific role characteristics, which are useful for ensuring quality care (James & Zarrett, 2006; Westerhof et al., 2017).

Ego integrity, or the integration of life cycles for older people that embraces death, is recognized as something that even older people who are unhealthy or near to death may pursue. Eco integrity emphasizes a traditional focus on establishing relationships with others, aiming for a mature and harmonious life until the very end of life. Thus, there is a growing need to promote ego integrity in older people who are spending the last days of their lives in nursing homes. In fact, the management of their ego integrity is a part of nurses' responsibilities and, thus, must be clearly identified to organize nursing care services properly, to promote continuity of interventions, and to check on the effects of interventions. As nurses are in a position to evaluate the physical, sociopsychological, and mental status of residents, they are in an optimal position to design personalized care and play an important role in managing residents' ego integrity. Thus, residents' quality of life in their final months and the quality of nurse/resident relationships may be improved.

Previous studies of ego integrity have focused primarily on older adults living in the community (Dezutter et al., 2016; Jo & Song, 2015; Tahreen & Shahed, 2014). Few studies have explored ways of helping older adults make this transition and integrate into nursing homes. Recently, Lim and Chang (2018a) studied the ways in which nurses perceive ego integrity in residents of nursing homes. They observed that nurses held subjective perceptions and that they should reflect on the concept as part of their care activities. This finding suggests that nurses are well positioned to manage residents' ego integrity effectively. This emerging phenomenon is worth exploring, given that nursing may significantly improve residents' quality of life. This study clarifies and conceptualizes the ways in which nurses manage the ego integrity of residents of nursing homes in their daily practice.

Methods

Study Design

This concept-development study adopted the hybrid model, which is used extensively to clarify, create, develop, and extend concepts, particularly in nursing. The hybrid model clarifies concepts to create new and more comprehensive definitions. At times, definitions emerge that differ completely from previous ones. The hybrid model combines inductive and deductive approaches, identifying the essential aspects of a concept and providing clarity through observation and interviews based on actual participant experiences. The main concept is derived (particularly when the data are ambiguous) through integrative literature analysis and fieldwork study (Schwartz-Barcott & Kim, 2000). Thus, the hybrid model consists of three phases: theoretical, fieldwork, and final analysis.

Data Collection and Procedure

Theoretical phase

"Management" refers to the process of dealing with or controlling things or people (Oxford University Press, n.d.). The development of knowledge about nurses' management belongs within the practice domain for enacting assessment and treatment activities (Schwartz-Barcott & Kim, 2000). The concept of nurses' management of residents' ego integrity was developed by dividing this phenomenon into two aspects: assessment and intervention.

A literature search was carried out using the following keywords: "nursing home," "nursing-home residents," "ego integrity," "management," "assessment," "intervention," and "strategy." Electronic databases including PubMed, CINAHL, MEDLINE, and ProQuest were searched for articles published between 1963 and March 31, 2018, using the search options provided by each database and EndNote software. Articles were included only if they had at least one keyword in the title, abstract, or list of key words. An initial search yielded 120 articles. After eliminating duplicate titles, 78 articles remained. Of these, 21 articles were excluded, leaving 57 articles available to review (Figure 1), including nine on psychology, three on social welfare, two on education, and 43 on nursing. The dimensions and attributes deemed most significant in articles of a theoretical nature are presented in Table 1. The important issues related to the assessment and intervention for the literature review are as follows. The assessment uncovered meanings of ego-integrity management, which help determine how residents

Figure 1

A Flowchart of Data Selection and Data Extraction in the Theoretical Phase

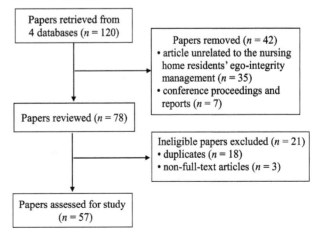

Table 1

Contents of Major Literature Review From a Theoretical Phase

Study Author (Year)	Conceptual Dimension and the Attribute of Ego-Integrity Management
Lim & Chang (2018a)	Nurses confirmed that, when residents identified new solutions to problems, flexible acceptance of a new lifestyle could be inferred. Here, ego integrity could be assessed through group activities and confirmed through stories retold by other residents. Identifying clues to the residents' positive acceptance of their whole life spans; identifying residents' ways of enjoying their current lives, referencing residents' attitudes toward and ability to form harmonious relationships; and identifying residents' integrated efforts to establish self-esteem. Wisdom helps individuals recognize experiences they can use to reconstruct their lives; this process is akin to the way in which individuals reconcile important social relationships in old age.
Park, Lim, Kim, Lee, & Chang (2018)	To help residents make the most of their remaining functional abilities, nurses must help them adjust to certain internal and external constraints. This could include having residents use spoons whenever possible to maximize their remaining capacities.
Harrison & Frampton (2017)	Identifying the residents' friendly relationships with others allowed nurses to assess how well the residents were adjusting to life in the nursing home.
Friedman et al. (2017)	Strengthening and maintaining high-quality relationships with the residents' families and friends outside the nursing home is another important factor for achieving ego integrity.
Hung et al. (2016)	Reducing problematic behaviors through safe environmental controls is essential. Specifically, it is important to provide a "home-like" atmosphere within the nursing home.
Drageset, Eide, Dysvik, Furnes, & Hauge (2015)	Identifying how residents create a harmonious view of life requires a meaningful self-image. Self-esteem is a key component of this dimension among residents.
Roberts & Bowers (2015)	This leads to good relationships between nurses, families, and other residents. Such relationships have a positive effect on residents' ability to articulate problems and reduce distress.
Haugan (2014)	Helping residents generate a positive view of life was best accomplished by creating calm experiences through everyday comforts. The residents often achieved ego integrity by enjoying small tasks.
Lim et al. (2014)	Harmonious relationships with other residents; the will for self-actualization; the spiritual needs required when actualizing and using ego integrity; the palliative care needed in nursing homes. To help residents accept death objectively as an extension of life, nurses must facilitate transcendental thinking about end-of-life issues. This task illustrates the nature of nursing science in relation to managing a peaceful death.
Vitale, Shaffer, & Acosta Fenton (2014)	The quality of a resident's relationship with his or her family and transcendent thoughts help to actualize ego integrity, leading to successful aging; this is a significant responsibility for nurses.
Brandburg, Symes, Mastel-Smith, Hersch, & Walsh (2013)	It is crucial to improve the residents' quality of life by analyzing and managing their physical, mental, and social status and interacting with them accordingly. Continuously confirming gratitude for life has been shown to be important. Those who positively express this gratitude have integrated the end of life well.
Aleksandrova-Yankulovska & ten Have (2015)	Preparing for the process of ego-integrity actualization and the positive acceptance of death: reflections and a positive attitude toward life and management are important for a positive death.
Ali & Ayoub (2010)	Importantly, spiritual peace and acceptance of a peaceful death are phases of ego-integrity actualization for the residents. Participation in religious activities can often lead to spiritual peace. Such activities can provide social benefits, aid with functional limitations, and assist with managing death anxiety. In the context of terminal care, a peaceful death can be advocated, while residents focus on physical, cognitive, social, and spiritual functions that mediate the integrity of their remaining abilities. In essence, spirituality can contain wider and deeper meanings above and beyond functional recovery or rehabilitation.

achieve friendly relationships with others and how each resident creates a harmonious view of his or her life. Interventions that were found to relate to managing the ego integrity of residents included those designed to help patients develop a positive view of life and to make the best use of their remaining functional abilities.

Fieldwork phase

The participants were eight nurses working at six nursing homes in Seoul and three other provinces. The selection criterion was being a nursing home nurse with more than 3 years of experience since 2008, when the long-term Korean care insurance was enacted and when nursing homes began to be formally evaluated. The participants had professional experience with residents of nursing homes. Before data collection, the director of each nursing institution was contacted to approve the data collection procedures. The participants, all volunteers, signed a written agreement stating that they were willing to be interviewed and could refuse to participate at any time. Interview questions were formulated, and the researcher personally conducted interviews based on the theoretical assessment and intervention areas. Each interview took 1–2 hours, and each participant completed one to three audiotaped interviews.

The interview data were transcribed, coded, and reviewed. Interviews and field observations were transcribed verbatim, and the content of transcripts was analyzed to identify and classify categories relevant to the key research questions. Each transcript was read several times to allow for full immersion. When all of the data had been coded and the categories were condensed, each category was assessed to determine data saturation.

Final analytic phase

The results, which reflected the essence of ego-integrity management among residents of nursing homes, were analyzed and compared with results obtained during the fieldwork phase. The key concepts derived from a review of the literature during the theoretical phase and the elements of concepts identified during fieldwork were reexamined, compared, synthesized, and analyzed to arrive at a final definition of ego-integrity management in the context of residents.

Ethical Considerations

This study was approved by the institutional review board of the authors' institution (Certificate Number: KU-IRB-16-276-A-1), and permission to conduct the research was obtained from each facility. The purpose of the study was explained to all participants, who were informed that their involvement was voluntary. Participants were assured that the information they provided would remain confidential.

Results

Theoretical Phase: Review of the Literature

A working definition of the ego-integrity management attributes and dimensions of residents of nursing homes was elicited theoretically using the experiences of the nurses. The concept of ego integrity includes various attributes, qualities, and meanings. Additional concept dimensions were defined by analyzing and classifying attributes. The nurses' management of residents' ego integrity was classified using attributes from the assessment and intervention dimensions.

Definition of the concept

The Oxford English Dictionary (2018) defines the ego as "the part of the mind that mediates between the conscious and the unconscious and is responsible for reality testing and a sense of personal identity," whereas integrity is defined as "the state of being whole and undivided," and management is defined as "the process of dealing with or controlling things or people" (Oxford University Press, n.d.). Thus, "ego-integrity management" may be defined as intervention and coaching to lead a subject toward a balanced and harmonious goal rather than as a subclassification of the ego.

No precise definition of ego-integrity management currently exists for residents of nursing homes. However, related assessments and interventions have been used with people experiencing profound disabilities, diseases, and injuries (Korean Ministry of Health and Welfare, 2018). In these cases, ego-integrity management has helped subjects accept their lives without remorse, be content with their present lives, have a harmonious view of the past and future, and have no fear of death (Erickson, 1963). In addition, ego-integrity management may refer to the process by which nurses help residents achieve this actualized goal using systematic assessments and individualized interventions. From the perspective of nurses, no precise definition of ego-integrity management exists for residents of nursing homes. Using assessment and intervention, ego-integrity management guides residents into a state in which they do not fear death but rather accept their lives with satisfaction and without regret, experiencing harmony between past, present, and future. The systematic assessment and personalized interventions provided by nurses help residents achieve as much ego integrity as possible.

Concepts related to ego integrity

The concepts of successful aging and gerotranscendence are used in similar ways in nursing. Successful aging involves maximizing positive and minimizing negative outcomes. Efforts to organize and integrate one's whole life in old age may be less comprehensive than ego integrity (Rylands & Rickwood, 2001). Gerotranscendence refers to the transformation of an older adult worldview that is universal and rational rather than materialistic and rational (Erikson, 1998). However, neither concept expresses the essence of ego integrity, which refers to positive sociopsychological adaptation in old age.

Ego-Integrity Management for Residents of Nursing Homes: Assessment

The assessment in this study uncovered two distinct meanings of ego-integrity management: (a) determining how residents achieve friendly relationships with others (with four attributes) and (b) determining how each resident creates a harmonious view of his or her life (with three attributes).

Determining how residents achieve friendly relationships with others

Attributes include residents' flexibility in accepting new ways of life, their active acceptance of others' ways of life, the strengthening of social relationships using the transition process, and wisdom based on accumulated experience.

The first step in identifying residents' social relationships is assessing how well residents have adjusted to life in the nursing home (Harrison & Frampton, 2017). Nurses have confirmed that, when residents come up with new solutions to problems, flexible acceptance of a new lifestyle may be inferred. Here, ego integrity may be assessed through group activities and confirmed through stories retold by other residents (Lim & Chang, 2018a).

A resident's social relationships may be strengthened within the new context even before admission to a nursing home. Afterward, emotional bonds emerge through communication and contact with others living in the facility (Björk et al., 2017). The maintenance of quality relationships with family and friends outside the nursing home (Friedman et al., 2017) and lifetime wisdom, based on accumulated experience, both help actualize ego integrity among residents. Wisdom helps individuals recognize experiences that they may use to reconstruct their lives. This process is akin to the way in which individuals reconcile important social relationships in old age (Lim & Chang, 2018a).

Determine how each resident creates a harmonious view of his or her life

Attributes for this dimension include residents' abilities to recognize themselves as individuals, their acceptance of death as an extension of a worthy life, and their continuous confirmation of gratitude. To create a harmonious view of life, residents must envision their own self-image as meaningful. Self-esteem is a key component of this dimension (Drageset et al., 2015). Residents must also accept the inevitability of death and frame it as an extension of a worthwhile life. To those living life as an extension of the past, accepting the reality of their current situation may bring comfort and fulfillment (Meier et al., 2010). Furthermore, continuously confirming gratitude for life has been shown to be important. Those who positively express this gratitude have integrated end of life well (Brandburg et al., 2013; Lim & Chang, 2018a).

Ego-Integrity Management for Residents of Nursing Homes: Intervention

Interventions reveal two reasons for managing the ego integrity of residents: (a) to help them develop a positive view of life (with four attributes) and (b) to make the best use of their remaining functional abilities (with four attributes).

Helping residents develop a positive view of life

Attributes included inducing a feeling of calmness through everyday comforts, which led to good relationships with nurses, family members, and other residents. Residents also found it easier to accept their past lives and view death as an extension of life.

The best way to help residents generate a positive view of life is to create calm experiences within a comfortable and satisfying living environment. For instance, residents often achieve ego integrity by carrying out small tasks (Haugan, 2014; Lim & Chang, 2018a). This feeling may lead to quality relationships that have a positive effect on residents' abilities to articulate problems and reduce their own distress (Roberts & Bowers, 2015). To help residents accept death objectively as an extension of life, nurses must facilitate transcendental thinking about end-of-life issues. This task illustrates the nature of nursing science in relation to managing a peaceful death (Ali & Ayoub, 2010; Lim et al., 2014). Finally, a comprehensive acceptance of the past helps residents reconcile their successes and failures, which fosters wisdom (James & Zarrett, 2006).

Helping residents make the best use of their remaining functional abilities

To develop this dimension, nurses encourage residents to use their remaining physical capacities, promoting increased mobility, spiritual comfort, and stability. Moreover, nurses guide residents to perceive their environment as safe.

To help residents make the most of their remaining functional abilities, nurses help residents adjust to internal and external constraints. For example, residents use spoons whenever possible to maximize their remaining capacities (Park et al., 2018). Movement may also be encouraged even among residents who are bedridden. Nursing homes in the United States have adopted "function-focused care" and "functional restorative care" in accordance with regulations for maintaining the functional capacities of residents who are bedridden. These interventions aim not only to maintain functional abilities but also to make these abilities last as long as possible. They serve as a method of assessing physical functioning within a nursing home context (Boltz et al., 2011; Resnick et al., 2007).

Participation in religious activities often leads to spiritual peace. Such activities may provide social benefits, ameliorate functional limitations, and assist with managing death anxiety. In the context of terminal care, a peaceful death may be advocated, while residents focus on physical, cognitive, social, and spiritual functions that mediate the integrity of their remaining abilities. In essence, spirituality contains wider and deeper meanings that are above and beyond functional recovery or rehabilitation (Ali & Ayoub, 2010; Lim et al., 2014). Reducing problematic behaviors through safe environmental control is a key factor. Specifically, it is important to provide a "home-like" atmosphere in nursing homes (Hung et al., 2016) to help residents feel as safe and autonomous as possible. Home-like interiors and music have been shown to reduce residents' problematic behaviors (Amella et al., 2008).

Management by nurses of the ego integrity of residents of nursing homes has been defined in the literature as follows.

A working definition of the process of managing the ego integrity of residents: In the theoretical phase of this study, nurses were found to manage the ego integrity of residents in ways that could be categorized into assessment and intervention components. A working definition of this process must include ways of determining whether a resident is showing friendly relationships with others through flexible acceptance of a new way of life and active acceptance of others' new ways of life, strengthening social relationships, and showing wisdom through accumulated experience. This definition must include the ways in which residents create a harmonious view of life, recognize that they are worthy people, accept death as an extension of a worthy life, and continuously confirm gratitude. The definition should also recognize that residents seek peace through life comforts; maintain good relationships with nurses, family members, and other residents; accept death positively; and accept their own life. Finally, ego integrity should be developed through interventions that help residents make the best possible use of their remaining functional abilities, encourage the use of physical capacities and increased mobility, promote spiritual comfort and stability, and guide residents to maintain a safe environment.

Fieldwork Phase

During the fieldwork phase of the assessment, the literature was reviewed to elicit a working definition of managing the ego integrity of residents of nursing homes. In addition, a new dimension was added. During the intervention phase, the first dimension (helping residents develop a positive view of life) was derived from one theoretical attribute. During the fieldwork phase, each attribute was broken down into a detailed guide to the meaning of residents' interpersonal relationships, particularly with regard to family members.

The assessment and intervention components are outlined, respectively in Tables 2 and 3, indicating how attributes were revealed in detail by nurses during the fieldwork phase. This section describes a novel dimension that was newly discovered during the assessment and presents aspects in a new way.

Ego-Integrity Management for Residents: Assessment

Identify the extent to which residents' basic needs are fulfilled

Minimal self-care meets a resident's basic physiological needs. According to the nurses, residents who could manage their basic needs for defecation, urination, toothbrushing, eating, and dressing and who wanted to engage in self-care were more likely to achieve positive self-realization and self-esteem outcomes.

There are times when the residents try to perform self-care. For example, even with difficulties, they still insist on eating or brushing their teeth by themselves. This reminds me of Maslow's Hierarchy of Needs Theory. If basic physiological needs are not met, one cannot achieve higher level needs such as those in the emotional, intellectual, and spiritual dimensions. These older adults often show a higher level of self-esteem and are more tolerant of others, which is part of those higher-level needs.

Psychological acceptance of self-management limits: Residents who accept the reality of their limitations without frustration and ask for help when they need it show better psychological acceptance of ego integrity, leading to a more comfortable attitude toward death.

I think those who accept their limits have a better chance of adapting their ego integrity, as they demonstrate better emotional control, showing no anger or impatience even when the situation is aggravating.

Willingness to engage in physical activity: According to the nurses, residents who show willingness to participate actively in everyday physical activities (e.g., cooperating during diaper changes and during transfers from bed to wheelchair) are more contented and accept the present reality in a more positive way.

Some residents cooperate when we try to transfer them from the bed to a wheelchair for a walk instead of just staying still. Even though they cannot move exactly as they want anymore, the will to actively participate in everyday physical activities makes them feel content.

Ego-Integrity Management for Residents: Intervention

Helping residents develop a positive view of life

Helping residents discover meaning in interpersonal relationships: According to the nurses, relationships with staff members, other residents, and visiting friends play an important role in supporting the residents' ego integrity. Helping residents maintain these relationships is a key feature of the nurses' ego-management activities.

We suggest that the residents smile at their roommates once in a while even when having to stay in bed. Getting along with people around them is critical for alleviating loneliness and depression, which is what they need to do to build good relationships with others. You cannot feel the same amount of happiness as when you smile together with others when you just smile alone.

Helping residents construct meaningful relationships with family: The nurses felt that helping residents in this way was an important intervention to support their ego integrity.

Table 2

Summary of Major Assessment Dimensions and Attributes From the Fieldwork Phase

Dimension/Attribute	Content Described	Relevant Quotation From Interviews (Nurse No.)
1. Determine how residents develop friendly relationships with others		
(a) Residents' flexible acceptance of a new way of life	According to the nurses, residents who showed no resistance to living in an unfamiliar environment and got along well with others achieved a comfortable daily routine by positively adapting to the environment (i.e., through more smiles and positive facial expressions).	*"When an older adult has an easygoing attitude, it's clear that he or she is adapting better. Making friends in a nursing home is so critical, especially when you are not feeling so well, for the friends you make are going to be your family. Those who have a good relationship with others are often more content with their lives."* (Nurse 6)
(b) Residents' active acceptance of others' ways of life	Residents who think of others first, as well as listening to and helping others, tend to have better relationships with others, showing thoughtful consideration.	*"There are residents sharing the same room with individuals with severe Alzheimer's disease, who cannot eat without having food falling out of their mouths. However, those residents help clean such individuals, even before we ask and call for residents who have been lying in bed for too long. They even celebrate each other's birthdays and give gifts."* (Nurse 2)
(c) Residents' strengthening social relationships	Residents who are usually self-regulated are constantly striving not to disturb others. They try not to complain, listening to (and respecting) others for who they are. This helps residents build stable relationships with those around them.	*"There are some residents who are concerned about many friends and family members. These residents show gratitude by saying how much they appreciate the help they get when their diapers are changed. That really warms our hearts."* (Nurse 3)
(d) Residents' wisdom, based on accumulated experience	Residents' wisdom is usually revealed through their attitudes or actions. Those with wisdom often are more considerate and build quality relationships. A solid interpersonal organizational style that reflects wisdom gained over one's life is an important factor when assessing ego integrity.	*"When their families are not able to visit often, some residents do not seem to be upset. Instead, they just have more small talks with their roommates or take the lead in having a fun time. Surprisingly, they tend to call their families to tell them they are really having a good time, are having no trouble with eating or sleeping, and the family does not have to visit the nursing home if they are too busy."* (Nurse 4)
2. Determine how residents create a harmonious view of their own lives		
(a) Residents recognizing themselves as worthy people	When the residents look back on their lives, they value their volunteer jobs, make efforts to build a better life, and respect their accomplishments and what they wanted to do, instead of having regrets and hatred. Those are the criteria for a meaningful life mentality, with which they judge their own ego integrity.	*"Some residents have helped others who are weak and not as materially sufficient, and that is what made their life meaningful. That kind of thought is really where grace comes from. For instance, there is a charity organization called 'The Green Umbrella.' We have a resident who's been a member of that organization since 1948, and now her son and grandson are actively volunteering in the organization."* (Nurse 4)
(b) Residents' acceptance of death as an extension of a worthy life	The acceptance of death is shown by residents overcoming anxiety and developmental crises surrounding death; this helps to determine the residents' quality of life.	*"'I will not have any regrets, even if I die while I am sleeping tonight.' Those who say things like that are really the ones who have lived their lives to the fullest; you can really feel the weight of their words. Also, even when Cheyne–Stokes respiration occurs during a resident's final hours, the peaceful facial expression explains everything."* (Nurse 3)

(continues)

Table 2

Summary of Major Assessment Dimensions and Attributes From the Fieldwork Phase, Continued

Dimension/Attribute	Content Described	Relevant Quotation From Interviews (Nurse No.)
(c) Residents' continuous confirmation of life gratitude	The residents who show gratitude whenever a visitor or staff member helps are the embodiment of gratitude. Even when a resident was born in a difficult time, he or she is still grateful for living a positive life.	*"There are some residents who really show their gratitude everywhere. They thank the physical therapist for the comfort provided and thank other staff members for their work, appreciate the nursing home program, and even stay till the end to help clean up an area after an activity. They really do not hold back on their gratitude."* (Nurse 8)

We always try our best to help the residents maintain good relationships with their families, while not forgetting the fact that we (nurses) are also a part of their family at the nursing home. We always suggest that residents take the medicine their families have bought, complete the physical therapy their families want them to complete, and tell their families how everything is going during visits.

The fieldwork phase produced a working definition of ego-integrity management. This definition included helping residents meet their basic needs (including minimal self-care to meet physiological needs, psychological acceptance of their own self-management limits, and willingness to engage in physical activity), maintain positive relationships with others,

create a harmonious view of life, and make the best use of their remaining functional abilities.

Final Analytic Phase

During the final analytic phase, the nurses' management of ego integrity was assessed across the theoretical and fieldwork phase results, distinguishing between attributes (Figure 2). First, the management concept was developed during the theoretical and fieldwork phases. Next, the dimensions and attributes of each phase were derived. The theoretical-phase results were defined more clearly during the fieldwork phase. The final analysis was performed after attributes from the theoretical phase were sufficiently saturated in the fieldwork phase.

Figure 2

Concept of Nurses' Management of Residents' Remaining Functional Abilities

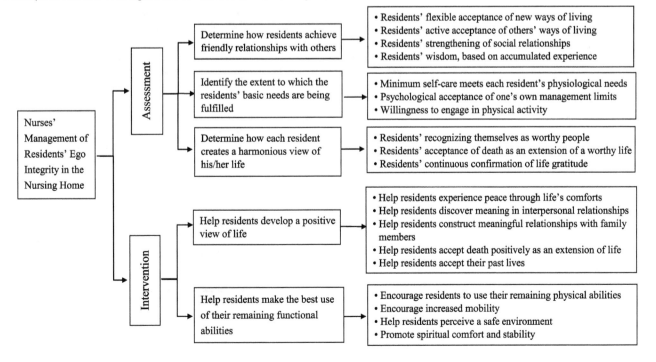

Table 3

Summary of Major Intervention Dimensions and Attributes From the Fieldwork Phase

Dimension/Attribute	Content Described	Relevant Quotation From Interviews
1. Help residents adopt a positive view of life		
(a) Help residents experience calm through the comforts of life	The nurses intervene with the residents by helping them recognize seasonal changes and what the residents do best and enjoy. Eventually, they emphasize composure and acceptance of death.	*"Helping residents realize this 'season of change' is really effective. We help them feel this change by showing different pictures or changes to the garden art. Showing them movies can really enrich their cultural life. When they see some classic movies starring Audrey Hepburn, whose grace is widely appreciated, their memories about the good old days come across."* (Nurse 2)
(b) Help residents accept death objectively as an extension of life	The nurses realize that accepting death in the continuum of life is critical when intervening to foster ego integrity. Especially when dying well is considered, combining the idea of death with religion or emotions to make the acceptance of death easier for each individual is an important factor when intervening to foster ego integrity.	*"We often see that residents of the same religion find peace when singing or listening to spiritual songs together. They also seem to accept death more peacefully, even when they are just talking about their religion."* (Nurse 6)
(c) Help residents accept their past lives	According to the nurses, when residents have regrets or negative attitudes about the past, it is important to help them accept the past through a positive intervention, which allows residents to live the rest of their lives (and accept death) more peacefully.	*"As most of the residents had difficult lives, the way they think about their past affects how they accept death. There are some residents who changed their attitude toward the past through reminiscence therapy."* (Nurse 3)
2. Help residents make the best use of their remaining functional abilities		
(a) Encourage the use of remaining physical abilities	The nurses emphasized the importance of allowing residents to use their remaining physical functional abilities with the least amount of help possible.	*"It's better for us to wait for the residents to use utensils and eat by themselves. That allows the residents to feel better about themselves, for they can still eat using their hands at will. Things they can do with their hands, like using the remote controller to change the TV channel and using a hand fan for 10 minutes as a punishment for losing a roshambo game, are helpful. It's also good to give the residents wet wipes to let them clean up themselves."* (Nurse 1)
(b) Encourage increased mobility	The nurses emphasized to residents that movement, considering a resident's level of mobility in bed, is important for helping residents use their remaining functional abilities.	*"We try to let the residents use their remaining functional abilities; however, for those who cannot leave their beds, we encourage them to use the bedside rails to help them get up, lie down, or rotate. In order to maintain their remaining physical functional abilities, we also train residents to use their hips when changing positions. For ladies with severe hemiplegia, we suggest that they try their best to manipulate their own legs."* (Nurse 2)
(c) Help residents perceive a safe environment	The nurses emphasized that residents should perceive their environment as safe and comfortable, similar to a home, so as to adapt to the new environment faster.	*"It's important to make the residents feel at home. That's why we ask their families to bring things the residents really appreciate from home. There are some residents who enjoy folk songs, so we ask their families to bring folk-song cassette tapes for the residents to listen to."* (Nurse 4)

(continues)

Table 3

Summary of Major Intervention Dimensions and Attributes From the Fieldwork Phase, Continued

Dimension/Attribute	Content Described	Relevant Quotation From Interviews
(d) Promote spiritual comfort and stability	The nurses said that it was important to assess each resident's spiritual needs and help him or her find spiritual comfort and stability.	*"There's no emotional bond greater than religion. However, we need to assess each resident's spiritual needs instead of just putting them all together, as if they had the exact same religion to begin with. Helping residents find their own spiritual comfort and stability, individual by individual, is the key."* (Nurse 8)

In the final analytic phase, the theoretical and fieldwork results were compared to redefine and establish the attributes of ego-integrity management by nursing home nurses.

Definition of ego-integrity management, carried out by nursing home nurses

The ways in which nurses managed the ego integrity of residents were defined as follows: The nurses' management of the residents' ego integrity included the following tasks: determining the extent to which residents' basic needs (such as minimum self-care) were fulfilled; understanding both the residents' psychological acceptance of their own self-management limits and their willingness to engage in physical activity; and determining whether the residents had friendly relationships with others, could flexibly accept new ways of life, could actively accept others' way of life, could strengthen social relationships through a new life process, and actualize wisdom through accumulated experience. This definition also describes how residents worked to create a harmonious view of their whole life's course by recognizing themselves as worthy people, accepting death as an extension of a worthy life, and continuously confirming gratitude.

In terms of interventions, nurses should help residents develop a positive view of life (e.g., by promoting feelings of peace through everyday comforts), discover meaning in interpersonal relationships, construct meaningful relationships with their families, accept death positively as an extension of life, and accept their past lives. Finally, the definition includes helping residents make the best use of their remaining functional abilities by using those abilities to work toward increased mobility. The nurses promote spiritual comfort and stability and help residents perceive their environment as safe.

Discussion

Sustaining ego integrity is a major task for older adults approaching the end of life (Erikson, 1963) and is a very important concept in nursing homes (Lim & Chang, 2018a). As essential care providers, nurses focus on managing the ego integrity of residents of nursing homes (Brandburg et al., 2013; Roberts & Bowers, 2015). Most previous studies have explored the ego-integrity achievement characteristics of community-dwelling older adults. By contrast, this study assesses ego-integrity issues in a nursing home to determine how nurses play a key role in managing this important life task.

As shown in the findings, managing the ego integrity of residents is different from other concepts related to successful aging that emphasize the positive aspects of old age. Successful aging involves managing sociopsychological integrity, particularly among older people who are healthy and maintain relatively competent physical and cognitive functions (Chodzko-Zajko et al., 2009; Martineau & Plard, 2018). Nurses working in nursing homes offer a different approach to maintaining ego integrity that focuses on relationships with others and helping individuals pursue a mature and harmonious life (Torges et al., 2008; Westerhof et al., 2017). In this context, nurses manage the ego integrity of residents by helping them establish more harmonious and positive relationships with others.

The relevant features of nurses' ego-integrity management were identified but not fully confirmed in the theoretical phase. The fieldwork phase provided insights from actual nursing home nurses and helped to identify key nursing practices (e.g., assessing how residents fulfill basic needs) that sustain the ego integrity of residents. The attributes discovered in this study provide a tutorial on the development of ego-integrity-management training resources.

The theoretical and fieldwork phases confirmed that acceptance of death was part of a continuum that reflected a valuable life—a factor now considered important in palliative care. Acceptance of death does not necessarily mean that a person is prepared for the exact moment of death. Rather, this concept represents the ability to look back on one's past with a positive, peaceful attitude, achieving contentment for the rest of one's life through actualized ego integrity (Kim et al., 2014). This kind of acceptance focuses on physical, cognitive, social, and spiritual functions—all characteristics that underpin peace in palliative care and also highlight the deeper meaning of nursing science (Ali & Ayoub, 2010; Lim et al., 2014).

Previous studies on the ways in which nurses manage the ego integrity of residents of nursing homes have derived concepts exclusively from literature reviews (Lim & Chang, 2018b), a technique that is quite limiting. By contrast, combining a literature review with analytic techniques provides a more comprehensive outline of the dimensions and attributes of a particular concept. The approach of this study was developed to improve both theoretical and fieldwork applicability by constructing a conceptual framework via a combined systematic review and interviews with actual nursing professionals. In this study, features that are highly relevant to the nursing workplace were extracted. By producing a body of nursing knowledge that fits well with current nursing home contexts in South Korea, this study contributes to building a foundation of evidence for an outline of ego-integrity management concepts in nursing home practice.

Conclusions

Identifying the concept of ego-integrity management in nursing home environments is useful as a way to help residents build quality social relationships and experience fulfilling end-of-life experiences. Ego-integrity management is a useful concept for nursing home practice because it has the potential to improve quality of care for a burgeoning older adult population. According to the findings of this study, strategies for managing the ego integrity of residents are a practical component of the professional, caring role of nurses. This management study focused on the role of nurses in nursing homes. The findings also confirmed the effectiveness of previous intervention studies that examined assessment tools and developed guidelines for ego-integrity management. This study paves the way for developing and implementing interventions for residents of nursing homes by clearly distinguishing the positive aspects of concepts related to ego-integrity management (i.e., successful aging and gerotranscendence).

Acknowledgments

This research was supported by a Basic Science Research Program grant from the National Research Foundation of Korea (NRF), which was funded by the Ministry of Education, Science and Technology (NRF-2017R1A2B4007896). We thank all the participants of the study.

Author Contributions

Study conception and design: SOC
Data collection: SYL, SOC
Data analysis and interpretation: SYL, SOC
Drafting of the article: SYL, SOC
Critical revision of the article: SYL, SOC

References

Aleksandrova-Yankulovska, S., & ten Have, H. (2015). Survey of staff and family members of patients in Bulgarian hospices on the concept of "good death". *American Journal of Hospice and Palliative Medicine, 32*(2), 226–232. https://doi.org/10.1177/1049909113516185

Ali, W. G. M., & Ayoub, N. S. (2010). Nurses' attitudes toward caring for dying patients in Mansoura university hospitals. *Journal of Medicine and Biomedical Sciences, 1*(1), 16–23.

Amella, E. J., Grant, A. P., & Mulloy, C. (2008). Eating behavior in persons with moderate to late-stage dementia: Assessment and interventions. *Journal of the American Psychiatric Nurses Association, 13*(6), 360–367. https://doi.org/10.1177/1078390307309216

Björk, S., Lindkvist, M., Wimo, A., Juthberg, C., Bergland, Å., & Edvardsson, D. (2017). Residents' engagement in everyday activities and its association with thriving in nursing homes. *Journal of Advanced Nursing, 73*(8), 1884–1895. https://doi.org/10.1111/jan.13275

Boltz, M., Capezuti, E., & Shabbat, N. (2011). Nursing staff perceptions of physical function in hospitalized older adults. *Applied Nursing Research, 24*(4), 215–222. https://doi.org/10.1016/j.apnr.2010.01.001

Brandburg, G. L., Symes, L., Mastel-Smith, B., Hersch, G., & Walsh, T. (2013). Resident strategies for making a life in a nursing home: A qualitative study. *Journal of Advanced Nursing, 69*(4), 862–874. https://doi.org/10.1111/j.1365-2648.2012.06075.x

Chodzko-Zajko, W., Schwingel, A., & Park, C. H. (2009). Successful aging: The role of physical activity. *American Journal of Lifestyle Medicine, 3*(1), 20–28. https://doi.org/10.1177/1559827608325456

Dezutter, J., Toussaint, L., & Leijssen, M. (2016). Forgiveness, ego-integrity, and depressive symptoms in community-dwelling and residential elderly adults. *Journals of Gerontology, Series B, 71*(5), 786–797. https://doi.org/10.1093/geronb/gbu146

Drageset, J., Eide, G. E., Dysvik, E., Furnes, B., & Hauge, S. (2015). Loneliness, loss, and social support among cognitively intact older people with cancer, living in nursing homes—A mixed-methods study. *Clinical Interventions in Aging, 10,* 1529–1536. https://doi.org/10.2147/CIA.S88404

Erikson, E. H. (1963). *Childhood and society* (2nd ed.). United States: Norton.

Erikson, E. H. (1998). *The lifecycle completed. Extended version with new chapters on the ninth stage by Joan M. Erikson.* Norton.

Friedman, E. M., Ruini, C., Foy, R., Jaros, L., Sampson, H., & Ryff, C. D. (2017). Lighten UP! A community-based group intervention to promote psychological well-being in older adults. *Aging & Mental Health, 21*(2), 199–205. https://doi.org/10.1080/13607863.2015.1093605

Harrison, J., & Frampton, S. (2017). Resident-centered care in 10 U.S. nursing homes: Residents' perspectives. *Journal of Nursing Scholarship, 49*(1), 6–14. https://doi.org/10.1111/jnu.12247

Haugan, G. (2014). Meaning-in-life in nursing-home patients: A valuable approach for enhancing psychological and physical well-being? *Journal of Clinical Nursing, 23*(13–14), 1830–1844. https://doi.org/10.1111/jocn.12402

Hung, L., Chaudhury, H., & Rust, T. (2016). The effect of dining room physical environmental renovations on person-centered care practice and residents' dining experiences in long-term care facilities. *Journal of Applied Gerontology, 35*(12), 1279–1301. https://doi.org/10.1177/0733464815574094

James, J. B., & Zarrett, N. (2006). Ego integrity in the lives of older women. *Journal of Adult Development, 13*(2), 61–75.

Jo, H., & Song, E. (2015). The effect of reminiscence therapy on depression, quality of life, ego integrity, social behavior function, and activities of daily living in elderly patients with mild dementia. *Educational Gerontology*, *41*(1), 1–13. https://doi.org/10.1080/03601277.2014.899830

Kim, S. J., Kim, M. S., Kim, H. J., Choi, J. E., & Chang, S. O. (2014). Nursing home nurses' ways of knowing about peaceful deaths in end-of-life care of residents: Personal knowledge and strategies. *Journal of Hospice & Palliative Nursing*, *16*(7), 438–445. https://doi.org/10.1097/NJH.0000000000000093

Kojima, G. (2015). Prevalence of frailty in nursing homes: A systematic review and meta-analysis. *Journal of the American Medical Directors Association*, *16*(11), 940–945. https://doi.org/10.1016/j.jamda.2015.06.025

Korean Ministry of Health and Welfare. (2018). *2018 senior medical welfare facilities of Welfare of the Aged Act*. http://www.law.go.kr/LSW/lsSc.do?tabMenuId=tab18&p1=&subMenu=1&nwYn=1&section=&tabNo=&query=%EB%85%B8%EC%9D%B8%EB%B3%B5%EC%A7%80%EB%B2%95 (Original work published in Korean)

Korean Statistical Information Service. (2018). Key population indicators. http://kosis.kr/statHtml/statHtml.do?orgId=101&tblId=DT_1BPA002&vw_cd=&list_id=&scrId=&seqNo=&lang_mode=ko&obj_var_id=&itm_id=&conn_path=E1 (Original work published in Korean)

Lim, S. Y., & Chang, S. O. (2018a). Nursing home staff members' subjective frames of reference on residents' achievement of ego integrity: A Q-methodology study. *Japan Journal of Nursing Science*, *15*(1), 17–30. https://doi.org/10.1111/jjns.12166

Lim, S. Y., & Chang, S. O. (2018b). Ego-integrity management of nursing-home residents: A concept analysis based on the method by Walker and Avant. *Journal of Korean Gerontological Nursing Society*, *20*(2), 97–108. https://doi.org/10.17079/jkgn.2018.20.2.97 (Original work published in Korean)

Lim, S. Y., Chang, S. O., Kim, S. J., Kim, H. J., Choi, J. E., & Park, M. S. (2014). Nurses' management of nursing-home residents' remaining functional ability: Concept development. *Journal of Korean Academy of Fundamentals of Nursing*, *21*(1), 57–68. https://doi.org/10.7739/jkafn.2014.21.1.57 (Original work published in Korean)

Martineau, A., & Plard, M. (2018). Successful aging: Analysis of the components of a gerontological paradigm. *Geriatrie et Psychologie Neuropsychiatrie du Vieillissement*, *16*(1), 67–77. https://doi.org/10.1684/pnv.2018.0724 (Original work published in French)

Meier, D. E., Lim, B., & Carlson, M. D. (2010). Raising the standard: Palliative care in nursing homes. *Health Affairs (Project Hope)*, *29*(1), 136–140. https://doi.org/10.1377/HLTHAFF.2009.0912

Oxford University Press. (n.d.). Ego-integrity management. In *Oxford English Dictionary*. Retrieved March 1, 2018. https://oxforddictionaries.com/

Paek, S. C., Zhang, N. J., Wan, T. T., Unruh, L. Y., & Meemon, N. (2016). The impact of state nursing home staffing standards on nurse staffing levels. *Medical Care Research and Review*, *73*(1), 41–61. https://doi.org/10.1177/1077558715594733

Park, M. S., Lim, S. Y., Kim, E. Y., Lee, S. J., & Chang, S. O. (2018). Examining practical nursing experiences to discover ways in which to retain and invigorate the remaining functions of the elderly with a demented and complex disability in nursing homes. *Japan Journal of Nursing Science*, *15*(1), 77–90. https://doi.org/10.1111/jjns.12174

Resnick, B., Rogers, V., Galik, E., & Gruber-Baldini, A. L. (2007). Measuring restorative care provided by nursing assistants: Reliability and validity of the Restorative Care Behavior Checklist. *Nursing Research*, *56*(6), 387–398. https://doi.org/10.1097/01.NNR.0000299854.52429.ac

Roberts, T., & Bowers, B. (2015). How nursing home residents develop relationships with peers and staff: A grounded theory study. *International Journal of Nursing Studies*, *52*(1), 57–67. https://doi.org/10.1016/j.ijnurstu.2014.07.008

Rylands, K. J., & Rickwood, D. J. (2001). Ego-integrity versus ego-despair: The effect of "accepting the past" on depression in older women. *The International Journal of Aging and Human Development*, *53*(1), 75–89. https://doi.org/10.2190/1LN2-J92C-2168-THPH

Schwartz-Barcott, D., & Kim, H. S. (2000). An expansion and elaboration of the hybrid model of concept development. In B. L. Rodgers & K. A. Knafl (Eds.), *Concept development in nursing: Foundations, techniques, and applications* (2nd ed., pp. 161–192). United States: Saunders.

Tahreen, S. F., & Shahed, S. (2014). Relationship between ego integrity, despair, social support and health related quality of life. *Pakistan Journal of Social and Clinical Psychology*, *12*(1), 26.

Torges, C. M., Stewart, A. J., & Duncan, L. E. (2008). Achieving ego integrity: Personality development in late midlife. *Journal of Research in Personality*, *42*(4), 1004–1019. https://doi.org/10.1016/j.jrp.2008.02.006

Vitale, S. A., Shaffer, C. M., & Acosta Fenton, H. R. (2014). Self-transcendence in Alzheimer's disease: The application of theory to practice. *Journal of Holistic Nursing*, *32*(4), 347–355. https://doi.org/10.1177/0898010114531857

Westerhof, G. J., Bohlmeijer, E. T., & McAdams, D. P. (2017). The relation of ego integrity and despair to personality traits and mental health. *Journals of Gerontology, Series B*, *72*(3), 400–407. https://doi.org/10.1093/geronb/gbv062

Wong, G. H., & Yap, P. L. (2016). Active ageing to gerotranscendence. *Annals of Academy of Medicine Singapore*, *45*(2), 41–43.

7

Development Trajectories and Predictors of the Role Commitment of Nursing Preceptors

Wei-Fang WANG[1] • Chich-Hsiu HUNG[2]* • Chung-Yi LI[3]

ABSTRACT

Background: The commitment of nursing preceptors to their role is an important driving force that supports their clinical teaching and affects teaching quality. Role commitment undergoes dynamic development and thus changes over time. Existing studies have utilized only cross-sectional study designs and have not analyzed the changes in commitment trajectories with related factors.

Purpose: This study aimed to investigate the development trajectories of the commitment of preceptors and to examine the predictors between the trajectories of role commitment among nursing preceptors.

Methods: A single-group, repeated-measures design was adopted, and 59 participants completed the Commitment to the Preceptor Role Scale and the Preceptor's Perception of Support Scale. The latent class growth analysis method was used to estimate the trajectory class patterns. The Wilcoxon rank-sum test, a nonparametric method, was used to compare the differences in demographic characteristics between the trajectories of commitment among nursing preceptors. Predictors were examined using binary logistic regression analysis.

Results: The two-class model was the best-fitting model to describe the trajectories of nursing preceptor commitment. The two classes in this model were "low commitment," which accounted for 90.3% of all the participants, and "high commitment," which accounted for 9.7%. A significant difference was found between the two classes in terms of motivation for being a preceptor ($p = .048$). Neither demographic characteristics nor organizational support had a predictive effect on the trajectories of commitment development.

Conclusions/Implications for Practice: This study found a low level of role commitment among new preceptors. Moreover, internal motivation was found to be a significant factor affecting the trajectories of this commitment. Therefore, institutions should foster an appropriate environment to enhance the role identity of preceptors as well as cultivate and stimulate their commitment to this role.

KEY WORDS:
nursing preceptor, commitment, trajectory.

Introduction

Insufficient nursing manpower is a global problem. The various clinical requirements and increases in work-related stress have had significant impacts on new nurses, making it difficult for healthcare providers to retain nursing talent, leading to a serious shortage of manpower. Therefore, it is necessary to provide a learning and development-friendly environment to attract new nursing personnel. Nursing preceptors play an essential role in the processes of recruiting and retaining new nurses (Beecroft, Dorey, & Wenten, 2008; Hautala, Saylor, & O'Leary-Kelley, 2007). In addition to providing clinical training to new nurses, preceptors serve as role models to help new nurses reduce their time spent exploring the unknown and making mistakes. Furthermore, preceptors play a supportive role in terms of helping familiarize newcomers with the workplace, creating harmonious working relationships, and facilitating the professional growth and development of these nurses.

Background

The preceptor system is a bridge between clinical practice and professional education that helps new nurses enhance their confidence in practice and the transition into their new role (Usher, Nolan, Reser, Owens, & Tollefson, 1999). Preceptors play multiple roles and have various responsibilities. They are clinicians as well as teachers and mentors; they are responsible for educating and counseling new nurses, helping them become familiar with the working environment when they graduate from schools or change jobs, and developing their social and professional capabilities (Beecroft et al., 2008; McCarty & Higgins, 2003). In the professional capability development ladder for nursing personnel, the Taiwan Nurses Association classifies the capabilities of nurses into the subcategories of clinical practice, academic, teaching, and administrative. Hence, during the professional development of nursing personnel, preceptors should take on the responsibility and mission of teaching, and all nurses with Clinical ladder level 3 (N3) must possess adequate teaching abilities (Taiwan Nurses Association, 2012). A study by Yeh (2009) showed that, although 89.0% of investigated preceptors agreed that they played an important role in the

[1]MSN, RN, Vice Director, Nursing Department, and Education Center, National Cheng Kung University Hospital, College of Medicine, National Cheng Kung University, and Doctoral Candidate, School of Nursing, Kaohsiung Medical University, Taiwan, ROC •
[2]PhD, RN, Professor, School of Nursing, Kaohsiung Medical University, and Adjunct Research Professor, Department of Medical Research, Kaohsiung Medical University Hospital, Taiwan, ROC •
[3]PhD, Professor, Department of Public Health, College of Medicine, National Cheng Kung University, Taiwan, ROC.

training and development of new nurses, only 29.4% believed that they had an adequate amount of time to instruct newcomers and only 55.2% exhibited a willingness to serve as preceptors. Ho, Yu, Chen, and Liu (2012) discovered that only 41.66% of preceptors were willing to serve in this role, indicating that the huge clinical workload and responsibilities had affected the commitment of preceptors to their role as well as their willingness to teach.

Commitment is defined as the intent to achieve goals with meaning through participation in life events (Lambert, Lambert, & Yamase, 2003). In addition, commitment reflects one's loyalty to a given role (Dibert & Goldenberg, 1995). Commitment and compassion toward teaching are two aspects of the same subject as well as the foundation of being a teacher. Whereas the professional capabilities of teachers may be developed by studying teaching methods and education-related knowledge, positive teaching attitudes and values are not easy to develop (Lin, 2012). A highly committed teacher is less likely to become a pedagogue as he or she will not only provide students with care but also continue to improve his or her own professional skills and knowledge and seek ways to enhance the learning effectiveness of students (Lin, 2012). On that account, the commitment of a preceptor to his or her role affects the quality of nursing education and thereby influences the learning processes and development of capabilities of new nurses. Therefore, nursing preceptors should be motivated and enthusiastic to teach to maintain their devotion to clinical teaching and improve teaching quality. Role commitment is a critical factor that supports the teaching practice of preceptors and furthermore reflects their belief in the professional role, their recognition of its values and goals, their positive evaluation of preceptor as a career, and their intention to stay in the position (Lu, Chang, & Wu, 2007).

Preceptors face various levels of stress at each stage, and their job commitment is likely to change because of excessive impacts and challenges. Studies have shown that job commitment tends to change with length of service (Fox, Henderson, & Malko-Nyhan, 2006; Lu, Chang, & Chiou, 2001). Hautala et al. (2007) emphasized that the major stressors of a preceptor originate from workload and lack of organizational support. The sense of commitment of preceptors is likely influenced by long-lasting workloads and stress, while organizational support such as training opportunities, teaching resources, promotions, and institutional recognitions and rewards may enhance this commitment and identification (Cloete & Jeggels, 2014; Dibert & Goldenberg, 1995; McCarty & Higgins, 2003; Usher et al., 1999).

Hyrkäs and Shoemaker (2007) analyzed the perceived support of preceptors and found that a Top 3 source of support was colleagues within the institutions, which sequentially included the following comments: "My co-workers in the nursing unit are supportive of the goals of the preceptor program," "I feel the nursing coordinators and nursing managers are committed to the success of the preceptor program," and "My goals as a preceptor are clearly defined." Ho et al. (2012) assessed the causes of decline in teaching willingness

among preceptors and proposed strategies to improve organizational support policies such as the simplification of learning passports, the organization of regular education and training, the provision of paid leave and paid trainings, improvements to the incentive system, the development of a counseling mechanism, and the establishment of teaching guidelines. After the implementation of these strategies, the teaching willingness of nursing preceptors increased from 41.66% to 73.33%. The studies of Dibert and Goldenberg (1995) and Usher et al. (1999) showed similar results, suggesting a positive correlation between sense of commitment and perceived support from the organization, with higher perceived support from the organization resulting in a stronger sense of commitment. Other studies have also confirmed that, as they receive more perceived benefits, rewards, and support from the organization, their commitment becomes more prominent (Cloete & Jeggels, 2014; Hallin & Danielson, 2009; Hyrkäs & Shoemaker, 2007).

In addition, personal factors and relevant teaching experience affect the ability and attitude of nursing preceptors to handle difficult teaching situations and therefore may influence the development of commitment (Dibert & Goldenberg, 1995; Usher et al., 1999; Wilson & Laschinger, 1994). These personal factors of influence include age, job seniority, level of education, motivation, and work unit (Dibert & Goldenberg, 1995; Wilson & Laschinger, 1994). Prior teaching experience includes experience as a preceptor for new nurses as well as the types of learners instructed (Dibert & Goldenberg, 1995; Usher et al., 1999). In their study on commitment, Wilson and Laschinger (1994) discovered that age and job seniority positively correlated with nursing preceptor role commitment. Dibert and Goldenberg (1995) found that those who lack motivation to be preceptors tend not to remain in their position. The commitment of nursing preceptors to their role and the frequency of instructing newly hired nurses have been positively correlated; however, no significant correlation has been found between commitment and the number of clinical practicums for nursing students instructed. Furthermore, the commitment of nursing preceptors has not been correlated with job seniority, level of education, or age. Usher et al. (1999) showed that frequency of precept and experience with learners of various backgrounds correlated positively with role commitment, whereas educational background, age, and gender did not. Hyrkäs and Shoemaker (2007) conducted a study among nursing preceptors participating in a preceptor workshop and found no correlation between commitment and personal factors such as age, job seniority, possession of a nursing certification, workplace, education, or precepting experience.

Given that the role commitment of nursing preceptors develops dynamically, this commitment changes over time. However, most of the existing studies only utilized cross-sectional study designs to explore the perceptions and responses of preceptors at a given moment (Hautala et al., 2007; Usher et al., 1999; Yonge, Krahn, Trojan, Reid, & Haase, 2002) and did not track changes in commitment over time. Hallin and Danielson (2009) conducted two cross-sectional surveys with a 6-year interval to investigate preceptors' perceived readiness and support received. However, the results represent two different study groups at two different time points because the participants at the data collection points were different. Thus, this study aimed to investigate the development trajectories of preceptor role commitment among Taiwanese nursing preceptors over a 6-month period and to examine the correlations among the development trajectory patterns of role commitment, personal factors, and perceived organizational support.

Methods

Design and Participants

This study adopted a single-group, repeated-measures design to explore the changes in sense of commitment among new preceptors before and 6 months after participating in an official preceptor training program. Data were collected every 2 months, and four repeated measures were conducted. Convenience sampling was used to recruit participants from a medical center in southern Taiwan. The inclusion criterion was being a preceptor candidate with a unit manager recommendation. The sample size was estimated based on Barcikowski and Robey's (1985) formula and Lu et al.'s (2001) suggested correlation coefficient of .35 for changes in nursing preceptor commitment in a repeated-measures study. Thus, this study set a repeated-measures benchmark effect size of 0.30 (medium level), a statistical power level of 0.80, and a threshold of significance level of .05. Given that the repeated measures of this study were conducted four times, the sample size was estimated to be 35 (Barcikowski & Robey, 1985). The statistical power analysis program G*Power 3.1.7 was used, and the same sample size was estimated. Latham, Hogan, and Ringl (2008) reported a 10% rate of attrition in their longitudinal research on establishing a mentoring program to create a positive workforce environment. Thus, this study set an attrition rate of 15%, giving a minimum sample size of 41.

Instruments

The study included three structured questionnaires: the demographic questionnaire, the Commitment to the Preceptor Role Scale (CPRS), and the Preceptor's Perception of Support Scale (PPSuS). The demographic questionnaire included the age, education, on-job education, job seniority, work unit, motivation to be a preceptor, past experience as an unofficial preceptor, and background of the previous preceptees.

The CPRS was developed by the researchers to measure the commitment of Taiwanese nurses to the preceptor role. Items on the CPRS were generated based on the researchers' clinical practice, a literature review, and Dibert and Goldenberg's (1995) original scale. The validity of the scale for this study was tested using a double-loop expert validity method. A group of 10 nursing preceptors with similar demographic backgrounds to the study participants was invited to review the first version of the scale, and the semantics of six items were revised according to their feedback. Then, another group of 10 preceptors was invited to review the second version of the scale. On the basis of their suggestions, the semantics of five items were modified, and one negatively phrased item was changed to be positively phrased. Finally, the third version was given to 10 experts from the previous two groups, and no further revision was required. The content validity index of the scale was between .89 and 1.0, indicating good validity. The CPRS uses a 6-point Likert scale (1 = strongly disagree, 2 = disagree, 3 = somewhat disagree, 4 = somewhat agree, 5 = agree, and 6 = strongly agree). The 10 items on the CPRS, which include three that are negatively phrased and counter-indicative, have a total possible score range between 10 and 60, with higher scores associated with a stronger sense of role commitment. The internal consistency reliability (Cronbach's α) of the scale was .90.

The items on the PPSuS were generated according to the researchers' clinical practice, a literature review, and Dibert and Goldenberg's (1995) original scale to measure the level of organizational support that is perceived by Taiwanese nursing preceptors. A double-loop expert validity method was used to test the validity of the scale. The first version was reviewed by a group of 10 nursing preceptors with similar backgrounds to the study participants. The semantics of six items were revised based on their recommendations. The second version was reviewed by another group of 10 nursing preceptors, and the wording of three items was revised based on their suggestions. Finally, the third version was given to 10 experts from the previous two groups, and one item was modified. The content validity index of this scale was between .89 and .99, indicating good validity. This 11-item scale includes three negatively phrased and counter-indicative items. Total possible scores for the PPSuS ranged from 11 to 66, with higher scores indicating more perceived support. The Cronbach's α of the scale in this study was .75.

Study Procedures

This study was approved by the institutional review board of the study hospital (No. B-ER-102-370). The period of data collection was from April to October 2014. After potential participants were introduced to the research purpose, they decided on their own whether to participate or not. Once a potential participant agreed to participate, he or she was asked to sign an informed consent form. All of the participants were asked to complete the three structured questionnaires, the demographic questionnaire, the CPRS, and the PPSuS, before they received preceptor training. Then, the CPRS was completed again in the second, fourth, and sixth months after the first data collection. The questionnaires were put in an envelope and given to the participants by the research assistant. After completing the questionnaires, each participant put them in the designated envelope, which was collected either by the file transfer mechanism of the research institution or by the research assistant. A telephone call was made to remind participants who had not submitted their completed questionnaires within 1 week to complete the survey. All of the participants had completed and submitted the questionnaires after the reminder calls had been made.

Data Analyses

SAS 9.4 and PASW 19.0 were used for the data analysis. This study applied a longitudinal and repeated-measures design to explore the trajectories of the role commitment of new nursing preceptors within the first 6 months and to examine the relationships between their sense of commitment, perceived organizational support, and demographic characteristics. The latent class growth analysis method was used to estimate trajectory class patterns (Andruff, Carraro, Thompson, & Gaudreau, 2009). This semiparametric statistical technique, which is based on classes, was adopted to analyze changes in longitudinal data (Nagin, 1999), allowing the present research to identify trajectory models and role commitment trends.

Fifty-nine participants were enrolled in the first survey. However, one participant missed the third survey. Therefore, 234 points of data over the four survey times were available for analysis. SAS 9.4 was adopted to analyze the trajectory classification, the Proc Traj command was executed, and the option "Poisson" was selected (Jones, Nagin, & Roeder, 2001; Nagin, 1999) to identify the classes and patterns of the trajectory. The linear model utilized the minimum values for the Bayesian information criterion (BIC; Schwarz, 1978) and for the Akaike information criterion (AIC; Akaike, 1987). The smaller the BIC value, the better the fit to the model. PASW 19.0 was employed for the descriptive analysis of demographic characteristics. Interval variables were presented with a mean and a standard deviation, whereas nominal variables were presented using a percentage. Then, the Wilcoxon rank-sum test, a nonparametric method, was used to compare the differences in demographic characteristics between the patterns of trajectory of nursing preceptor commitment. Finally, a binary logistic regression analysis was utilized to examine the predictors of the trajectories of role commitment, with the statistical significance (p value) set at < .05.

Results

Demographic Characteristics and Perceived Organizational Support

Fifty-nine participants agreed to participate in this study and signed the informed consent form. Fifty-eight completed the questionnaires at all of the four survey points, with one participant failing to complete the questionnaires at the third and fourth survey points, resulting to an attrition rate of 1.7% (1/59). The data of all 59 participants were included in the statistical analysis. The ages of participants ranged from 24.08 to 44.25 years (M = 26.82 years, SD = 2.90 years), with job seniority ranging between 2 and 14 years and

7 months (M = 3.76, SD = 2.10). A large majority of the participants had graduated from a university (94.9%), and 23.7% were studying through an on-job educational program. Only 23.7% of the participants reported "internal factors" as a motivation to be a preceptor. These internal factors included fondness for teaching, feeling of honor, and the belief that being a preceptor was beneficial for promotion. By contrast, most of the participants (76.3%) attributed their motivations to external factors such as adherence to institutional assignment decisions. A minority of participants (40.7%) worked in the emergency room, intensive care units, and special, nonward units, whereas most (59.3%) worked in general wards. Approximately one quarter of the participants had previous experience working as nursing preceptors for newly hired nurses (25.4%). In addition, 33.9% had prior experience precepting nursing students, whereas 32.2% had prior experience precepting nurses. The average score of perceived organizational support was 43.57 (SD = 4.37; Table 1).

Trajectories of Nursing Preceptor Role Commitment

The trajectories of nursing preceptor role commitment were analyzed, and two, three, and four classes were identified using stepwise selection. By identifying the minimum BIC

TABLE 1.

Demographic Characteristics and Perceived Organizational Support (N = 59)

Variable	n	%
Age (years; *M, SD*)	26.82	2.90
Years of working experience (*M, SD*)	3.76	2.10
Education		
Bachelor's degree	56	94.9
Master's degree	3	5.1
On-job education		
No	45	76.3
Yes	14	23.7
Motivation to be a nursing preceptor		
Internal factors	14	23.7
External factors	45	76.3
Unit		
Special ward	24	40.7
General ward	35	59.3
Experience as unofficial preceptor for newly hired nurses		
No	44	74.6
Yes	15	25.4
Previous preceptee's role		
Not available	20	33.9
Nursing students	20	33.9
Nurses	19	32.2
Organizational support (score; *M, SD*)	43.57	4.37

TABLE 2.
The Trajectories of Nursing Preceptor Role Commitment at the Four Time Points

Time	Class 1 (n = 54)			Class 2 (n = 5)			Total (N = 59)		
	95% CI for Mean Traj 1			95% CI for Mean Traj 2			95% CI for Mean Traj All		
	Mean	Lower	Upper	Mean	Lower	Upper	Mean	Lower	Upper
T1	40.23	38.45	42.01	52.35	45.79	58.91	41.41	39.75	43.06
T2	40.11	38.35	41.86	53.70	46.51	60.89	41.42	39.77	43.08
T3	40.61	38.82	42.39	49.15	43.12	55.17	41.45	39.78	43.12
T4	41.00	39.21	42.79	52.71	45.68	59.74	42.16	40.47	43.84

Note. Traj = trajectories. T1 = baseline; T2 = 2 months; T3 = 4 months; T4= 6 months.

and AIC values, the analysis indicated that the two-class model provided the best fit (BIC = −734.84, AIC = −719.24). The two classes were then named "low commitment" (Class 1), which accounted for 90.3% of the total participants, and "high commitment" (Class 2), which accounted for 9.7%. The mean scores for role commitment at the 4-point measures for the two classes are indicated in Table 2. The results showed that the sense of commitment for all of the participants was on an upward development trend.

The mean score of Class 1 was 40.23 (of 60) at the first time point, declined slightly to 40.11 at the second time point, and then rose steadily to 41.00 at the fourth time point. The mean score of Class 2 was initially 52.35, rose to 53.70 at the second time point, dropped to 49.15 at the third time point, and then rose to 52.71 at the fourth time point. Although the mean scores of Class 2 fluctuated, its mean score curve remained above that of Class 1 (Figure 1).

The Relationships Between Demographic Characteristics and Perceived Organizational Support and Trajectories of Commitment

The differences in the demographic characteristics of participants and the perceived support between the two classes of

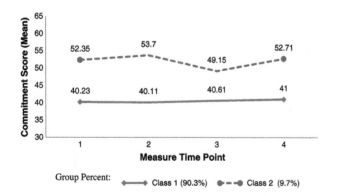

Group Percent: ◆——→ Class 1 (90.3%)   ●- -● Class 2 (9.7%)

Figure 1. Changes in role commitment for the two groups (Classes 1 and 2) at the four time points. *Note.* 1 = Time 1. before preceptor training; 2 = Time 2. after preceptor training 2 months; 3 = Time 3. after preceptor training 4 months; 4= Time 4. after preceptor training 6 months.

commitment trajectory were analyzed using the Wilcoxon rank-sum test. The result showed a significant difference in motivation for being a preceptor between the two classes (*p* = .048), with a greater proportion of "high commitment" (Class 2) participants motivated by internal factors than "low commitment" (Class 1) participants. However, no other significant differences were found between the two classes (Table 3).

Predictors of Role Commitment Trajectories

Binary logistic regression analysis was used to examine the predictors of participant role commitment trajectories using the "low commitment" (Class 1) group as the reference group to conduct a univariate regression followed by a multivariable regression analysis. A forward stepwise selection was adopted to add independent variables to the model. The result indicated that demographic characteristics and perceived support from the organization did not differ significantly. In other words, neither demographic characteristics nor organization support was able to predict the trajectories of nursing preceptor role commitment (Table 4).

Discussion

After repeated measures and analyses, this study indicates that the trajectories of the role commitment of new nursing preceptors change dynamically and may be distinguished into two classes: low commitment (Class 1) and high commitment (Class 2). Moreover, the motivation of nurses to be a preceptor differed significantly between these two classes. Interestingly, internal motivation accounted for a higher proportion of Class 2 participants. However, neither demographic characteristics nor perceived organizational support was a significant predictor of commitment trajectories.

A large majority (90.3%) of the participants were classified as "low commitment" (Class 1) individuals, whereas only 9.7% were classified as "high commitment" (Class 2) individuals. This indicates that the sense of role commitment is nascent in new nursing preceptors. Further development through learning, practice, experience, reflection, and internalization is needed. Over the course of the 6-month study period, the commitment trajectory of the Class 1 group showed a slight decline at the second time point and an upward trend

TABLE 3.

Comparisons of Demographic Characteristics and Perceived Organizational Support Between the Commitment Trajectories of the Two Classes of Nursing Preceptors (N = 59)

Variable	Class 1 (n = 54)		Class 2 (n = 5)		p
	n	%	n	%	
Age (years; M, SD)	26.93	3.01	25.68	0.82	.157
Years of working experience (M, SD)	3.93	2.31	3.18	0.64	.540
Education					
Bachelor's degree	51	94.4	5	100.0	.592
Master's degree	3	5.6	0	0	
On-job education					
No	42	77.8	3	60.0	.375
Yes	12	22.2	2	40.0	
Motivation to be a nursing preceptor					
Internal factors	11	20.4	3	60.0	.048*
External factors	43	79.6	2	40.0	
Unit					
Special ward	23	42.6	1	20.0	.329
General ward	31	57.4	4	80.0	
Experience as unofficial preceptor for newly hired nurses					
No	41	75.9	3	60.0	.438
Yes	13	24.1	2	40.0	
Previous preceptee's role					
Not available	18	33.3	2	40.0	.544
Nursing students	20	37.0	0	0.0	
Nurses	16	29.6	3	60.0	
Organizational support (score; M, SD)	43.48	3.63	46.60	9.56	.555

Note. Analysis with Wilcoxon's rank sum test.
*$p < .05$.

for other points of time. Thus, the overall commitment trajectory for this group tended to rise slowly. The trajectory of the Class 2 group manifested a substantial drop at the third time point that fell even below the first time point, gradually climbing back at the fourth time point and showing an overall fluctuating pattern. More studies with a larger sample size are needed to confirm the development pattern of role commitment in nursing preceptors.

The mean score for role commitment at the first time point was 41.41, which is lower than the mean score of 48.75 that was found in Hyrkäs and Shoemaker's (2007) study. Moreover, most of our participants were categorized into the low commitment group. The differing findings may be due to differences in demographic characteristics of participants between the two studies. In Hyrkäs and Shoemaker's study, the average age of the participants was 46.11 years, and the average job seniority was 16.8 years. Both are greater than the average age of 26.82 years and job seniority of 3.67 years for our participants. The average length of experience as preceptors was 7.5 years in Hyrkäs and Shoemaker, whereas the participants in this study were all newly appointed nursing preceptors. The age, job seniority, and past experience

as preceptors of participants in these two studies were completely different. The overall trajectory of role commitment showed a growing trend over the 6-month study period in this study. Future studies should expand the duration of the study period to explore the long-term impact of demographic characteristics on nurse commitment to the preceptor role.

Furthermore, this study found that internal motivation differed significantly between the two classes, with a higher proportion of nurses in the high commitment group (Class 2) motivated by internal factors. This result is similar to the findings of Luhanga, Billay, Grundy, Myrick, and Yonge (2010) and Carlson, Pilhammar, and Wann-Hansson (2010). Dibert and Goldenberg (1995) and Usher et al. (1999) showed that motivation is an important factor that affects the role commitment of preceptors. Some participants in this study took over the role of preceptor because of their own wishes or needs, including enjoyment of teaching, the honor of being a preceptor, and the perceived positive impact on future promotion prospects. In addition, most internally motivated participants were in the high commitment group. As most of our participants were recommended by their working units to take over the role of preceptors, most noted "adherence

TABLE 4.
Predictors of the Commitment Trajectories of Participants (N = 59)

Variable	Class 2 (n = 5) vs. Class 1 (n = 54)		
	OR	95% CI	p
Age (years)	0.511	[0.170, 1.535]	.232
Years of working experience	0.703	[0.257, 1.924]	.493
Education			
Bachelor's vs. master's	0.002	0.000	.999
On-job education			
No vs. yes	0.429	[0.064, 2.867]	.382
Motivation to be a nursing preceptor			
Internal vs. external factors	5.864	[0.870, 39.511]	.069
Unit			
Special vs. general	0.337	[0.035, 3.218]	.345
Experience as unofficial preceptor for newly hired nurses			
No vs. yes	0.476	[0.072, 3.164]	.442
Previous preceptee's role			
Not available vs. nurses	0.593	[0.088, 4.009]	.592
Student nurses vs. nurses	0.000	0.000	.998
Organizational support	1.137	[0.957, 1.349]	.144

Note. Class 1 is the reference class.

to institutional assignment decisions" as their primary motivation, which may be the reason most of the participants were classified in the low commitment group. Thus, it is important to assess the internal motivation of nurses when selecting future preceptors in addition to assessments of seniority and professional capabilities. In terms of human resources, many medical institutions consider teaching as a task for a preceptor that is performed in addition to his or her normal clinical duties. This situation may affect the willingness of nurses to accept the role of a preceptor. Therefore, how to create a teaching environment and supportive atmosphere that elicits the internal motivations of nursing preceptors is an important issue.

Because of the impact of the 2003 SARS epidemic on Taiwan's clinical care sector and the high demand for professional personnel, medical team education and training have received great attention (Ministry of Health and Welfare, Executive Yuan, Taiwan, ROC, 2012). The Teaching Quality Improvement Program for Teaching Hospitals has been included in the training standards for nursing preceptors since 2007 (Yin, 2013) and has recently been incorporated into training programs for clinical medical personnel and used as a critical indicator for teaching hospital accreditation (Chan, 2015). Today's teaching hospitals have set up clinical training programs and incentive policies for nursing preceptors such as offering teaching subsidies, offering opportunities to attend conferences, rewarding attendance at faculty development classes, and obtaining advantages for training and education.

These programs and policies focus on creating teaching-oriented organizational cultures that encourage newly appointed preceptors to perceive the importance of their role and the

support from the organization, thereby facilitating their role commitment. Previous studies have shown that greater perceived support from the organization correlates with a stronger sense of commitment in preceptors (Cloete & Jeggels, 2014; Hyrkäs & Shoemaker, 2007; Usher et al., 1999). However, this study indicates that perceived organizational support did not differ significantly between the two groups of nursing preceptors. Future research should collect the perceived organizational support of preceptors at various time points to explore the changes in perceived support as well as the impact of these changes on overall role commitment.

Conclusions

Nursing preceptors play a critical role in passing down professional nursing knowledge and skills. Commitment is an important element that supports their teaching quality. This study indicates that a low level of role commitment exists among new preceptors in Taiwan. Moreover, internal motivation was found to be a significant factor affecting the role commitment of preceptors. Therefore, institutions should create an environment that enhances the role identity of their preceptors as well as cultivates and stimulates their role commitment.

Time and interaction with others are required for new preceptors to develop a sense of commitment. Learning and practice experiences may be internalized and shaped into the role. Therefore, tracking the role commitment of preceptors is a long-term task. Future research should expand the tracking period and increase the sample size to construct a development trajectory model of preceptor role commitment. Because the formation of sense of commitment requires professional identity, role play, and organizational cultivation, institutions must create a teaching-oriented atmosphere and utilize different strategies of encouragement and guidance to facilitate the internal motivation of nursing preceptors.

Acknowledgments

This study was funded by the Taiwan Nurses Association, ROC (TWNA-1032019). We thank Shang-Chi Lee for providing the statistical consulting services of the Biostatistics Consulting Center, National Cheng Kung University Hospital. We are also grateful for the time and effort committed by the participating preceptors.

References

Akaike, H. (1987). Factor analysis and AIC. *Psychometrika, 52*(3), 317–332. doi:10.1007/BF02294359

Andruff, H., Carraro, N., Thompson, A., & Gaudreau, P. (2009). Latent class growth modeling: A tutorial. *Tutorials in Quantitative Methods for Psychology, 5*(1), 11–24. doi:10.4135/97808 57020994.n9

Barcikowski, R. S., & Robey, R. R. (1985). *Sample size selection in single group repeated measures analysis*. The Annual Meeting of the American Educational Research Association, Chicago, IL.

Beecroft, P. C., Dorey, F., & Wenten, M. (2008). Turnover intention in new graduate nurses: A multivariate analysis. *Journal of Advanced Nursing, 62*(1), 41–52. doi:10.1111/j.1365-2648.2007.04570.x

Carlson, E., Pilhammar, E., & Wann-Hansson, C. (2010). Time to precept supportive and limiting conditions for precepting nurses. *Journal of Advanced Nursing, 66*(2), 432–441. doi:10.1111/j.1365-2648.2009.05174.x

Chan, C. Y. (2015). Indications of performance in the teaching quality improvement program for teaching hospitals—Review and experience. *Journal of Healthcare Quality, 9*(1), 17–23. (Original work published in Chinese)

Cloete, I. S., & Jeggels, J. (2014). Exploring nurse preceptors' perceptions of benefits and support of and commitment to the preceptor role in the Western Cape Province. *Journal of the Democratic Nursing Organisation of South Africa, 37*(1), 1–7. doi:10.4102/curationis.v37i1.1281

Dibert, C., & Goldenberg, D. (1995). Preceptors' perceptions of benefits, rewards, supports and commitment to the preceptor role. *Journal of Advanced Nursing, 21*(6), 1144–1151. doi:10.1046/j.1365-2648.1995.21061144.x

Fox, R., Henderson, A., & Malko-Nyhan, K. (2006). A comparison of preceptor and preceptee's of how the preceptor's role is operationalized. *Journal of Clinical Nursing, 15*(3), 361–364. doi:10.1111/j.1365-2702.2006.01329.x

Hallin, K., & Danielson, E. (2009). Being a personal preceptor for nursing students: Registered Nurses' experiences before and after introduction of a preceptor model. *Journal of Advanced Nursing, 65*(1), 161–174. doi:10.1111/j.1365-2648.2008.04855.x

Hautala, K. T., Saylor, C. R., & O'Leary-Kelley, C. (2007). Nurses' perceptions of stress and support in the preceptor role. *Journal for Nurses in Staff Development, 23*(2), 64–70. doi:10.1097/01.NND.0000266611.78315.08

Ho, C. H., Yu, C. C., Chen, C. W., & Liu, H. H. (2012). Improving the teaching willingness of preceptors. *Chang Gung Nursing, 23*(2), 186–196. (Original work published in Chinese)

Hyrkäs, K., & Shoemaker, M. (2007). Changes in the preceptor role: Revisiting preceptors' perceptions of benefits, rewards, support and commitment to the role. *Journal of Advanced Nursing, 60*(5), 513–524. doi:10.1111/j.1365-2648.2007.04441.x

Jones, B. L., Nagin, D. S., & Roeder, K. (2001). A SAS procedure based on mixture models for estimating developmental trajectories. *Sociological Methods and Research, 29*(3), 374–393. doi:10.1177/0049124101029003005

Lambert, V. A., Lambert, C. E., & Yamase, H. (2003). Psychological hardiness, workplace stress and related stress reduction strategies. *Nursing and Health Sciences, 5*(2), 181–184. doi:10.1046/j.1442-2018.2003.00150.x

Latham, C. L., Hogan, M., & Ringl, K. (2008). Nurses supporting nurses: Creating a mentoring program for staff nurses to improve the workforce environment. *Nursing Administration Quarterly, 32*(1), 27–39. doi:10.1097/01.NAQ.0000305945.23569.2b

Lin, M. C. (2012). Teachers' enthusiasm and sense of educational mission for the meaning of teacher education. *Taiwan Education Review, 676*, 2–9. (Original work published in Chinese)

Lu, K. Y., Chang, L. C., & Wu, H. L. (2007). Relationships between professional commitment, job satisfaction, and work stress in public health nurses in Taiwan. *Journal of Professional Nursing, 23*(2), 110–116. doi:10.1016/j.profnurs.2006.06.005

Lu, K. Y., Chang, Y. Y., & Chiou, S. L. (2001). Changes in nursing professional commitment among junior college graduates. *The Journal of Nursing Research, 9*(1), 28–38. (Original work published in Chinese)

Luhanga, F. L., Billay, D., Grundy, Q., Myrick, F., & Yonge, O. (2010). The one-to-one relationship: Is it really key to an effective preceptorship experience? A review of the literature. *International Journal of Nursing Education Scholarship, 7*, Article21. doi:10.2202/1548-923X.2012

McCarty, M., & Higgins, A. (2003). Moving to an all graduate profession: Preparing preceptors for their role. *Nurse Education Today, 23*(2), 89–95. doi:10.1016/S0260-6917(02)00187-9

Ministry of Health and Welfare, Executive Yuan, Taiwan, ROC. (2012). *Application guidelines for the teaching quality improvement program for teaching hospitals*. Retrieved from http://wd.vghtpe.gov.tw/mec/down1.jsp?id=721andtype=2 (Original work published in Chinese)

Nagin, D. S. (1999). Analyzing developmental trajectories: A semiparametric, group-based approach. *Psychological Methods, 4*(2), 139–177. doi:10.1037//1082-989X.4.2.139

Schwarz, G. (1978). Estimating the dimension of a model. *Annals of Statistics, 6*(2), 461–464. doi:10.1214/aos/1176344136

Taiwan Nurses Association. (2012). *Plan and guideline for basic nurses in the clinical nursing ladder system.* Retrieved from http://www.twna.org.tw/frontend/un10_open/welcome.asp# (Original work published in Chinese)

Usher, K., Nolan, C., Reser, P., Owens, J., & Tollefson, J. (1999). An exploration of the preceptor role—Preceptors' perceptions of benefits, rewards, supports and commitment to the preceptor role. *Journal of Advanced Nursing, 29*(2), 506–514. doi:10.1046/j.1365-2648.1999.00914.x

Wilson, B., & Laschinger, H. K. S. (1994). Staff nurses' perception of job empowerment and organizational commitment: A test of Kanter's theory of structural power in organizations. *Journal of Nursing Administration, 24*(4s), 39–45. doi:10.1097/00005110-199404011-00007

Yeh, L. Y. (2009). *Willingness and associated factors for preceptors to guide new staff nurses* (Unpublished master's thesis). China Medical University, Taichung City, Taiwan, ROC. (Original work published in Chinese)

Yin, Y. C. (2013). Two-year post graduate training program for nurses: Implementation status and personal perspectives. *The Journal of Nursing, 60*(3), 11–16. doi:10.6224/JN.60.3.11 (Original work published in Chinese)

Yonge, O., Krahn, H., Trojan, L., Reid, D., & Haase, M. (2002). Supporting preceptors. *Journal for Nurses in Staff Development, 18*(2), 73–77. doi:10.1097/00124645-200203000-00005

Attitude of Nursing Students Toward Scientific Research

Seher ÜNVER[1]* • Remziye SEMERCI[2] • Zeynep Kızılcık ÖZKAN[3] • İlker AVCIBAŞI[4]

ABSTRACT

Background: Nursing, a social applied science, is a dynamic profession. Professional nurses must be curious, investigative, and open to learning as well as practice critical and analytic thinking to sustain their professionalism.

Purpose: The aim of this study was to determine the attitudes of nursing students toward scientific research.

Methods: A descriptive and cross-sectional study design was used. This study was conducted at a nursing department of a university in Turkey. A sample of 375 nursing students participated. Data were collected using the "Personal Information Form" and "Attitude Scale towards Scientific Studies." Standard descriptive statistical methods, correlation, Mann–Whitney U, Kruskal–Wallis, and post hoc Bonferroni were used in data analysis.

Results: Nearly all (90.1%) of the participants were female, and 33.9% were sophomore (second-year) students. Junior (third-year) students held the most positive attitudes toward research, as compared with the participants in other academic years. Participants who had participated in scientific activities held more positive attitudes toward research than those who had not. Participants who had prior experience doing scientific research showed more positive attitudes toward research and researchers than those without this experience. Being older, having scientific research experience, following the continuous broadcasts related to nursing, and participating in scientific activities all significantly influenced attitude toward research ($p < .05$).

Conclusions/Implications for Practice: Although nursing students who participated in this study exhibited generally positive attitudes toward scientific research, they had relatively little experience participating in scientific activities. Therefore, to foster a positive scientific research culture among undergraduate students, grants should be provided that encourage wider participation in scientific activities and offer opportunities for undergraduate students to do scientific research.

KEY WORDS:
attitude, nursing, students, scientific research, education.

Introduction

Nursing is a dynamic profession that operates as a social, applied, and empirical science (Adıgüzel, Tanrıverdi, & Özkan, 2011; Karagözoğlu, 2005). Nursing studies investigate not only human beings but also their experiences and approach events and problems in a questioning manner, delivering rational and evidence-based solutions to problems in light of available information and science (Karagözoğlu, 2006). Basing nursing practices on scientific information brings professional identity to the profession (Korkmaz, 2011).

To sustain professionalism, the members of a profession must be curious, investigative, open to learning, innovative and creative, and independent; cooperate with the members of other professions; have critical, analytic thinking abilities; implement evidence-based care; and evaluate outcomes (Adıgüzel et al., 2011, Laaksonen, Paltta, von Schantz, Ylönen, & Soini, 2013). To bring scientific qualifications to a profession, its members should recognize the problems that they face, determine the problem and problem-related variables, and find solutions to these problems using scientific research processes (Adıgüzel et al., 2011; Bökeoğlu & Yılmaz, 2005; Rezaei & Zamani-Miandashti, 2013). Nurses have embraced the necessity of doing scientific research to respond to the expectations worldwide for rapid and continuous improvements (Aydın, Adıgüzel, & Topal, 2015).

Educational institutions promote and instill the professional cultural value of embracing and adhering to the scientific process (Büyüköztürk, 1997). Universities, in particular, are expected to lead scientific research and raise individuals with scientific attitudes and behaviors in addition to providing education services (Aydın et al., 2015; Korkmaz, Şahin, & Yeşil, 2011a). Thus, nursing students should be initiated into research culture and adopt positive attitudes toward scientific research during their undergraduate education to improve the nursing profession, to contribute to the professionalization of this profession, and to maintain quality of care, nurse autonomy, and power (Çelik, Önder, Durmaz, Yurdusever, & Uysal, 2014).

Determining the attitude of nursing students toward scientific research is very important, as these students will play a vital role in ensuring clinical research studies in the

[1]PhD, RN, Assistant Professor, Faculty of Health Sciences, Department of Surgical Nursing, Trakya University, Edirne, Turkey • [2]BSN, RN, Research Assistant, Faculty of Health Sciences, Department of Child Health and Disease Nursing, Trakya University, Edirne, Turkey • [3]PhD, RN, Research Assistant, Faculty of Health Sciences, Department of Surgical Nursing, Trakya University, Edirne, Turkey • [4]MSN, RN, Research Assistant, Faculty of Health Sciences, Department of Public Health Nursing, Trakya University, Edirne, Turkey.

future. Students in this field who do not show positive attitudes toward scientific research are likely not to contribute to the development of the nursing profession and not to provide evidence-based care that promotes high-quality health outcomes (Halabi, 2016). Therefore, it is important to understand the attitudes of nursing students toward scientific research. As undergraduate nursing education is a four-academic-year degree program in Turkey (Gerçek, Okursoy, & Dal, 2016), the purpose of this study was to determine the attitudes toward scientific research of nursing students in all four academic years.

Methods

This descriptive and cross-sectional study was performed on the 570 currently enrolled students at the Department of Nursing at Trakya University in Turkey during the spring term of the 2015–2016 academic year. The sample was composed of the 375 students (65.8% of the total number of enrolled students) who completed the self-administered personal information forms during mandatory basic nursing courses, including fundamentals of nursing, medical and surgical nursing, women's health and disease nursing, child health and disease nursing, mental health and diseases nursing, and public health nursing. The forms were administered to all of the students who had volunteered as participants and who attended class on the day of data collection during April and May 2016.

Data were collected using a personal information form and the Scale of Attitudes towards Scientific Research form. The personal information form, developed as a result of a literature review by the researchers, included student-related variables addressing introductive features and scientific study experience. This form was composed of seven questions, three of which related to introductive features (age, gender, and academic year) and four of which related to attitudes toward scientific studies (whether students take statistics/research courses, have scientific research experience, constantly follow publications about nursing, and participate in scientific meetings, congresses, symposiums, and/or other similar activities).

The Scale of Attitudes towards Scientific Research was developed by Korkmaz, Şahin, and Yeşil (2011b). This scale is a 5-point Likert-type scale and consists of 30 items, which were categorized under four factors. Participants were asked to rate each of the item using one of the following responses: 1 = *completely disagree*, 2 = *disagree*, 3 = *undecided*, 4 = *agree*, and 5 = *completely agree*. The factors and question distribution were as follows: "reluctance to be helpful to researchers" (Items 1–8), "negative attitude toward research" (Items 9–17), "positive attitude toward research" (Items 18–24), and "positive attitude toward researchers" (Items 25–30). The first and second subdimensions contained negative expressions, with high scores indicating negative attitude. The third and fourth subdimensions contained positive expressions, with high scores indicating positive attitude. Reliability coefficients (Cronbach's alpha) ranged from α = .77 to α =

.85 for the subdimensions in the original scale. In this study, the overall reliability was α = .77, and the subdimensions reliability coefficients ranged from α = .83 to α = .88, as follows: reluctance to be helpful to researchers (α = .85), negative attitude toward research (α = .83), positive attitude toward research (α = .86), and positive attitude toward researchers (α = .88).

Students were given information about the study before the application of the personal information form and the scale. The students who provided informed consent were asked to fill in the personal information form and the scale anonymously. Filling out the form and the scale took approximately 10 minutes.

The data of the study were analyzed using SPSS 19.0 (IBM Corp., Armonk, NY, USA) package program. The features of the students related to introductive and scientific studies were evaluated using the score, percentage, mean, and standard deviation. The relation between the age of the students and the subdimension points of the scale was tested using Spearman correlation analysis. The informative features of the students and the subdimension points of the scale were compared using the Mann–Whitney U, Kruskal–Wallis H, and post hoc Bonferroni tests. A $p < .05$ value was accepted as indicating statistical significance.

Written permission to conduct this study was obtained from the ethical committee of the Faculty of Medicine at Trakya University (Permission no. 07/19, dated April 7, 2016). Verbal consent was obtained from the participants before the personal information form and scale were applied, at which time they were told that they could withdraw from the study anytime and that the information obtained would be used for scientific purposes only.

Results

The average age of the participants was 20.4 ± 1.6 (range = 18–30) years. Nearly all (90.1%) were female, most were sophomore (second-year) students, 38.1% had taken at least one course on statistics/research, 13.6% had experience doing scientific research, 21.6% followed the continuous broadcast related to nursing, and 47.5% had participated in scientific meetings, congresses, symposiums, and/or other similar activities (Table 1).

A positive correlation was identified between the average age of the participants and the point averages of the "Positive Attitude towards Research" subdimension ($r = .119$, $p = .021$). Thus, it was determined that increasing age was positively associated with level of positive attitude toward research (Table 2).

After comparing the academic years of the participants against the subdimension points, the "Positive Attitude towards Research" point was statistically significantly different among the four academic-year groups ($p = .006$; Table 3). A post hoc Bonferroni test was performed to analyze this difference, with junior (third-year) students showing a more positive attitude toward research than freshman (first-year) students (Table 4).

TABLE 1.

Informative Features of Nursing Students (N = 375)

Introductive Feature	n	%
Age (*M* and *SD*)	20.40	1.6
Gender		
Female	338	90.1
Male	37	9.9
Academic year		
First	96	25.6
Second	127	33.9
Third	107	28.5
Fourth	45	12.0
Did you take a course on statistics/research?		
Yes	143	38.1
No	232	61.9
Do you have experience doing scientific research?		
Yes	51	13.6
No	324	86.4
Do you follow the continuous broadcast related to nursing?		
Yes	81	21.6
No	294	78.4
Do you participate in scientific activities, meetings, congresses, symposia, or other related activities?		
Yes	178	47.5
No	197	52.5

Note. Participants' age ranged from 18 to 30 years.

After comparing the scientific research experience of the participants with the subdimension points of the scale, the point averages for the "reluctance to be helpful to researchers" ($p = .004$) and "negative attitude toward research" ($p = .007$) of the participants with no scientific research experience were found to be high. Furthermore, the point averages of the "positive attitude toward research" ($p < .001$) and "positive attitude toward researchers" ($p = .016$) of the participants with prior scientific research experience were found to be significantly higher (Table 3).

After evaluating the students' status of following the continuous broadcast related to nursing and the subdimension points of the scale, the "positive attitude toward research" score of the participants who followed this broadcast was found to be significantly higher than that of those who do not ($p < .001$; Table 3).

Finally, participants who participated in activities had a significantly higher "positive attitude toward research" score than those who do not ($p < .001$; Table 3).

Discussion

This study found that 13.6% of the participants had scientific research experience, 21.6% followed the continuous

broadcast related to nursing, and 47.5% participated in scientific meetings, congresses, symposiums, and/or other similar activities. These findings parallel the data of several previous studies (Aydın et al., 2015; Çelik et al., 2014; Park, McGhee, & Sherwin, 2010). Gerçek et al. (2016) searched the awareness and attitudes of nursing students toward research and development in nursing and found that 42% participated in scientific meetings. Uysal Toraman, Hamaratçılar, Tülü, and Erkin (2017) determined that 51.6% of the nursing students had participated in a scientific meeting. Björkström, Johansson, Hamrin, and Athlin (2003) stated that 26.7% of the nursing students were interested in the research area of nursing. Blenkinsop (2003) stated that reading scientific research about nursing helped promote positive attitudes toward research. Pruskil, Burgwinkel, Georg, Keil, and Kiessling (2009) searched the attitudes of medical students toward science and their involvement in research activities, finding that 30% expressed that it was not difficult to reach and read scientific articles. In Park et al.'s (2010) study, 25% of the medical student participants had participated previously in scientific activities. Upon evaluating the data of the studies conducted, it was observed that students did not participate in scientific activities sufficiently and that few students had scientific research experience. As scientific research is known to affect the nursing profession in both the present and the future, it is important to equip students with sufficient scientific information and to allow them to participate in scientific activities, take part in research, and read scientific articles and studies. Nurse educators should encourage their students to do scientific research as well as provide opportunities to take part in research. In this way, nursing students may improve their abilities and acquire positive attitudes toward research.

This study found a positive relationship between student age and attitude, with junior (third-year) students showing the most positive attitudes toward research of all four academic-year groups. The National Core Curriculum for Nursing in Turkey has set standards that require nurses to take evidence-based decisions in their clinical practices and their education

TABLE 2.

The Age of Participants With Subdimension Scores of the Scale With Correlation Coefficients and Significance Levels (N = 375)

Subdimension	Age	
	r_s	p
Reluctance to be helpful to researchers	−.072	.162
Negative attitude toward research	−.033	.522
Positive attitudes toward research	.119	.021
Positive attitude toward researchers	−.020	.699

Note. r_s = Spearman correlation analysis.

TABLE 3.

Subdimension Scores of the Scale, According to the Introductive Features of Participants (N = 375)

Variable	Reluctance to be Helpful to Researchers		Negative Attitude Toward Research		Positive Attitudes Toward Research		Positive Attitude Toward Researchers	
	M	*SD*	*M*	*SD*	*M*	*SD*	*M*	*SD*
Academic year								
First	19.95	5.47	19.27	5.30	23.55	4.54	23.78	4.17
Second	20.86	5.76	19.68	5.30	24.24	4.98	24.21	3.98
Third	19.73	6.25	19.16	5.78	25.36	4.89	24.27	3.17
Fourth	20.44	5.43	18.51	3.86	23.51	4.60	23.67	3.95
KW	2.686		1.870		12.523		1.619	
p	.443		.600		.006		.655	
Do you have experience doing scientific research?								
Yes	17.98	6.53	17.24	4.51	27.14	4.51	25.20	3.73
No	20.61	5.59	19.60	5.23	23.85	4.52	23.87	3.80
U	6220.500		6317.00		4874.500		6546.500	
p	.004		.007		< .001		.016	
Do you follow the continuous broadcast related to nursing?								
Yes	19.96	6.02	18.71	4.41	26.51	3.88	25.89	3.02
No	20.33	5.73	19.44	5.39	23.68	4.90	23.82	3.97
U	11588.00		11079		7448.500		10287	
p	.711		.337		< .001		.059	
Do you participate in scientific activities, meetings, congresses, symposia, or other related activities?								
Yes	20.17	6.13	18.69	5.14	25.38	4.85	24.26	3.90
No	20.32	5.48	19.82	5.20	23.31	4.62	23.87	3.71
U	17200.500		15509.500		13092.500		16262.500	
p	.751		.053		< .001		.222	

Note. KW = Kruskal–Wallis H test; *U* = Mann–Whitney *U* test.

(Erdil et al., 2014). According to the nursing education curriculum, 2–3 hours per week of research/statistics courses are required (Uysal Toraman et al., 2017). These courses are given to students to encourage them to do nursing research, to teach them the phases of research, and to increase their desire to participate in scientific activities (Halabi & Hamdan-Mansour, 2012). On the other hand, in Turkey, senior (fourth-year) nursing students take an examination at the end of their undergraduate degree program to be able to start working in state hospitals. As a result, during their fourth year of education, students usually prepare to pass this examination, and this may have an effect on their scientific activities and attitudes toward research. At the institution where this study was conducted, students take research courses during their third (junior) academic year. Thus, these students showed a more positive attitude toward research. Similarly in the literature, Meraj et al. (2016) stated that older medical students showed more positive attitudes than their younger peers. In addition, it has been shown that older students are more aware of research and of the different phases of research. Hence, we recommend that nursing research courses be performed as early as possible during the nursing education curriculum so that nursing students may be prepared to do nursing research. This may improve their research skills in clinical practice settings and may further help improve their attitudes toward nursing research at an earlier phase in their studies.

TABLE 4.

Positive Attitudes Toward Research Scores of Participants, According to Academic Year

Academic Year	*n*	Mean	*df*	χ^2	*p*
First	96	168.32	3	12.523	.006[a]
Second	127	185.20			
Third	107	217.18			
Fourth	45	168.50			

Note. χ^2 = Kruskal–Wallis H test.
[a]After Bonferroni correction, there was a significant difference between the first and third academic-year groups.

In this study, the participants with scientific research experience earned a higher score for positive attitude toward research and researchers than those without. The results of a study that was conducted in Turkey showed that nursing students who wrote a scientific research-based as a master's thesis showed more positive attitudes toward research and became more aware of the conduct and reading of scientific research (Uysal Toraman et al., 2017). In Akdolun Balkaya et al.'s (2013) study, 66.9% of nursing and midwifery students said that they improved their skills in critical thinking and problem solving by doing research. Ryan (2016) stated that undergraduate nursing students showed positive attitudes toward research but that they did not have enough experience related to support and opportunity. Abu-Zaid and Alnajjar (2014) stated that medical students with prior scientific research experience showed more positive attitudes toward scientific research than those without. In a study conducted in Saudi Arabia, results showed that 44.4% of the undergraduate medical students had positive attitudes toward health research because of a belief that their previous experiences and skills in doing research had facilitated their personal development (Al-Hilali et al., 2016). These results gathered from the literature show that having research experience enhanced nursing students, contributed to their professional identity, and improved their thought and decision-making processes. The research experiences of students affect their perspective on doing research and help them acquire a positive attitude. Finally, these affect their future and professional role after graduation. Hence, to develop the ability of nursing students to conduct research, school directors may organize and support student participation in scientific activities and educators may encourage students to read scientific nursing journals and to take part in scientific research/projects. These activities may encourage nursing students to search more scientific research and to read the findings from other cultures, which will increase their awareness of new developments and trends in national and international nursing.

In this study, the participants who followed the continuous broadcast related to nursing and those who had participated in scientific activities had more positive attitudes toward research than those who did not follow these broadcasts or had not participated in scientific activities. In one study that was conducted in Turkey, Çelik et al. (2014) determined that nursing students who had scientific research experience, who followed periodical publications, or who regularly read the scientific research held more positive attitudes toward scientific research. Demir et al. (2012) stated that 37.8% of the nurses in their study were aware of nursing-related scientific research and that 70.7% of them desired to participate in scientific research work. Nel, Burman, Hoffman, and Randera-Rees (2014) surveyed the attitudes of medical students toward research and stated that 72% held positive attitudes toward research and believed that participating in scientific meetings was important to their education. Murdoch-Eaton et al. (2010)

stated that medical students who participate in scientific meetings and who read scientific publications showed positive attitudes toward research and had acquired better skills for conducting and evaluating research. In accordance with these findings, encouraging students to do scientific research and supporting their participation in scientific activities are important to helping them develop positive attitudes toward research and researchers.

A limitation of this study is that it was carried out on nursing students in only one region in Turkey. Therefore, the findings may not be generalized to all nursing students in Turkey or to those in other countries. We recommend that future studies examine factors that influence the attitudes of nursing students toward scientific research using larger randomized sample sizes and that investigations be conducted into the attitudes of clinical nurses.

In conclusion, the attitudes of Turkish nursing students toward scientific research were found to be positive. Being older, having scientific research experience, following the continuous broadcast related to nursing, and participating in scientific activities all significantly and positively influenced the attitudes of the participants toward research. As scientific activities play an important role in further developing the nursing profession, nurse educators should emphasize the role of nursing students as researchers during their courses and give them opportunities to participate in scientific activities. Acquiring research abilities gives nurses the power and capacity to improve the quality of nursing care.

Acknowledgment

Special thanks to the students who participated in this study and donated their time.

References

Abu-Zaid, A., & Alnajjar, A. (2014). Female second-year undergraduate medical students' attitudes towards research at the College of Medicine, Alfaisal University: A Saudi Arabian perspective. *Perspectives on Medical Education, 3*(1), 50–55. https://doi.org/10.1007/s40037-013-0093-9

Adıgüzel, O., Tanrıverdi, H., & Özkan, D. S. (2011). Occupational professionalism and the case of nurses as the members of the profession. *Journal of Administrative Sciences, 9*(2), 239–259. (Original work published in Turkish)

Akdolun Balkaya, N., Demirtaş Çevik, N. Ö., Atik Nalbant, M., Murat Öztürk, D., Ağartan, E., & Önder, A. (2013). Why nursing and midwifery students do research and participate in scientific activities? *Journal of Düzce University Health Sciences Institute, 4*(3), 1–6.

Al-Hilali, S. M., Al-Kahtani, E., Zaman, B., Khandekar, R., Al-Shahri, A., & Edward, D. P. (2016). Attitudes of Saudi Arabian undergraduate medical students towards health research. *Sultan Qaboos University Medical Journal, 16*(1), e68–e73. https://doi.org/10.18295/squmj.2016.16.01.012

Aydın, Y., Adıgüzel, A., & Topal, E. A. (2015). Determination of attitudes of midwives and nurses towards scientific studies. *Journal Human Rhythm, 1*(4), 168–175. (Original work published in Turkish)

Björkström, M. E., Johansson, I. S., Hamrin, E. K. F., & Athlin, E. E. (2003). Swedish nursing students' attitudes to and awareness of research and development within nursing. *Journal of Advanced Nursing, 41*(4), 393–402. https://doi.org/10.1046/j.1365-2648.2003.02557.x

Blenkinsop, C. (2003). Research: An essential skill of a graduate nurse? *Nurse Education Today, 23*(2), 83–88. https://doi.org/10.1016/S0260-6917(02)00168-5

Bökeoğlu, O. Ç., & Yılmaz, K. (2005). The relationship between attitudes of university students towards critical thinking and research anxieties. *Education Management of Theory and Practice, 41*(1), 47–68. (Original work published in Turkish)

Büyüköztürk, Ş. (1997). Development of anxiety scale for research. *Education Management, 3*(4), 453–464. (Original work published in Turkish)

Çelik, S., Önder, G., Durmaz, K., Yurdusever, Y., & Uysal, N. (2014). Determination of anxiety and attitude towards doing scientific research of nursing students. *Journal of Health Sciences and Professions, 1*(2), 23–31. (Original work published in Turkish)

Demir, Y., Ak, B., Bilgin, N. Ç., Efe, H., Albayrak, E., Çelikpençe, Z., & Güneri, N. (2012). Barriers and facilitating factors to research utilization in nursing practice. *Journal of Contemporary Medicine, 2*(2), 94–101. (Original work published in Turkish)

Erdil, F., Başer, M., Kaya, H., Özer, N., Duygulu, S., Orgun, F., … Işık, B. (2014). *The national core training program for nursing.* Ankara, Turkey: Gulhane Military Medical Academy Press. (Original work published in Turkish)

Gerçek, E., Okursoy, A., & Dal, N. A. (2016). Awareness and attitudes of Turkish nursing students towards research and development in nursing. *Nurse Education Today, 46*(11), 50–56. https://doi.org/10.1016/j.nedt.2016.08.015

Halabi, J. O. (2016). Attitudes of Saudi nursing students toward nursing research. *Saudi Journal for Health Sciences, 5*(3), 118–124. https://doi.org/10.4103/2278-0521.195813

Halabi, J. O., & Hamdan-Mansour, A. (2012). Attitude of Jordanian nursing students towards nursing research. *Journal of Research in Nursing, 17*(4), 363–373. https://doi.org/10.1177/1744987110379782

Karagözoğlu, Ş. (2005). Nursing as a scientific discipline. *Journal of Cumhuriyet University School of Nursing, 9*(1), 6–14. (Original work published in Turkish)

Karagözoğlu, Ş. (2006). Science, scientific research process and nursing. *Journal of Hacettepe University School of Nursing, 2006,* 64–71. (Original work published in Turkish)

Korkmaz, F. (2011). Professionalism and nursing in Turkey. *Hacettepe University Faculty of Health Sciences Nursing Journal, 2011,* 59–67. (Original work published in Turkish)

Korkmaz, Ö., Şahin, A., & Yeşil, R. (2011a). Teachers' opinion regarding scientific researches and researchers. *Journal of Theoretical Educational Science, 4*(2), 109–127 (Original work published in Turkish)

Korkmaz, Ö., Şahin, A., & Yeşil, R. (2011b). Study of validity and reliability of scale of attitude towards scientific research. *Elementary Education Online, 10*(3), 961–973. (Original work published in Turkish)

Laaksonen, C., Paltta, H., von Schantz, M., Ylönen, M., & Soini, T. (2013). Journal club as a method for nurses and nursing students' collaborative learning: A descriptive study. *Health Sciences Journal, 7*(3), 285–292.

Meraj, L., Gul, N., Zubaidazain, Akhter, I., Iram, F., & Khan, A. S. (2016). Perceptions and attitudes towards research amongst medical students at Shifa College of Medicine. *Journal of the Pakistan Medical Association, 66*(2), 165–169.

Murdoch-Eaton, D., Drewery, S., Elton, S., Emmerson, C., Marshall, M., Smith, J. A., … Whittle, S. (2010). What do medical students understand by research and research skills? Identifying research opportunities within undergraduate projects. *Medical Teacher, 32*(3), e152–e160. https://doi.org/10.3109/01421591003657493

Nel, D., Burman, R. J., Hoffman, R., & Randera-Rees, S. (2014). The attitudes of medical students to research. *South Africa Medical Journal, 104*(1), 32–36. https://doi.org/10.7196/samj.7058

Park, S. J. K., McGhee, C. N. J., & Sherwin, T. (2010). Medical students' attitudes towards research and a career in research: An Auckland, New Zealand study. *The New Zealand Medical Journal, 123*(1323), 34–42.

Pruskil, S., Burgwinkel, P., Georg, W., Keil, T., & Kiessling, C. (2009). Medical students' attitudes towards science and involvement in research activities: A comparative study with students from a reformed and a traditional curriculum. *Medical Teacher, 31*(6), e254–e259. https://doi.org/10.1080/01421590802637925

Rezaei, M., & Zamani-Miandashti, N. (2013). The relationship between research self-efficacy, research anxiety and attitude toward research: A study of agricultural graduate students. *Journal of Educational and Instructional Studies in the World, 3*(4), 69–78.

Ryan, E. J. (2016). Undergraduate nursing students' attitudes and use of research and evidence-based practice—An integrative literature review. *JCN: Journal of Clinical Nursing, 25*(11–12), 1548–1556. https://doi.org/10.1111/jocn.13229

Uysal Toraman, A., Hamaratçılar, G., Tülü, B., & Erkin, Ö. (2017). Nursing students' attitudes towards research and development within nursing: Does writing a bachelor thesis make a difference? *International Journal of Nursing Practice, 23*(2), e12517. https://doi.org/10.111/ijn.12517

9

Effects of Nursing Education Using Films on Perception of Nursing, Satisfaction with Major and Professional Nursing Values

Hyangjin PARK[1] • Haeryun CHO[2*]

ABSTRACT

Background: Cinenurducation, a film-based approach to nursing education that incorporates student-centered, problem-solving, experiential, and reflective learning strategies, allows students to experience a variety of indirect experiences and improves critical thinking and self-reflection through discussion.

Purpose: The aims of this study were, first, to employ a cinenurducation approach to help instill a proper professional nursing identity in second-year nursing students and, second, to examine the effects of this approach on the perception of nursing, satisfaction with major, and professional nursing values of the participants.

Methods: An experimental, pretest-and-posttest design was used to test the primary variables, including perception of nursing, satisfaction with major, and professional nursing values. The nursing educational program was developed based on the learning concepts of cinenurducation and the core concepts of nursing. The program, which included six films, addressed the following concepts: *Me Before You* (problem solving and professionalism), *Testament of Youth* (nursing management and professionalism), *Girl, Interrupted* (interpersonal skills and nursing knowledge), *Hungry Heart* (interpersonal skills and problem solving), *Iris* (nursing knowledge and problem solving), and *Chronic* (nursing knowledge and cooperation). The experimental group ($n = 14$) participated in the 8-week educational program, and the control group ($n = 15$) did not.

Results: Perception of nursing, satisfaction with major, and professional nursing values all improved significantly more in the experimental group than in the control group, with large effects observed.

Conclusions: Cinenurducation is an effective approach to promoting professional nursing identity in nursing students. Educators should incorporate films into nursing education. In addition, nursing education should incorporate a variety of educational materials to provide students with opportunities for reflective learning.

KEY WORDS:
films, nursing education, nursing students, satisfaction.

Introduction

Professional nursing identity refers to the awareness of the functions and roles that professional nurses are expected to perform in clinical contexts (Dadich & Doloswala, 2018). Developing a positive professional nursing identity is critical for nursing undergraduate students (Browne et al., 2018). Nursing students who are not satisfied with their major may neglect their studies, hold a negative perception of nursing (Admi et al., 2018; Feng et al., 2016), and fail to establish a proper professional nursing identity, which may negatively affect their development of professional competencies (Mazhindu et al., 2016). Having a proper professional nursing identity enables nurses to examine and judge clinical situations comprehensively (Heldal et al., 2019). Thus, nursing students must be provided with a nursing education that promotes the development of a proper professional nursing identity. In other words, professional nursing identity may be connected to perception of nursing, satisfaction with major, and professional nursing values (Woo & Park, 2017).

Perception of nursing refers to beliefs regarding the traditional, social, and professional impressions of nurses and nursing prospects (de Braganca & Nirmala, 2018; Emeghebo, 2012). Nursing students who hold positive perceptions of nursing display high levels of self-esteem, professional intuition, and professional identity. Furthermore, these students are highly likely to become good nurses in the clinical field (de Braganca & Nirmala, 2018; Woo & Park, 2017). Therefore, developing a positive perception of nursing is essential to improving nursing identity.

Satisfaction with major refers to students' satisfaction with meeting their expectations related to their academic major. A good understanding of the career associated with one's

[1]PhD, RN, Associate Manager, Department of Prevention and Public Relations & Research and Development Team, Korea Center on Gambling Problems, Seoul, Republic of Korea • [2]PhD, RN, Associate Professor, Department of Nursing, Wonkwang University, Iksan, Republic of Korea.

major increases this satisfaction (Feng et al., 2016). In particular, nursing students' satisfaction with their major promotes dedication to studies, helps them develop positive values about their major, and affects their nursing-related knowledge and attitudes (Feng et al., 2016). Thus, nursing students with high levels of satisfaction with their major are more likely to become good nurses with a clear nursing identity (Admi et al., 2018).

Professional nursing values are the overall beliefs that encompass views on nurses' activities and roles as well as opinions on nurses as professionals (Ayla et al., 2018; Bijani et al., 2019). As the starting point of nursing students' development into professional nurses, professional nursing values relate directly to excellent nursing (Bijani et al., 2019; Pickles et al., 2019). These values are important because they improve the quality of nursing, understanding of patients, and job satisfaction (Bijani et al., 2019; Parandeh et al., 2014).

Positive professional values are developed continuously in nursing students through their education and learning experience (Kantek et al., 2017; Kaya et al., 2017; Parandeh et al., 2014). These values affect their satisfaction with major and their perception of nursing (Ahn & Song, 2015; Cho & Kim, 2016; Lim & Jo, 2016). Having well-established professional nursing values helps nurses make better decisions and develop a positive professional nursing identity, which can help them avoid moral pain and provide quality care (Parandeh et al., 2014; Posluszny & Hawley, 2017; Woo & Park, 2017).

Films have been reported to be effective in helping students experience a variety of learning including emotions, feelings, knowledge, actions, skills, and attitudes (J. Oh, Kang, et al., 2012; J. Oh & Steefel, 2016; Zeppegno et al., 2015). When selecting a film, the film content must match the learning objectives and, if students are able to understand and discuss the film, then any kind and characteristic of the film can be used (J. Oh, Kang, et al., 2012; J. Oh & Steefel, 2016). Therefore, using films as an educational tool helps students understand nursing situations that they cannot otherwise fully experience (J. Oh, Shin, et al., 2012; J. Oh & Steefel, 2016).

Cinenurducation is an approach to nursing education that has recently attracted significant attention (Klemenc-Ketis & Kersnik, 2011; J. Oh, Kang, et al., 2012; Zeppegno et al., 2015). Cinenurducation, based on the experiential learning theory of Kolb (1984), involves the student-centered, problem-solving, experiential, and reflective types of learning (J. Oh, Kang, et al., 2012; J. Oh & Steefel, 2016). One advantage of this educational method is that it provides opportunities to discuss and debate issues raised through films. The film format allows learners to discuss issues concisely and calmly, which promotes students' problem-solving and creative thinking capabilities (Kim, 2014; J. Oh, Kang, et al., 2012). In addition, studies have shown that students clarify their knowledge and attitudes by watching films, discussing films in group settings, and talking about one another's reactions, thereby developing critical thinking and self-reflection (J. Oh, Shin, et al., 2012; J. Oh & Steefel, 2016). In other words, cinenurducation stimulates the visual areas of the learner's brain, allowing learners to experience a situation, emotionally empathize, and formulate solutions while actively participating in the class and discussing solutions (Edmonds, 2011; Kolb, 1984; J. Oh, Kang, et al., 2012).

Research related to cinenurducation has focused on understanding patients and health promotion in nursing (Briggs, 2011), multicultural nursing and multicultural competence enhancement (Edmonds, 2011), and shedding light on mental illness and mental health nursing (Zauderer & Ganzer, 2011). However, in these studies, students were not able to gain a comprehensive understanding of nursing because of the reliance on using film clips and excerpted scenes rather than complete film content. Films may need to be viewed in full to maximize learning efficacy. J.-A. Oh (2010) suggested that learners should watch films in their entirety to gain a comprehensive understanding of the situation and content of the main character, which will maximize opportunities for discussion and creative learning. Therefore, the educational effects of cinenurducation in which full film content is used remain to be verified.

Some studies have indicated that third-year nursing students with clinical practice experience tend to have a negative perception of nursing, low satisfaction with their major, and inadequate professional nursing values (Emeghebo, 2012; Lee, 2004; Woo & Park, 2017). These tendencies have been attributed to their experiencing clinical practicum before their professional nursing identity had fully formed. Therefore, this study was designed to use films in nursing education to establish a proper professional nursing identity in second-year nursing students and to examine the effects of this education on perception of nursing, satisfaction with major, and professional nursing values. The research questions addressed in this study were as follows: (a) "Did the intervention improve perception of nursing?", (b) "Did the intervention improve nursing major satisfaction?", and (c) "Did the intervention improve nursing professional values?"

Conceptual Framework

The conceptual framework in this study is shown in Figure 1. The intervention method in this study was developed using the learning concepts of cinenurducation (J. Oh, Kang, et al., 2012), which include student-centered, problem-solving, experiential, and reflective learning. In terms of student-centered learning, the learning objectives were introduced briefly before film viewing, and the wide degree of freedom allowed to the participants to analyze and reflect was guaranteed. In terms of problem-solving learning, students were introduced to discussion topics related to the core concepts of nursing, which were communicated through various situations in the films, before watching the film (Park et al., 2013). Furthermore, six films related to nursing core concepts were used to provide experiential learning, which induced indirect experiences of various situations. Finally, in terms of reflective learning, students shared their feelings and engaged in a discussion on the topics raised after each film was screened.

Figure 1
Conceptual Framework of this Study Based on Conceptual Metaphor of Cinenurducation by J. Oh, Kang, et al. (2012)

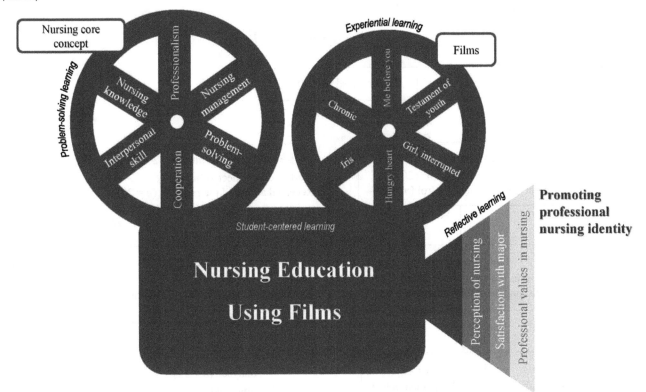

To promote professional nursing identity by improving perception of nursing, satisfaction with major, and professional nursing values, the contents of nursing education were organized using the nursing core concepts proposed by Park et al. (2013), which represent the most common and basic nursing tasks in clinical settings.

Methods

Study Design

An equivalent control group was used in this study. A pretest/posttest, nonsynchronized design was used to examine the effect of the intervention on participants' perception of nursing, satisfaction with major, and professional nursing values (Figure 2).

Participants and Setting

The participants in this study were nursing students in their second year of a 4-year undergraduate program of a university located in Iksan City. In undergraduate nursing programs in South Korea, first-year students take an introductory course on nursing, second-year students take a basic major course and laboratory practicum, and third- and fourth-year students take a major course and clinical practicum. Nursing students are expected to establish their professional nursing identity before completing their nursing major course (Ayla et al., 2018). Therefore, the inclusion criteria for participants were (a) second-year nursing student and (b) voluntarily agreeing to participate, whereas the exclusion criteria were (a) having previously received nursing education via artwork such as films, paintings, or literature or (b) being absent from the intervention more than twice.

The educational intervention in this study was formatted as an extracurricular class that was not compulsory and was not graded. The researchers publicly posted the syllabus, overall purpose of the research, and participant criteria, and 40 students applied as volunteers to participate in the class and research.

G*Power 3.1.3 (Faul et al., 2007) was used to calculate the sample size required (significance level = .05, effect size = 1.0, power = .80). The effect size reported in previous studies (Kim, 2014; Zeppegno et al., 2015) was 1.0. As the required sample size estimated for this study was 14 nursing students per group, the total number of participants required was 28. After estimating the potential dropout rate, 20 students were recruited per group. In the control group, five participants withdrew, including three who did not attend the posttest and two who provided invalid answers on the questionnaire. In the experimental group, six participants withdrew, including three who were absent from two or

Figure 2
Participant Recruitment Process

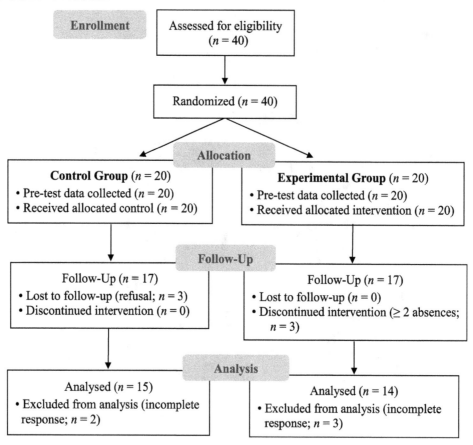

more sessions and three who provided invalid answers on the questionnaire (Figure 2). Thus, the data of 29 participants (experimental group = 14, control group = 15) were available for analysis, which met the required number of subjects for this study.

Nursing Education Using Films

Films were selected for the intervention that were appropriate to the purpose of this study and in line with the criteria described by J. Oh, Shin, et al. (2012). These criteria are as follows: (a) absent of controversial issues related to sexuality and addressing only generally accepted concepts related to culture, emotion, ideology, or philosophy; (b) a popular genre (not an educational material or a documentary) that may be watched in a relaxed manner; and (c) having the strong potential to generate sufficient discussion questions on the nursing core concepts proposed by Park et al. (2013). Eleven films were initially selected based on literature reviews and data from previous research and on a list of films screened at a nursing film festival held by the Korean Nurses Association (2015). Of these 11 films, three were not available on digital video disk and were excluded. After watching the remaining eight films, the researchers excluded two films with content deemed as difficult for students to understand. The final six films were used in this study. The

researchers arranged the film screenings based on the nursing core concepts, from general to specific contents, and then developed discussion topics. The six films and the concepts addressed were as follows: *Me Before You* (problem solving and professionalism), *Testament of Youth* (nursing management and professionalism), *Girl, Interrupted* (interpersonal skills and nursing knowledge), *Hungry Heart* (interpersonal skills and problem solving), *Iris* (nursing knowledge and problem solving), and *Chronic* (nursing knowledge and cooperation; Table 1).

J. Oh and Steefel (2016) suggested that cinenurducation allows nursing students to approach discussion topics from various angles, helping them better understand the characters and background of the film. Thus, in this study, the films were screened in full. The researchers identified topics and set up discussions to enable the students to deduce the core concepts of nursing after viewing the films. For example, the main character of the film *Chronic*, a hospice nurse, shared a relationship with his patients similar to that of a wife or siblings. Moreover, a patient with cancer demanded that he kill her. The discussion topics for this film, which were selected to help students derive nursing core concepts, included "What are chronic diseases and what is your understanding of hospice care?" and "What is patient-centered care, and what is an appropriate therapeutic relationship between nurses and patients?"

Table 1

Contents of Nursing Education Using Films

Session	Nursing Core Concept	Content	Film	Running Time (Min)	Country (Years)	Discussion Topics	Method (Time)
1	–	Orientation	–	–	–	• Information about this course and schedule	• Orientation (5 min) -Introduce movie -Discussion topics • Movies (90–120 min) • Break (10 min) • Discussion (30–40 min) -Sharing thoughts on topics • Wrap-up (10 min) - Feedback
2	• Problem solving • Professionalism	Critical thinking Ethical issue	*Me Before You*	110	United States (2016)	• Discussion about bioethics and ethical concepts (principles of autonomy) • What is well-dying? • Pros and cons of death with dignity as a health professional	
3	• Nursing management • Professionalism	Leadership Ethical value oriented	*Testament of Youth*	129	England (2014)	• The role of nurses in contributing to national crises • Discussion about ethical concepts (principles of precedence, justice, and sincerity) • Ethical dilemma: national profit versus maintenance of individual life	
4	• Interpersonal skill • Nursing knowledge	Communication Mental health	*Girl, interrupted*	127	United States (1999)	• Understanding the patients with mental health problems • Critique of therapeutic communication in film • Cases related to mental health such as depression, anxiety, and social adaptation in film	
5	• Interpersonal skill • Problem solving	Patient understanding Nursing process	*Hungry Heart*	112	United States (2014)	• Understanding the various health beliefs of family members • The influence of family belief and value on health • Applying the nursing process for family health	
6	• Nursing knowledge • Problem solving	Dementia Nursing process	*Iris*	90	United States (2001)	• What is dementia? • The influence of dementia on the family • Applying the nursing process for dementia patients and their family	
7	• Nursing knowledge • Cooperation	Chronic disease Patient-centered care	*Chronic*	94	Mexico (2015)	• Understanding chronic diseases and hospice care • What is patient-centered care? • Establishing the therapeutic relationship between nurses and patients as professionals	
8		Wrap up	–	–	–	• Sharing feelings about this course	

Note. Min/min = minutes.

The intervention was conducted once per week for 8 weeks. Each session took approximately 3 hours and was organized as follows: 5 minutes of orientation, 90–120 minutes of film viewing, 10 minutes of break time, 30–40 minutes of discussion to share feelings and thoughts on the discussion topics, and 10 minutes of feedback and summary. The content validity of this program with regard to the core concepts of nursing and the discussion topics were verified twice by three professors of nursing after watching the six films together.

Measurements

Demographic variables

To test homogeneity, information on gender, age, satisfaction with major, perceived difficulty of major, and motivation for selecting major was collected from the participants. A 5-point Likert scale was used to score satisfaction with major, with higher scores indicating greater satisfaction. Perceived difficulty of major included lecture class, practice class, others, or none. Motivation for selecting major included suggestion of acquaintance, fitting aptitude, or high employment rate.

Perception of nursing

The 20-item checklist of Kang et al. (2003) was used to measure perception of nursing. Of these 20 items, six were related to professional perception, six were related to traditional perception, three were related to forecast about nursing, and five were related to social perception. All items were scored using a 5-point Likert scale, with higher scores indicating a more positive perception of nursing. The measurement reliability, as measured using Cronbach's alpha, was .94 in Kang et al. and .78 in this study.

Satisfaction with major

Satisfaction with major was measured using an 18-item scale that was revised by Lee (2004) from a 34-item instrument by Ha (1999). Items were measured using a 5-point Likert scale, with higher total scores indicating greater satisfaction. Satisfaction with major included general satisfaction about nursing, satisfaction with social awareness related to the nursing major, content satisfaction with the classes of the nursing major, and satisfaction with the relationship between professors and students (Lee, 2004). The measurement reliability, as measured using Cronbach's alpha, was .94 in Lee and .86 in this study.

Professional nursing values

To measure professional nursing values, the 29-item scale developed by Yeun et al. (2005) was used. This scale covers the five dimensions of professional self-concept (nine items), social recognition (eight items), nurse professionalism (five items), practical nursing role (four items), and nursing identity (three items), and items are scored using a 5-point Likert scale, with higher scores indicating stronger nursing professional values. The measurement reliability, as measured by Cronbach's alpha, was .92 in Yeun et al. and .85 in this study.

Data Collection and Ethical Considerations

This study was conducted after approval for the ethical consideration of participants was obtained from the institutional review board of the researchers' institution (IRB No. WKIRB-201703-SB-015). For blinding purposes, the first author and second author were separately involved, respectively, in collecting the study data and conducting the intervention. Using SPSS, the participants were randomly assigned to the experimental and control groups in two classes of 20 students. Only the data collector knew the designation of each group to ensure that the instructor and the participants remained blinded.

Data were collected from August 28 to December 13, 2017. Pretest and posttest data were collected first from the control group and then from the experimental group. The control group took the pretest between August 28 and 30, 2017, with the posttest conducted between October 18 and 20, 2017, after conclusion of the intervention. The experimental group took the pretest on October 25, 2017, with the posttest conducted on December 13, 2017, after conclusion of the intervention.

Informed consent forms, general information on the study, study research aims, and information on voluntary consent/withdrawal were provided to potential participants. After providing informed consent, the participants were enrolled and completed the questionnaires, which took about 5 minutes. A small gift was presented to each participant upon questionnaire completion.

The control group had received no film teaching or other supplemental teaching interventions. For ethical considerations, the intervention was given to the control group after all study data had been collected.

Data Analysis

The collected data were analyzed using IBM SPSS Statistics 24.0 (IBM, Inc., Armonk, NY, USA). The general characteristics, perception of nursing, satisfaction with major, and professional values were estimated by number, percentage, mean, and standard deviation. The skewness of these variables was between –0.73 and 0.52, and kurtosis was between –0.57 and 0.33. As the skewness and kurtosis were both < ±1.965, the collected data were interpreted as normally distributed. Homogeneity between the experimental and control groups was verified using a chi-square test and an independent t test. To identify the effects of nursing education using films, an independent t test was used, and the effect size was calculated using Cohen's d formula. Dependent variables that were not homogeneous in the pretest were controlled by covariance, analyzed using analysis of covariance, and were assessed for effect size using the eta-squared formula.

Results

Homogeneity Test

No significant difference was observed between the two groups in terms of gender, age, general satisfaction with major, perceived difficulty of their major, motivation for selecting major, satisfaction with major, or professional nursing values (Table 2). However, a significant intergroup difference in the pretest score of perception of nursing was found and subsequently analyzed by controlling covariance to verify the effect.

Effects of Nursing Education Using Films

The effects of nursing education using films are shown in Table 3. The independent t test of the mean difference between posttest and pretest scores showed that the intervention had a significant effect on satisfaction with major ($t = 2.59$, $d = 0.97$, $p = .018$) and professional nursing values ($t = 2.92$, $d = 0.93$, $p = .007$) in the experimental group. Analysis of covariance, which controlled for the perception of nursing pretest scores by covariance, showed that the intervention had a significant effect on perception of nursing ($F = 6.88$, $\eta^2 = 0.55$, $p = .014$), with large effects observed (Cohen, 1988).

Discussion

This study was conducted to verify the effect in nursing students of a film-based nursing educational intervention on perception of nursing, satisfaction with major, and professional nursing values. To evaluate the effects of the program,

the changes in pretest and posttest results were examined between the experimental and control groups.

After the completion of the intervention, a larger increase in the mean score for perception of nursing was observed in the experimental group than in the control group, with a large effect size of 0.55 (Cohen, 1988). This result supports that nursing students' perception of nursing may be improved by educating them about nursing knowledge, skills, attitudes, beliefs, values, and ethical standards (Ayla et al., 2018; de Braganca & Nirmala, 2018). In particular, nursing students who meet professional nurses during hospital visits or clinical practice may be highly affected by the experience (de Braganca & Nirmala, 2018). In this study, participants in the experimental group engaged in 30–40 minutes of group discussion on each film with an instructor who was an expert in nursing. This interactivity provided opportunities for participants to share opinions with a nursing expert on related knowledge, ethical dilemmas, nursing roles, and beliefs and values related to patients and their families. Regardless of teaching style, an instructor's guidance and questions during discussion or reinforcement of students' opinions may help students think deeper about the core concepts that underlie nursing. The discussion, participated in jointly by the instructor and students, contributed to enhancing the participants' perception of nursing. The learning experience of watching and discussing films in groups has been reported to improve the effectiveness of reflective learning through the sharing of reactions and opinions with others (J. Oh, Shin, et al., 2012; J. Oh & Steefel, 2016). In this study, the film-based nursing education intervention effectively improved the participants'

Table 2

Intergroup Test for Homogeneity (N = 29)

Characteristic	Experimental Group ($n = 14$)		Control Group ($n = 15$)		t/χ^2	p
	n	%	n	%		
Gender					3.12	.077
Male	0	0.0	3	20.0		
Female	14	100.0	12	80.0		
Age (years; M and SD)	19.79	0.80	19.60	0.83	0.61	.545
General satisfaction with major (M and SD)	3.64	0.63	3.87	0.92	0.76	.454
Perceived difficulty of major					3.42	.331
Lecture class	7	50.0	12	80.0		
Practice class	2	14.3	1	6.7		
Others	1	7.1	1	6.7		
None	4	28.6	1	6.7		
Motivation for selecting major					4.96	.084
Suggestion of acquaintance	4	28.6	6	40.0		
Fitting aptitude	1	7.1	5	33.3		
High employment rate	9	64.3	4	26.7		
Prescore (M and SD)						
Perception of nursing	3.59	0.27	3.89	0.27	2.91	.007
Satisfaction with major	3.91	0.33	3.97	0.40	0.43	.673
Professional values in nursing	3.49	0.34	3.65	0.32	1.33	.195

Table 3

Effects of Nursing Education Using Films (N = 29)

Variable	Experimental Group (n = 14), M ± SD		Control Group (n = 15), M ± SD		t	p	Cohen's d
	Pretest	Posttest	Pretest	Posttest			
	Difference Between Posttest and Pretest		Difference Between Posttest and Pretest				
Perception of nursing	3.59 ± 0.27	4.06 ± 0.57	3.89 ± 0.27	3.78 ± 0.27			
	0.48 ± 0.56		−0.10 ± 0.21		6.88 [a]	.014	0.55 [b]
Satisfaction with major	3.91 ± 0.33	4.27 ± 0.35	3.97 ± 0.40	3.95 ± 0.39			
	0.37 ± 0.50		−0.02 ± 0.23		2.59	.018	0.97
Professional nursing values	3.49 ± 0.34	3.88 ± 0.46	3.65 ± 0.32	3.60 ± 0.38			
	0.40 ± 0.48		−0.05 ± 0.34		2.92	.007	0.93

[a] Analysis of covariance (pretest score). [b] Eta squared (η^2).

perception of nursing because the group and discussion activities with the instructor were excellent venues for promoting participant reflection. Therefore, nursing education using a variety of teaching methods is necessary to allow students to reflect fully on their learning.

Furthermore, satisfaction with major was found to have improved significantly in the experimental group, with a large effect size of 0.97 (Cohen, 1988). As few studies have focused on whether films for nursing students affect satisfaction with major, it is difficult to conduct a comparison of other study results with this study. The core concepts of nursing, including professionalism, nursing management, problem solving, cooperation, interpersonal skills, and nursing knowledge, were dealt with in this intervention, with nursing students having the opportunity to think deeply about their perceptions of nursing science. In previous studies, clear awareness of nursing science has been found to relate to satisfaction with the nursing major (Ahn & Song, 2015; Cho & Kim, 2016; Kaya et al., 2017). In this study, the intervention helped the participants establish the value of nursing science, which may promote nursing major satisfaction. In addition, this study, which applied cinenurducation to promote student-centered, experiential, and reflective learning, empowered the participants to discuss freely on nursing topics with instructors rather than limiting them to listening to traditional lectures (J. Oh, Kang, et al., 2012; Zeppegno et al., 2015). This aspect may have had a positive effect on nursing major satisfaction by building closer relationships between instructors and students. Many studies suggest that nursing students should be provided with various experiences that promote increased satisfaction with their major, because students with higher levels of satisfaction showed higher academic achievement and nursing professionalism (Bijani et al., 2019; Pickles et al., 2019; Woo & Park, 2017). Therefore, the intervention in this study may be used as an effective educational strategy to increase nursing students' satisfaction with their major, which may ultimately improve their professional nursing identity.

In addition, nursing education using films was found to be effective in improving professional nursing values, with a large effect size of 0.93 (Cohen, 1988). According to Zeppegno et al. (2015), film-based education for medical students positively affects attitudes toward psychiatry including social distance from a patient with a mental disorder and interpersonal reactivity, such as dispositional empathy. Klemenc-Ketis and Kersnik (2011) reported that education using films positively influences communication, empathy, and attitude in medical students. The results of this study are similar. The viewing of films in their entirety helped the participants better understand nursing situations (J.-A. Oh, 2010; Zeppegno et al., 2015). In-depth discussions after watching the films helped the participants clarify their attitudes and knowledge and reinforced their professional nursing values while accepting others' opinions (J. Oh & Steefel, 2016). In this study, the indirect experience of nursing scenarios through the films, including situations that promoted problem-solving and reflective learning, gave the participants a deeper understanding of various situations. Moreover, the participants discussed topics related to nursing core concepts and shared opinions, which helped enhance their professional nursing values. Therefore, the intervention in this study may be an effective strategy for developing positive professional nursing values and, subsequently, improving professional nursing identity in nursing students.

Nursing education using films was developed based on the learning concepts of cinenurducation suggested by J. Oh, Kang, et al. (2012) and the core concepts of nursing (Park et al., 2013). The films screened in this study were selected to introduce discussion topics related to the core concepts of nursing. Because the selected film reflects the core concept of nursing, nursing education using films can be regarded as effective in promoting professional nursing identity. The purpose of watching films was to engage in indirect experiential learning on the core concepts of nursing. Participants watched films in their entirety, which made it easier to understand the situations, characters, and contexts in their entirety. To facilitate understanding of the nursing core concepts in nursing students, discussions with an instructor and peers were conducted after watching the films. An educator who understands the nursing core concepts participated in the discussion, providing a role model for the nursing students. Furthermore, even films, which could be difficult at the level of second-year students, were able to reflect through discussions in which all peer students participated.

Although this program helped nursing students understand the content of the films and organize their opinions, one limitation was the length of time required for each session. Therefore, a teaching method that requires less time per session is needed. Educators may provide orientation and discussion topics on the films via online sources, and then students could watch the film in advance and discuss the topics offline. Meanwhile, the films in this study were selected from Western countries only. Thus, the selection lacked consideration of possible differences/discrepancies between Eastern and Western cultural settings. Therefore, further research is needed to account for cultural contexts in films. In addition, as this study was conducted on second-year nursing students, the nursing professional identity formed before the clinical practicum may conflict with the experience in the clinical setting. Therefore, longitudinal research should be conducted to confirm the persistence of intervention effects through graduation.

Conclusions

This study was conducted to verify whether nursing education using films affected the perception of nursing, satisfaction with major, and professional nursing values in nursing students. The results showed that the intervention was effective in these three aspects. Therefore, it is suggested that the intervention developed in this study be used as a strategy to improve the professional nursing identity of nursing students.

On the basis of this study, the implications of nursing education in undergraduate programs are as follows. First, nursing students' indirect experience through using films may promote learning of the core concepts of nursing. Therefore, educators should actively attempt nursing education using films. Second, this intervention was meaningful in terms both of using films as an educational resource and of promoting reflective learning through in-depth discussions. In the future, nursing education should be designed to provide students with opportunities for reflective learning using various educational materials. Finally, to help better establish the professional nursing identity of undergraduate students, educators should offer various supplementary courses such as the intervention attempted in this study in addition to the standard curriculum.

Acknowledgment

This research was supported by a 2021 research grant from Wonkwang University.

Author Contributions

Study conception and design: HC
Data collection: HP, HC
Data analysis and interpretation: HP
Drafting of the article: HP, HC
Critical revision of the article: HP, HC

References

Admi, H., Moshe-Eilon, Y., Sharon, D., & Mann, M. (2018). Nursing students' stress and satisfaction in clinical practice along different stages: A cross-sectional study. *Nurse Education Today, 68*, 86–92. https://doi.org/10.1016/j.nedt.2018.05.027

Ahn, T., & Song, Y. A. (2015). Affecting factors of nursing professionalism perceived by nursing students. *Journal of East-West Nursing Research, 21*(1), 10–17. https://doi.org/10.14370/jewnr.2015.21.1.10 (Original work published in Korean)

Ayla, I. A., Ozyazicioglu, N., Atak, M., & Surenler, S. (2018). Determination of professional values in nursing students. *International Journal of Caring Sciences, 11*(1), 254–261.

Bijani, M., Tehranineshat, B., & Torabizadeh, C. (2019). Nurses', nursing students', and nursing instructors' perceptions of professional values: A comparative study. *Nursing Ethics, 26*(3), 870–883. https://doi.org/10.1177/0969733017727153

Briggs, C. L. (2011). Engaging students using feature films. *The Journal of Nursing Education, 50*(6), Article 360. https://doi.org/10.3928/01484834-20110519-06

Browne, C., Wall, P., Batt, S., & Bennett, R. (2018). Understanding perceptions of nursing professional identity in students entering an Australian undergraduate nursing degree. *Nurse Education in Practice, 32*, 90–96. https://doi.org/10.1016/j.nepr.2018.07.006

Cho, J. A., & Kim, J. S. (2016). Factors affecting nursing college students' satisfaction with their department. *Journal of the Korea Academia-Industrial Cooperation Society, 17*(4), 587–595. https://doi.org/10.5762/kais.2016.17.4.587 (Original work published in Korean)

Cohen, J. (1988). *Statistical power analysis for the behavioral sciences* (2nd ed.). Lawrence Erlbaum Associates.

Dadich, A., & Doloswala, N. (2018). What can organisational theory offer knowledge translation in healthcare? A thematic and lexical analysis. *BMC Health Services Research, 18*, Article No. 351. https://doi.org/10.1186/s12913-018-3121-y

de Braganca, A. V., & Nirmala, R. (2018). Perceived public image of a nurse and work meaningfulness among nurses. *International Journal of Nursing Education, 10*(3), 1–5. https://doi.org/10.5958/0974-9357.2018.00056.9

Edmonds, M. L. (2011). Use of film in teaching multiculturalism to future nurse educators. *The Journal of Nursing Education, 50*(9), Article 544. https://doi.org/10.3928/01484834-20110819-02

Emeghebo, L. (2012). The image of nursing as perceived by nurses. *Nurse Education Today, 32*(6), e49–e53. https://doi.org/10.1016/j.nedt.2011.10.015

Faul, F., Erdfelder, E., Lang, A. G., & Buchner, A. (2007). G*Power 3: A flexible statistical power analysis program for the social, behavioral, and biomedical sciences. *Behavior Research Methods, 39*(2), 175–191. https://doi.org/10.3758/BF03193146

Feng, D., Zhao, W., Shen, S., Chen, J., & Li, L. (2016). The influence of perceived prejudice on willingness to be a nurse via the mediating effect of satisfaction with major: A cross-sectional study among Chinese male nursing students. *Nurse Education Today, 42*, 69–72. https://doi.org/10.1016/j.nedt.2016.04.012

Ha, H. S. (1999). *A study of department satisfaction and school satisfaction of undergraduate students* [Unpublished master's thesis]. Seoul National University, Republic of Korea. (Original work published in Korean)

Heldal, F., Kongsvik, T., & Haland, E. (2019). Advancing the status of nursing: Reconstructing professional nursing identity through patient safety work. *BMC Health Services Research, 19*(1), Article No. 418. https://doi.org/10.1186/s12913-019-4222-y

Kang, H. Y., Go, M. H., Yang, J. J., & Kim, S. M. (2003). Nurses' image perceived by academic and vocational high school teachers in Korea. *Journal of Korean Academy of Nursing, 33*(6), 792–801. (Original work published in Korean)

Kantek, F., Kaya, A., & Gezer, N. (2017). The effects of nursing education on professional values: A longitudinal study. *Nurse Education Today, 58*, 43–46. https://doi.org/10.1016/j.nedt.2017.08.004

Kaya, H., Işik, B., Şenyuva, E., & Kaya, N. (2017). Personal and professional values held by baccalaureate nursing students. *Nursing Ethics, 24*(6), 716–731. https://doi.org/10.1177/0969733015624488

Kim, S. Y. (2014). Effects of biomedical ethics education using movies on biomedical ethics awareness of nursing students. *The Journal of the Korea Contents Association, 14*(7), 281–290. https://doi.org/10.5392/JKCA.2014.14.07.281 (Original work published in Korean)

Klemenc-Ketis, Z., & Kersnik, J. (2011). Using movies to teach professionalism to medical students. *BMC Medical Education, 11*, Article No. 60. https://doi.org/10.1186/1472-6920-11-60

Kolb, D. A. (1984). *Experiential learning: Experience as the source of learning and development.* Prentice-Hall.

Korean Nurses Association. (2015). *Nursing association, nursing film festival opening ceremony.* https://www.koreanurse.or.kr/board/board_read.php?board_id=press&member_id=admin&exec=&no=78&category_no=&step=0&tag=&sgroup=76&sfloat=&position=0&mode=&find=stitle&search (Original work published in Korean)

Lee, D. J. (2004). *The relationships among satisfaction in major, gender identity, and gender stereotypes of male nursing students* [Unpublished master's thesis]. Yonsei University, Seoul, Republic of Korea. (Original work published in Korean)

Lim, K.-M., & Jo, E.-J. (2016). Influence of satisfaction with clinical practice and image of nurses on nursing professionalism of nursing students. *Journal of the Korea Academia-Industrial Cooperation Society, 17*(4), 556–566. https://doi.org/10.5762/KAIS.2016.17.4.556 (Original work published in Korean)

Mazhindu, D. M., Griffiths, L., Pook, C., Erskine, A., Ellis, R., & Smith, F. (2016). The nurse match instrument: Exploring professional nursing identity and professional nursing values for future nurse recruitment. *Nursing Education in Practice, 18*, 36–45. https://doi.org/10.1016/j.nepr.2016.03.006

Oh, J., Kang, J., & de Gagne, J. C. (2012). Learning concepts of cinenurducation: An integrative review. *Nurse Education Today, 32*(8), 914–919. https://doi.org/10.1016/j.nedt.2012.03.021

Oh, J., Shin, H., & de Gagne, J. C. D. (2012). QSEN competencies in pre-licensure nursing education and the application to cinenurducation. *Journal of Korean Academic Society of Nursing Education, 18*(3), 474–485. https://doi.org/10.5977/jkasne.2012.18.3.474 (Original work published in Korean)

Oh, J., & Steefel, L. (2016). Nursing students' preferences of strategies surrounding cinenurducation in a first year child growth and development courses: A mixed methods study. *Nurse Education Today, 36*, 342–347. https://doi.org/10.1016/j.nedt.2015.08.019

Oh, J.-A. (2010). Review of literature and implication for nursing education: Cinemeducation. *The Journal of Korean Academic Society of Nursing Education, 16*(2), 194–201. (Original work published in Korean)

Parandeh, A., Khaghanizade, M., Mohammadi, E., & Mokhtari Nouri, J. (2014). Factors influencing development of professional values among nursing students and instructors: A systematic review. *Global Journal of Health Science, 7*(2), 284–293. https://doi.org/10.5539/gjhs.v7n2p284

Park, Y. I., Kim, J. A., Ko, J.-K., Chung, M. S., Bang, K.-S., Choe, M.-A., Yoo, M. S., & Jang, H. Y. (2013). An identification study on core nursing competency. *Journal of Korean Academy Society of Nursing Education, 19*(4), 663–674. https://doi.org/10.5977/jkasne.2013.19.4.663 (Original work published in Korean)

Pickles, D. P., Lacey, S., & King, L. (2019). Conflict between nursing student's personal beliefs and professional nursing values. *Nursing Ethics, 26*(4), 1087–1100. https://doi.org/10.1177/0969733017738132

Posluszny, L., & Hawley, D. A. (2017). Comparing professional values of sophomore and senior baccalaureate nursing students. *Journal of Nursing Education, 56*(9), 546–550. https://doi.org/10.3928/01484834-20170817-06

Woo, C. H., & Park, J. Y. (2017). Specialty satisfaction, positive psychological capital, and nursing professional values in nursing students: A cross-sectional survey. *Nurse Education Today, 57*, 24–28. https://doi.org/10.1016/j.nedt.2017.06.010

Yeun, E. J., Kwon, Y. M., & Ahn, O. H. (2005). Development of a nursing professional values scale. *Journal of Korean Academy Nursing, 35*(6), 1091–1100. (Original work published in Korean)

Zauderer, C. R., & Ganzer, C. A. (2011). Cinematic technology: The role of visual learning. *Nurse Educator, 36*(2), 76–79. https://doi.org/10.1097/NNE.0b013e31820b4fbf

Zeppegno, P., Gramaglia, C., Feggi, A., Lombardi, A., & Torre, E. (2015). The effectiveness of a new approach using movies in the training of medical students. *Perspectives on Medical Education, 4*(5), 261–263. https://doi.org/10.1007/s40037-015-0208-6

10

Nurses' Knowledge on Sepsis Related to Mechanical Ventilation: An Intervention Study

Emmanuel Zamokwakhe HLUNGWANE[1] • Wilma TEN HAM-BALOYI[2*] • Portia JORDAN[3] •
Benedict Raphael OAMEN[1]

ABSTRACT

Background: Sepsis is a leading cause of mortality and morbidity worldwide. South African adult public critical care units experience incidences of sepsis on an ongoing basis. Nurses caring for mechanically ventilated adult patients in intensive care units (ICUs) need to base their nursing care on "surviving sepsis campaign" (SSC) guidelines to properly manage sepsis. Adequate knowledge on sepsis guidelines remains crucially indicated for nurses as they endeavor to maintain asepsis in critically ill patients.

Purpose: This study was conducted to assess the effect of an educational intervention on nurses' knowledge and practices of sepsis in mechanically ventilated adult patients in public ICUs.

Methods: An intervention study, with quasi-intervention two-group, pretest–posttest design, was used to collect data using a self-administered, structured, pretest and posttest questionnaire designed to measure nurses' knowledge and practices on sepsis related to mechanical ventilation. The study was conducted between June and October 2018. An educational intervention was developed and validated. Five purposively selected public ICUs in the Eastern Cape, South Africa, were selected and assigned to three groups: Intervention Group 1 (ICUs 1 and 2), which received the full intervention (containing a 20-minute PowerPoint presentation, printed materials based on sections of the SSC guidelines, and monitoring visits bimonthly for 3 months); Intervention Group 2 (ICUs 3 and 4; receiving the same as Intervention Group 1 but with no monitoring visits); and the control group (ICU 5; receiving no intervention).

Results: One hundred seventeen nurses completed the questionnaires at pretest, and 94 completed the questionnaires at posttest, producing a response rate of 79% and 80%, respectively. The results revealed a significant knowledge score increase between pretest and posttest for both Intervention Group 2 (53.28 ± 14.39 and 62.18 ± 13.60, respectively; $p = .004$) and the control group (56.72 ± 13.72 and 70.05 ± 12.40, respectively; $p = .001$). Similarly, a recommended practice score increase was shown for Intervention Group 2 (58.8 ± 9.63 and 62.80 ± 9.52, respectively), and a significant increase was shown for the control group (56.72 ± 7.54 and 63.29 ± 5.89, respectively; $p = .002$). Intervention Group 1 showed a detectable but not significant decline in knowledge (57.72 ± 13.99 and 54.61 ± 12.15, respectively) and recommended practice (61.22 ± 8.66 and 60.33 ± 7.83, respectively) scores.

Conclusions: The availability of SSC guidelines was found to have increased knowledge on sepsis related to mechanical ventilation, although including monitoring visits as part of the educational intervention was not found to have a positive effect on increasing knowledge and practices. Further studies are required to explore factors contributing to improving knowledge and practices on sepsis related to mechanical ventilation and the effect that various educational interventions have in this context.

KEY WORDS:
critical care unit, sepsis, surviving sepsis campaign guidelines, nurses, mechanical ventilation.

Introduction

From the limited data available in Africa, up to 50% of patients in intensive care units (ICUs) have been reported to acquire healthcare-associated infections (Mahomed et al., 2017; Ndadane & Maharaj, 2019). Furthermore, there is a paucity of data on the burden of sepsis in adult critical care units in the public sector in South Africa. Clinical practice guidelines for sepsis management such as the 2016 surviving sepsis campaign (SSC) guidelines (Rhodes et al., 2017) have been developed to eradicate sepsis globally. However, no evidence has yet been published related to the implementation of sepsis guidelines in public adult ICUs in South Africa. Furthermore, it is unclear from observation whether nurses have sufficient knowledge regarding sepsis and related guidelines and whether their practices related to managing sepsis in adult mechanically ventilated patients are evidence based.

Globally, sepsis is a major public health problem for healthcare professionals. Sepsis has been associated with approximately 28.6%–30% of mortality in the United States, although there are no information estimates related to sepsis

[1]BSN, RN, Master Student, Department of Nursing Science, Nelson Mandela University, Port Elizabeth, South Africa • [2]PhD, RN, Research Associate, Faculty of Health Sciences, Nelson Mandela University, Port Elizabeth, South Africa • [3]PhD, RN, Professor, Faculty of Medicine and Health Sciences, Department of Nursing and Midwifery, Stellenbosch University, South Africa.

in ICUs (Saldanha & Messias, 2017; Sinha et al., 2018; Vincent et al., 2019). The number of sepsis cases per annum was approximately 15–19 million cases worldwide, whereas, in Europe, approximately 30%–38% of patients in critical care units have had at least one healthcare-associated infection (Vincent et al., 2019).

Both developed and developing countries are affected by sepsis. However, with improved technologies (such as digital alerting and electronic warning systems) being used for at-risk patient detection in the ICU, appropriate hygiene protocols, and adequate nutrition, sepsis has been successfully minimized, especially in developed countries (Downing et al., 2019; Joshi et al., 2019; Westphal et al., 2018).

Sepsis-related morbidity and mortality in developing countries are believed to be disproportionately high compared with developed countries (Westphal et al., 2018). Although a number of research studies of sepsis have been conducted in sub-Saharan countries such as Kenya, Uganda, and Tanzania, its epidemiology in these countries remains poorly described, especially for adult ICUs (Tupchong et al., 2015).

Clinical practice guidelines are described as statements that include recommendations intended to optimize patient care. These guidelines should be informed by a systemic review of the evidence and an assessment of the benefits and harms of alternative care options (Kredo et al., 2016). Guidelines have a range of purposes, including improving effectiveness and quality of care. In addition, guidelines aim to decrease variations in clinical practice and decrease costly and preventable mistakes and adverse events, thus increasing patient safety (Jordan, 2011; Kredo et al., 2016).

Patients on mechanical ventilators are at a greater risk of sepsis because of the interference with normal processes during intubation and artificial/assisted ventilation. Patients managed through the use of clinical practice guidelines are more likely to have reduced incidences of developed sepsis. Reducing incidences of sepsis further decreases the incidences of other complications such as sepsis-induced acute respiratory distress syndrome, prolonged hospital stays, and mortality (Kim & Hong, 2016).

According to Mpasa (2017), noncompliance by nurses to clinical practice guidelines is a barrier to the management of mechanically ventilated patients in critical care units. Nurses are at the bedside of these patients and must therefore be knowledgeable in their field and associated practice, according to the latest evidence related to sepsis. Nurses have a fundamental role in surveilling sepsis, recording data correctly, and reporting information to provide relevant data that will allow fellow nurses to improve their practice and more effectively monitor their actions (Kleinpell et al., 2013).

Purpose

The aim of this study was to investigate the effect of an educational intervention on nurses' sepsis-related knowledge and practices in mechanically ventilated adult patients in public ICUs in Eastern Cape Province, South Africa.

Methods

Study Design

An intervention study using a quasi-experimental, two-group, pretest–posttest design (Gray et al., 2016; Moule et al., 2017; Sidani, 2015) was conducted in three phases. These phases included Phase 1, the pretest questionnaire (collecting baseline data before the implementation of the educational intervention); Phase 2, the educational intervention (development, review, and implementation of the intervention, based on SSC guidelines); and Phase 3, the posttest questionnaire (evaluation of the educational intervention implemented in Phase 2 of the study). Phases 1 and 2 were conducted between June and September 2018, whereas Phase 3 was conducted between the second week of September to the third week of October 2018.

Study Setting

This study was conducted in ICUs in five tertiary public hospitals in Eastern Cape Province (two public hospitals in Nelson Mandela Bay, two in Buffalo City, and one in Oliver Tambo District). The total bed capacity of these ICUs was 56 beds, providing care for adult patients only. In these five ICUs, there were more nurse specialists (with formal college training) than nurses with in-hospital training.

Population and Sampling

Nurses working in the five targeted ICUs were purposively allocated to three groups: Intervention Group 1 (ICUs 1 and 2), which received the full intervention; Intervention Group 2 (ICUs 3 and 4), which received part of the intervention; and the control group (ICU 5), which received no intervention. Group allocation was done based on geographical location. To recruit the largest sample possible, convenience sampling was used to invite all nurses (diploma and degree nurses) working in the selected adult ICUs who were available and willing to participate.

Data Collection Instrument

As no previous validated questionnaire was available, self-administered, structured pretest and posttest questionnaires were developed based on the latest SSC guidelines (Rhodes et al., 2017). The questionnaires measured the items discussed in the following sections.

Demographic data of the participants (section A)

Demographic data were collected on participants' gender, age (in years), number of years worked in ICUs, position held by the participant in the unit, type of employment, specialized ICU training as an additional qualification, and highest professional qualification. Closed-ended questions were used to collect these data.

Knowledge related to sepsis in mechanically ventilated adult patients in intensive care units (section B)

This item included four subsections, of which three explored the availability and use of the guidelines. Subsection 4 explored the knowledge of nurses related to the guidelines. "True" or "false" responses were solicited.

Practices related to sepsis in mechanically ventilated adult patients in intensive care units (section C)

This item included three subsections. Subsection 1 had 12 questions, whereas the other two subsections had four questions each. Subsection 1 assessed nursing practices related to the guidelines in mechanically ventilated adult patients admitted in ICUs, Subsection 2 assessed the diagnosis of sepsis, and Subsection 3 assessed the practices of the guidelines. A 5-point Likert scale, ranging from (1) *never* to (5) *always*, was used.

The Intervention

The educational intervention was developed by the first author based on 2016 SSC guidelines (Rhodes et al., 2017). These guidelines include "The Sepsis in Resource Limited Nations Initiative," which was deemed by the first author to be suitable for inclusion in the educational intervention because of the limited resources available to the public health system in South Africa. The developed educational intervention consisted of a 20-minute PowerPoint presentation, printed materials based on the 2016 SSC guidelines, and, for Intervention Group 1, monitoring visits conducted twice per month over the 3 months after the implementation of the educational intervention. The purpose of the monitoring visits was to check if the guidelines were being used by the participants and whether any clarification regarding its use was required. Intervention Group 2 received the same educational intervention, but no monitoring visits were made. The control group did not receive any intervention.

Data Collection Process

After obtaining relevant ethical clearances and permissions, all of the eligible nurses at the five selected ICUs were invited to participate. The study was explained to these nurses to provide a broad understanding of the research and to enable them to make informed decisions. All of the nurses who agreed to participate completed consent forms before completing the pretest questionnaire, which was distributed by the first author. Participants were asked not to discuss the answers, and the questionnaires were collected by the first author immediately after completion.

The process of collecting the pretest data in all of the ICUs took 3 weeks, after which the educational intervention was immediately implemented, lasting for a period of 3 months. Posttest data were collected in the same manner as the pretest data upon completion of the intervention.

Data Analysis

A Microsoft Excel template was used by the first author to capture pretest/posttest results to obtain both knowledge and practice scores. A statistician assisted with the descriptive and inferential statistics, as these were calculated to obtain the measures of central tendency (i.e., mean, median, and dispersion). The chi-square test of independent variance was used to determine if there were significant relationships among the responses from the participants. A chi-square p value less than .005 was considered statistically significant. Cramer's V was calculated to produce a statistically significant result with a value greater than .01.

Validity and Reliability

The pretest and posttest questionnaires were evaluated by the statistician, and the pretest and posttest questionnaires and educational intervention were reviewed by five experts, including an intensivist, a critical care nursing educator at the local university, a nurse manager at a private college, a unit manager at a private hospital, and a unit manager at a public hospital. The reviewers considered the cost efficiency, user friendliness, and availability of the equipment used to implement the educational intervention based on the SSC guidelines as well as the educational intervention's relevancy in terms of context, scope of practice of the nurses, face validity, and internal and external validity. To ensure reliability, the pretest and posttest questionnaires and the educational intervention were piloted in ICU 3 on 14 participants. After the pilot study, five questions in Section B (Statements B4.3 and B4.4) and Section C (Statements C1.6, C1.8, and C1.12) were revised. The results of the pilot study were not included in the main study.

Study Permission and Ethical Clearance

The relevant ethical clearances were obtained from the university (Ref. No. H17-HEA-NUR-021) as well as the Eastern Cape Department of Health (Ref. No. EC_201801_005). Furthermore, hospital managers and unit managers in the selected ICUs granted permission for data collection. Written consent was obtained from all of the nurses who agreed to participate. After the conclusion of data collection, the control group (ICU 5) was given a copy of the PowerPoint presentation and the printed materials based on the 2016 SSC guidelines.

Results

In the pretest phase, questionnaires were distributed to 127 participants. One hundred twenty-one questionnaires were returned, with four discarded because of incompleteness, giving a response rate of 92%. In the posttest phase, questionnaires were distributed to 117 participants. One hundred one questionnaires were returned, with seven discarded because of incompleteness, giving a response rate of 80%.

Demographic Data

Demographic data for the group of participants at enrollment are presented in Table 1.

A predominant number of participants were female, with most between the ages of 40 and 59 years. Almost all of the participants were permanently employed and involved with patient care. More than half of the participants had more

than 10 years of experience in the ICU. Nearly 40% held a 4-year diploma in nursing science, and more than half had received specialized critical care training.

Knowledge Related to Sepsis in Mechanically Ventilated Adult Patients in Intensive Care Units

Descriptive statistics for the items on knowledge related to sepsis in mechanically ventilated adult patients in ICUs are presented in Table 2.

Table 1

Demographic Data of the Participants, Pretest (n = 117) and Posttest (n = 94)

| Characteristic | Number of Participants | | | | | |
| | Pretest (*n* = 117) | | Posttest (*n* = 94) | | Total (*N* = 211) | |
	n	%	*n*	%	*n*	%
Gender						
Male	14	12.0	10	10.6	24	11.4
Female	103	88.0	84	89.4	187	88.6
Age (years)						
< 25	2	1.7	1	1.1	3	1.4
25–29	10	8.5	12	12.8	22	10.4
30–39	25	21.4	22	23.4	47	22.4
40–49	27	23.1	29	30.8	56	26.5
50–59	46	39.3	26	27.7	72	34.1
≥ 60	7	6.0	4	4.2	11	5.2
Number of years worked in ICUs						
< 1	8	6.8	12	12.8	20	9.5
1–4	20	17.1	20	21.3	40	18.9
5–9	28	23.9	22	23.4	50	23.7
10–19	28	23.9	15	15.9	43	20.4
≥ 20	33	28.2	25	26.6	58	27.5
Position held by the participants						
Unit manager	3	2.6	0	0	3	1.4
Operational manager	3	2.6	0	0	3	1.4
Nurse involved with patient care	111	94.8	92	97.8	203	96.2
Clinical facilitator	0	0	1	1.1	1	0.5
Other	0	0	1	1.1	1	0.5
Type of employment						
Permanently employed	116	99.1	94	100.0	210	99.5
Agency employed	1	0.9	0	0	1	0.5
Specialized ICU training as an additional qualification						
Have specialized in ICU	72	61.5	56	59.6	128	60.7
Have not specialized in ICU	45	38.5	38	40.4	83	39.3
Highest professional qualification						
Diploma in general nursing	36	30.8	28	29.8	64	30.3
4-year diploma in nursing science	38	32.5	45	47.9	83	39.3
Bachelor of nursing/degree	39	33.3	18	19.1	57	27.0
Master's degree	4	3.4	2	2.1	6	2.8
Doctor of philosophy	0	0	0	0	0	0
Other	0	0	1	1.1	1	0.5

Note. ICU = intensive care unit.

Table 2

Knowledge Related to Sepsis in Mechanically Ventilated Adult Patients in Intensive Care Units: Pretest (n = 117) and Posttest (n = 94)

Statement	Correct Answers				Incorrect Answers			
	Pretest		Posttest		Pretest		Posttest	
	n	%	n	%	n	%	n	%
B4.1 [a]: Routine screening of potentially infected seriously ill patients allows earlier implementation of therapy.	114	97.4	93	98.9	3	2.6	1	1.1
B4.2 [a]: The goal of treatment is to administer IV antimicrobials within first hour of septic shock and severe sepsis without septic shock.	103	88.0	85	90.4	14	12.0	9	9.6
B4.3 [a]: Source control intervention should be undertaken < 24 hr after diagnosis.	107	91.5	79	84.0	10	8.5	15	16.0
B4.4: A fluid challenge technique cannot be applied where fluid administration continues as long as hemodynamic factors continue to improve.	38	32.5	42	44.7	79	67.5	52	55.3
B4.5 [a]: Vasopressor therapy initially to target mean arterial pressure of 70 mmHg.	81	69.2	58	61.7	36	30.8	36	38.3
B4.6 [a]: The head of the bed elevation is maintained at 30–45 degree to limit aspiration and prevent development of ventilator-associated pneumonia.	110	94.0	93	98.9	7	6.0	1	1.1

[a] Correct statements on knowledge.

Most of the items concerning participants' knowledge related to sepsis in mechanically ventilated adult patients in ICUs in both the pretest and posttest questionnaires were correctly answered by participants. Moreover, the rate of correctness of answers, with the exception of answers to Items B4.3 and B4.5, had improved on the posttest questionnaire. There was a medium significant difference on Item B4.3 at posttest, χ^2 ($df = 4$, $n = 94$) = 17.25, $p = .002$, $V = 0.30$ (medium).

Practices Related to Sepsis in Mechanically Ventilated Adult Patients in Intensive Care Units

Descriptive statistics for the answers to questions on the practices related to sepsis in mechanically ventilated adult patients in ICUs are shown in Table 3.

Statements C1.1–C1.12

The findings revealed that most participants gave correct answers for most items with an improvement in practices for the posttest, with the exception of Statements C1.2, C1.7, C1.8, and C1.12. Medium statistical differences were only noted for Statements C1.2 for both pretest, χ^2 ($df = 8$, $n = 117$) = 25.74, $p = .001$, $V = 0.33$ (medium), and posttest, χ^2 ($df = 8$, $n = 94$) = 18.55, $p = .017$, $V = 0.31$ (medium); C1.8 for the pretest only, χ^2 ($df = 8$, $n = 117$) = 16.20, $p = .040$, $V = 0.26$ (medium); and C1.12 for both pretest, χ^2 ($df = 8$, $n = 117$) = 20.09, $p = .010$, $V = 0.29$ (medium), and posttest, χ^2 ($df = 8$, $n = 94$) = 17.39, $p = .026$, $V = 0.30$ (medium).

Comparison Within the Three Groups During Pretest and Posttest

The results of the comparisons within Intervention Group 1, Intervention Group 2, and the control group in terms of the responses to questions on the knowledge and practices related to sepsis in mechanically ventilated adult patients in ICUs are presented in Table 4.

The knowledge score was higher in the pretest (57.72) than the posttest (54.61) in Intervention Group 1, although the difference was not significant. A significant increase in knowledge score was seen in the scores for both Intervention Group 2 (62.18 vs. 53.28) and the control group (56.72 vs. 70.05). With regard to practice scores, similar results were noted, but with a significance only for the control group ($p = .002$).

Discussion

This study was designed to assess the effect of an educational intervention on nurses' knowledge and practices of sepsis in mechanically ventilated patients in adult public ICUs. The results study show that an educational intervention based on the SSC guidelines, including a 20-minute PowerPoint presentation and handing out of printed materials, may have some effect on sepsis knowledge related to mechanical ventilation of adult patients. Including monitoring visits as part of the educational intervention did not show a positive effect in terms of increasing knowledge or practice scores. Studies have been done to investigate the effect of educational interventions on healthcare professionals' knowledge in various healthcare contexts (Abu Farha et al., 2018; Melo E Lima et al., 2018; Patel et al., 2015). However, studies including an educational intervention on sepsis related to mechanical ventilation in the adult public ICUs are scarce. Therefore, further research is required to expand knowledge in the field of nursing education with respect to sepsis related to mechanically ventilated patients in the ICU context. This study is believed to be the first of its kind to be undertaken in South Africa.

Table 3

Practices Related to Sepsis in Mechanically Ventilated Adult Patients in Critical Care Units: Pretest (n = 117) and Posttest (n = 94)

Statement	Correct Answers				Incorrect Answers			
	Pretest		Posttest		Pretest		Posttest	
	n	%	n	%	n	%	n	%
C1.1 [a]: To reduce mortality, low tidal volume is applied.	59	50.4	56	59.6	58	49.6	38	40.4
C1.2 [a]: To reduce mortality, high positive end-expiratory pressure is applied to patients.	72	61.5	56	59.6	45	38.5	38	40.4
C1.3 [a]: Plateau pressures are measured to achieve the upper limit goal.	87	74.4	72	76.6	30	25.6	22	23.4
C1.4 [a]: Positive pressure is applied to avoid alveolar collapse at the end of expiratory.	104	88.9	91	96.8	13	11.1	3	3.2
C1.5 [a]: The head of the bed elevation is maintained to limit aspiration and prevent development of ventilator-associated pneumonia.	113	96.6	92	97.9	4	3.4	2	2.1
C1.6: Pulmonary artery catheter is used routinely.	73	62.4	69	73.4	44	37.6	25	26.6
C1.7 [a]: Recruitment maneuver in patient with refractory hypoxemia is not applied.	77	65.8	48	51.1	40	34.2	46	48.9
C1.8 [a]: Prone position is used in patient with FIO_2/PaO_2 of 200–300.	77	65.8	32	34.0	40	34.2	62	66.0
C1.9: Noninvasive ventilation is applied to patients with ARDS.	73	62.4	61	64.9	44	37.6	33	35.1
C1.10: Beta 2 agonist is routinely given to treat sepsis-induce ARDS.	49	41.9	52	55.3	68	58.1	42	44.7
C1.11: Conservative fluid strategy is applied in all ARDS patients irrespective of clinical presentation.	52	44.4	49	52.1	65	55.6	45	47.9
C1.12 [a]: Severe septic patient undergoes spontaneous trial regularly to evaluate ability to discontinue mechanical ventilation when aroused or hemodynamically stable.	99	84.6	78	83.0	18	15.4	16	17.0

Note. ARDS = acute respiratory distress syndrome.
[a] Correct statements on practices.

Table 4

Group Comparisons of Knowledge and Practices Related to Sepsis in Mechanically Ventilated Adult Patients in ICUs: Pretest (n = 117) and Posttest (n = 94)

Variable	Pre/Post	n	Mean	SD	Difference	t	df	p	Cohen's d
Intervention Group 1									
Knowledge score	Pre	46	57.72	13.99	3.11	1.03	77	.307	n/a
	Post	33	54.61	12.15					
Practice score	Pre	46	61.22	8.66	0.88	0.47	77	.643	n/a
	Post	33	60.33	7.83					
Intervention Group 2									
Knowledge score	Pre	46	53.28	14.39	−8.89	−2.93	84	.004	0.63
	Post	40	62.18	13.60					Medium
Practice score	Pre	46	58.89	9.63	−3.91	−1.89	84	.063	n/a
	Post	40	62.80	9.52					
Control group									
Knowledge score	Pre	25	56.72	13.72	−13.33	−3.43	44	.001	1.01
	Post	21	70.05	12.40					Large
Practice score	Pre	25	56.72	7.54	−6.57	−3.24	44	.002	0.96
	Post	21	63.29	5.89					Large

Note. ICU = intensive care unit; n/a = not applicable.

The pretest-to-posttest increases in knowledge scores were relatively high for all three intervention groups but increased most significantly in Intervention Group 2 and the control group. High overall knowledge scores may be attributed to educational level (Khalil et al., 2019). For example, 61% of the participants were ICU trained, with approximately 40% of the ICU trained nurses having completed their training recently. This may have been associated with the generally high knowledge scores as well as the knowledge improvement in the posttest, which is consistent with Elkalmi et al.'s (2014) study on motivation and obstacles for adverse drug reaction among healthcare professionals, which found a significant association between improvement in knowledge and the educational level of participants.

For Intervention Group 2, the increase in knowledge scores was attributed to the educational intervention, which included a PowerPoint presentation and printed materials (Abu Farha et al., 2018; Tahoon et al., 2020). Prior studies have reported a similar effect for educational interventions using PowerPoint presentations, videos, WhatsApp group sharing, guidelines, and clinical scenarios on knowledge improvement outcomes (Abu Farha et al., 2018; Prins & Human, 2019; Tahoon et al., 2020). In this study, for the control group, the significant improvement in knowledge scores may be attributed to participants' involvement in the study having enhanced their knowledge about sepsis.

The practice scores, which were generally higher than the knowledge scores in the pretest phase, also were higher at posttest for both Intervention Group 2 and, significantly, the control group. However, these increases were not as significant as the increases in knowledge scores. This finding is congruent with a similar study by Melo E Lima et al. (2018). Furthermore, an increase in knowledge scores may also translate into increased scores for practices at posttest.

The finding of this study regarding the increase in practice scores for Intervention Group 2, although not significant, is similar to that of other studies that found an improvement in health professionals' practice scores, especially in relation to the effectiveness of an educational intervention (Bisallah et al., 2018; Kissoon, 2014; Varallo et al., 2017). Therefore, it is recommended that training using up-to-date clinical practice guidelines such as SSC guidelines be incorporated into the daily routine of critical care nurses and that quality systems be implemented to ensure these guidelines are adhered to and are enforced for all nurses in ICUs. In addition, comparisons of the two intervention groups against the control group indicate a small, statistically significant improvement in knowledge and practices among nurses. However, when these results were analyzed separately, comparing knowledge and practice scores, practice scores were higher than knowledge scores on the pretest yet did not increase as significantly as knowledge scores. Furthermore, most of the participants gave correct answers during pretest and posttest questionnaires. Many factors may have contributed to the reported findings, including differences in the control group versus the intervention groups in terms of, for example, age, level of experience,

level of motivation, and bed occupancy rate in the ICU. Finally, a traditional approach of some nurses in the management of patients, including using their intuition, and information from their peers or colleagues, may have contributed to Intervention Group 1's performance (Jordan et al., 2016).

It is recommended that an observational study be conducted to describe the practices of nurses in relation to their knowledge of sepsis in mechanically ventilated adult patients in ICUs to better elucidate the findings highlighted in this study.

Furthermore, more studies on factors influencing the increase or decline in knowledge and practice scores should be conducted, especially in resource-constrained settings such as the South African public health system.

Limitations

This study was affected by several limitations. First, the study was conducted in the ICUs of public hospitals in Eastern Cape Province only. Thus, the results should not be generalized to private hospitals or to public hospitals in other provinces.

Second, convenience sampling was used in this study to enroll as many participants as possible. However, the anonymous nature of the questionnaire made it difficult to ensure that all of the participants completed the questionnaires at both time points.

Third, the researcher used a self-administered structured questionnaire to obtain responses regarding the practices related to sepsis treatment. This did not allow the truthfulness of reporting to be verified. This limitation would be addressed in an observational study format. Furthermore, the educational intervention could include a demonstration to enhance practices regarding sepsis related to mechanical ventilation in adult patients in ICUs.

Fourth, the posttest questionnaire was done 3 months after the start of the educational intervention. Although time frames of 3 months or less have been used in other educational intervention studies using a theory-based approach (Arrogi et al., 2017; Bosch et al., 2019), this time frame may be overly short for real uptake and usage by participants to take place. Furthermore, the methods (e.g., a 20-minute PowerPoint presentation) used in the educational intervention may not have had the same effect on all of the participants, and confounding variables such as employment of new staff, shortage of staff, and in-service education as well as uncontrolled demographic differences between the control and intervention groups may have influenced the implementation of the educational intervention and its effect on knowledge and practice scores. Finally, the study only targeted nurses working in ICUs. As nurses do not decide on the treatment plan alone, the guidelines should be adapted for and introduced to the entire team, including other stakeholders such as physicians and technicians. Therefore, it is recommended that both the educational intervention and the questionnaire be adapted and further tested with a more diverse sample. The educational intervention should use alternative methods of education, which may be implemented over a longer period to evaluate its impact on outcomes such as length of stay and patient prognosis.

Conclusions

The findings of this study indicate that the availability of SSC guidelines has a small but significant and positive effect on sepsis knowledge related to mechanical ventilation. However, including monitoring visits in the educational intervention had no effect on related knowledge or practices. Thus, the educational intervention used in this study should be further adapted and explored to improve efficacy.

The results of this study may be used by both hospital managers and nurses to improve adherence to best practices with regard to sepsis in adult mechanically ventilated patients in public ICUs. Furthermore, the results may be used in the training of intensive care nurses. Finally, more research is required, especially using more-diverse samples, to explore the factors that contribute to improving knowledge and practices and the differing effects that educational interventions using different teaching and implementation strategies have in the context of the management of sepsis in adult mechanically ventilated patients in public ICUs.

Acknowledgments

The authors would like to thank Vicki Igglesden for editing the article and the respondents for participating in the study.

Author Contributions

Study conception and design: EZH, WTHB, PJ
Data collection: EZH, BO
Data analysis and interpretation: EZH
Drafting of the article: EZH, WTHB, PJ
Critical revision of the article: WTHB, PJ

References

Abu Farha, R., Abu Hammour, K., Rizik, M., Aljanabi, R., & Alsakran, L. (2018). Effect of educational intervention on healthcare providers knowledge and perception towards pharmacovigilance: A tertiary teaching hospital experience. *Saudi Pharmaceutical Journal, 26*(5), 611–616. https://doi.org/10.1016/j.jsps.2018.03.002

Arrogi, A., Schotte, A., Bogaerts, A., Boen, F., & Seghers, J. (2017). Short- and long-term effectiveness of a three-month individualized need-supportive physical activity counseling intervention at

the workplace. *BMC Public Health, 17*(1), Article No. 52. https://doi.org/10.1186/s12889-016-3965-1

Bisallah, C. I., Rampal, L., Lye, M. S., Mohd Sidik, S., Ibrahim, N., Iliyasu, Z., & Onyilo, M. O. (2018). Effectiveness of health education intervention in improving knowledge, attitude, and practices regarding tuberculosis among HIV patients in General Hospital Minna, Nigeria—A randomized control trial. *PLOS ONE, 13*(2), Article e0192276. https://doi.org/10.1371/journal.pone.0192276

Bosch, M., McKenzie, J. E., Ponsford, J. L., Turner, S., Chau, M., Tavender, E. J., Knott, J. C., Gruen, R. L., Francis, J. J., Brennan, S. E., Pearce, A., O'Connor, D. A., Mortimer, D., Grimshaw, J. M., Rosenfeld, J. V., Meares, S., Smyth, T., Michie, S., & Green, S. E. (2019). Evaluation of a targeted, theory-informed implementation intervention designed to increase uptake of emergency management recommendations regarding adult patients with mild traumatic brain injury: Results of the NET cluster randomised trial. *Implementation Science, 14*(1), Article No. 4. https://doi.org/10.1186/s13012-018-0841-7

Downing, N. L., Rolnick, J., Poole, S. F., Hall, E., Wessels, A. J., Heidenreich, P., & Shieh, L. (2019). Electronic health record-based clinical decision support alert for severe sepsis: A randomised evaluation. *BMJ Quality Safety, 28*, 762–768. https://doi.org/10.1136/bmjqs-2018-008765

Elkalmi, R. M., Al-lela, O. Q., & Jamshed, S. Q. (2014). Motivations and obstacles for adverse drug reactions reporting among healthcare professionals from the perspective of Lewin's force field analysis theory: Analytic approach. *Journal of Pharmacovigilance, 2*(3), Article 130. https://doi.org/10.4172/2329-667.1000130

Gray, J. R., Grove, S. K., & Sutherland, S. (2016). *The practice of nursing research: Appraisal, synthesis, and generation of evidence.* Elsevier.

Jordan, P. J. (2011). *Evidence-informed clinical guidelines for nursing care practices related to the safety of the mechanically ventilated patient* [Unpublished doctoral dissertation]. Nelson Mandela Metropolitan University.

Jordan, P. J., Bowers, C. A., & Morton, D. (2016). Barriers to implementing evidence-based practice in a private intensive care unit in the Eastern Cape. *Southern African Journal of Critical Care, 32*(2), 50–54. https://doi.org/10.7196/SAJCC.2016.v32i2.253

Joshi, M., Ashrafian, H., Arora, S., Khan, S., Cooke, G., & Darzi, A. (2019). Digital alerting and outcomes in patients with sepsis: Systematic review and meta-analysis. *Journal of Medical Internet Research, 21*(12), Article e15166. https://doi.org/10.2196/15166

Khalil, A. I., Felemban, R., & Tunker, R. (2019). Impact of an educational intervention in enhancing nurses' knowledge towards psychiatric patients' ethical and legal rights. *Journal of Nursing Education and Practice, 9*(10), 1–14. https://doi.org/10.5430/jnep.v9n10p1

Kim, W.-Y., & Hong, S.-B. (2016). Sepsis and acute respiratory distress syndrome: Recent update. *Tuberculosis and Respiratory Diseases, 79*(2), 53–57. https://doi.org/10.4046/trd.2016.79.2.53

Kissoon, N. (2014). Sepsis guideline implementation: Benefits, pitfalls and possible solutions. *Critical Care, 18*, Article 207. https://doi.org/10.1186/cc13774

Kleinpell, R., Aitken, L., & Schorr, C. A. (2013). Implications of the new international sepsis guidelines for nursing care. *American Journal of Critical Care, 22*(3), 212–222. https://doi.org/10.4037/ajcc2013158

Kredo, T., Bernhardsson, S., Machingaidze, S., Young, T., Louw, Q., Ochodo, E., & Grimmer, K. (2016). Guide to clinical practice guidelines: The current state of play. *International Journal for Quality in Health Care, 28*(1), 122–128. https://doi.org/10.1093/intqhc/mzv115

Mahomed, S., Mahomed, O., Sturm, A. W., Knight, S., & Moodley, P. (2017). Challenges with surveillance of healthcare-associated infections in intensive care units in South Africa. *Critical Care Research and Practice, 2017*, Article ID 7296317. https://doi.org/10.1155.2017/7296317

Melo E Lima, T. R., Maia, P. F. C. M. D., Valente, E. P., Vezzini, F., & Tamburlini, G. (2018). Effectiveness of an action-oriented educational intervention in ensuring long term improvement of knowledge, attitudes and practices of community health workers in maternal and infant health: A randomized controlled study. *BMC Medical Education, 18*(1), Article No. 224. https://doi.org/10.1186/s12909-018-1332-x

Moule, P., Aveyard, H., & Goodman, M. (2017). *Nursing research: An introduction* (3rd ed.). SAGE.

Mpasa, F. (2017). *Management of endotracheal tube cuff pressure in mechanical ventilated adult patients in intensive care units in Malawi* [Unpublished doctoral dissertation]. Nelson Mandela Metropolitan University.

Ndadane, N., & Maharaj, R. C. (2019). The epidemiology of sepsis in a district hospital emergency centre in Durban, KwaZulu Natal. *African Journal of Emergency Medicine, 9*(3), 123–126. https://doi.org/10.1016/j.afjem.2019.02.001

Patel, S. V., Desai, C. K., Patel, P. P., & Dikshit, R. K. (2015). An impact of educational intervention on reporting of adverse drug reactions. *International Journal of Pharmacy, 5*(2), 485–492. https://doi.org/10.1016/j.afjem.2019.02.001

Prins, L., & Human, L. (2019). Early identification and referral of organ donors in five private hospitals: A survey to determine the knowledge and view of critical care professional nurses pre and post a PowerPoint training intervention. *South African Journal of Critical Care, 35*(2), 48–55. https://doi.org/10.7196/SAJCC.2019.v35i2.370

Rhodes, A., Evans, L. E., Alhazzani, W., Levy, M. M., Antonelli, M., Ferrer, R., Kumar, A., Sevransky, J. E., Charles, L., Sprung, C. L., Nunnally, M. E., Rochwerg, B., Rubenfeld, G. D., Angus, D. C., Annane, D., Beale, R. J., Bellinghan, G. J., Bernard, G. R., Chiche, J. D., … Dellinger, R. P. (2017). Surviving sepsis campaign: International guidelines for management of sepsis and septic shock: 2016. *Critical Care Medicine, 45*(3), 1–67. https://doi.org/10.1097/CCM.0000000000002255

Saldanha, C., & Messias, A. (2017). Sepsis needs follow-up studies in intensive care units—Another avenue for translational research. *Novel Approaches in Drug Designing & Development, 1*(1), 1–3. https://doi.org/10.19080/NAPDD.2017.01.555555

Sidani, S. (2015). *Health intervention research: Understanding research design and methods.* SAGE. http://dx.doi.org/10.4135/9781473910140

Sinha, M., Jupe, J., Mack, H., Coleman, T. P., Lawrence, S. M., & Fraleya, S. I. (2018). Emerging technologies for molecular diagnosis of sepsis. *Clinical Microbiology Reviews, 31*(2), e00089–e00017. https://doi.org/10.1128/CMR.00089-17

Tahoon, M. A., Khalil, M. M., Hammad, E., Morad, W. S., Awad, S. M., & Ezzat, S. (2020). The effect of educational intervention on healthcare providers' knowledge, attitude, and practice towards antimicrobial stewardship program at, National Liver Institute, Egypt. *Egyptian Liver Journal, 10*, Article No. 5. https://doi.org/10.1186/s43066-019-0016-5

Tupchong, K., Koyfman, A., & Foran, M. (2015). Sepsis, severe sepsis, and septic shock: A review of the literature. *African Journal of Emergency Medicine, 5*(3), 127–135. https://doi.org/10.1016/j.afjem.2014.05.004

Varallo, F. R., Planeta, C. S., & Mastroianni, P. C. (2017). Effectiveness of pharmacovigilance: Multifaceted educational intervention related to the knowledge, skills and attitudes of multidisciplinary hospital staff. *Clinics (Sao Paulo), 27*(1), 51–57. https://doi.org/10.6061/clinics/2017(01)09

Vincent, J.-L., Jones, G., David, S., Olariu, E., & Cadwell, K. K. (2019). Frequency and mortality of septic shock in Europe and North America: A systematic review and meta-analysis. *Critical Care, 23*, Article No. 196. https://doi.org/10.1186/s13054-019-2478-6

Westphal, G. A., Pereira, A. B., Fachin, S. M., Sperotto, G., Gonçalves, M., Albino, L., Bittencourt, R., Franzini, V. R., & Koenig, Á. (2018). An electronic warning system helps reduce the time to diagnosis of sepsis. *Revista Brasileira de Ter Intensiva, 30*(4), 414–422. https://doi.org/10.5935/0103-507X.20180059

11

Questionnaire Development of a Good Nurse and Better Nursing from Korean Nurses' Perspective

Mihyun PARK[1] • Eun-Jun PARK[2]*

ABSTRACT

Background: The concepts of "good nurse" and "better nursing" have changed over time and should be investigated from the perspective of nurses.

Purpose: The aim of this study was to develop and assess the psychometric properties of two questionnaires used to assess "good nurse" and "better nursing."

Methods: The interview data of 30 registered nurses (RNs) from a previous study were reviewed to develop the questionnaire items, and content validity was examined. One hundred seventeen RNs participated in a pilot survey for pretesting the constructs, 469 RNs participated in a main survey to explore these constructs using exploratory factor analysis (EFA), and 468 RNs participated in model refining and validation using confirmatory factor analysis.

Results: After a critical review of RN interview data and content validity evaluation, 73 of 124 statements on "good nurse" and 56 of 57 statements on "better nursing" were selected. In the pilot survey, the number of items was reduced to 45 for both questionnaires using an EFA. In the main survey, EFA was used to load 34 items on the five factors of the good nurse questionnaire and 26 items on the three factors of the better nursing questionnaire. In the confirmatory factor analysis, to obtain better fitting models, the good nurse questionnaire consisted of 17 items on the five factors of collaboration, professional competency, self-efficacy, a sense of achievement, and compassion, whereas the better nursing questionnaire consisted of 16 items on the three factors of person-centered nursing, proactive nursing, and expertise in caring. The construct reliability, convergent validity, and discriminant validity of the questionnaires were achieved.

Conclusions/Implications for Practice: The concept of "good nurse" from the perspectives of the nurses in this study was similar with those of patients in previous studies, while including individual traits such as sense of achievement. Better nursing is conceptualized with the exemplary performance of nursing focusing on the nature of nursing and leading excellence and power in clinical practice. The study findings inform what nursing education and workforce development should focus on for nursing to continuously progress. Furthermore, it is recommended that the concepts of a good nurse and better nursing be compared across different countries using the questionnaires.

KEY WORDS:
surveys and questionnaires, validation studies, nurses, nursing, nursing care.

Introduction

What makes a good nurse? Although the concepts of a good nurse vary in the nursing literature, "good nursing" is often referred to among the public and nursing professionals. According to the virtue ethics of Aristotle, a good nurse is one who possesses essential virtues to perform a nurse's function well. Nurse virtues have changed through history and differed depending on the identified function of a nurse as nurses' identity changes responding to changes in healthcare. Although a univocal definition of a good nurse across time and location seems to be impractical, it still requires a continuous inquiry among nursing scholars.

Since the beginning of modern nursing, nurses' identity has changed from assistants of physicians to providers of professional care to patients. This change has led to a paradigmatic shift in the concept of a good nurse (Begley, 2010). According to historical reviews (Begley, 2010; Fry, 2004), the notion of a good nurse has changed from an etiquette-oriented perspective to an ethics-oriented perspective and from a vocation to a professional. The virtue of a good nurse in the Nightingale period included assisting physicians with loyalty, obedience, and modesty. These are no longer generally considered virtues of current professional nurses, especially in many developed countries. Rather, accountability and autonomy may be the essential virtues of today's nursing professionals (Begley, 2010; Fry, 2004).

Nursing scholars who study the virtues and concept of a good nurse today often inquire the view of patients. This current trend in nursing studies is desirable because nurses identify their primary role as promoting the well-being of patients. Thus, nursing outcomes should reflect patients' experience with nurses. Patients commonly described a good nurse as having virtues such as being compassionate, kind, respectful, honest, and responsible in addition to having professional

[1]PhD, RN, Associate Professor, College of Nursing, The Catholic University of Korea, Seoul, ROK • [2]PhD, RN, Professor, Department of Nursing, Konkuk University, ROK.

knowledge and skills to promptly address their care needs (Gallagher et al., 2009; Rchaidia et al., 2009; Van der Elst et al., 2012). Although these virtues are common in both Western and Eastern countries, Asian patients reflect Asian values and culture in their perspectives of a good nurse. In Taiwanese (Chou et al., 2007) and Korean (Cho et al., 2006; Han et al., 2006) studies, patients expressed that a good nurse should treat them as family or as a relative, which reflects Asian culture recognizing their family members as ideal and primary caregivers. The patients in a Japanese study (Izumi et al., 2006) emphasized having good interpersonal relationship skills as a virtue of a good nurse, introducing the traditional meaning of the *kanji* character "Person-*hito*." Differences in the essential virtues of nurses across time and place may promote further study on a good nurse in various societies.

Furthermore, the perspectives of a good nurse must be learned from not only patients but also nurses. There are differences and similarities in the perspectives between patients and nurses (Aydin Er et al., 2017; Catlett & Lovan, 2011; Kim et al., 2019). Some virtues of a good nurse such as being compassionate, respectful, and responsible and having professional knowledge and skills were shared between patients and nurses. However, unlike patients, nurses identified collaboration or commitment to a relationship with colleagues or an organization as the virtues of a good nurse (Catlett & Lovan, 2011; Kim et al., 2019). Nurses do not limit their role in a patient–nurse relationship, although both patients and nurses often emphasize virtues required for the relationship. Accordingly, the perspectives of nurses on a good nurse need to be explored in addition to those of patients. The concept of a good nurse would reveal the critical virtues of nurses who are responding to rapidly changing healthcare environments, including patients' expectations. Thus, nursing education and evaluation should be consistent with the critical virtues of nurses to enhance the quality of the nursing workforce.

Korean scholars conducted a qualitative study to learn nurses' perspectives of a good nurse and better nursing for the first time in 2015 (Um et al., 2017). They investigated the concept of better nursing to develop a good nursing practice in terms of positive change and improvement in nursing. The participating nurses were asked to describe some anecdotes in narrative form based on their direct or indirect experiences of being a good nurse and promoting a better nursing practice. In the study, the definition of a good nurse or better nursing was not given to the nurses, and nurses were asked to provide their own perspectives by asking questions such as "Who is a good nurse?" and "What is your experience or observation about better nursing practice for patients?" The identified characters of a good nurse in the study were not very different from those in previous studies. For example, the nurses described good nurses as those who showed observation and assessment skills based on knowledge, compassion for their patients in pain and difficulties, and attitudes of helping or treating other nurses well. Better nursing was described using anecdotes of providing outstanding patient care with excellence and power, as

emphasized in Benner (1984). For example, one of the study participants illustrated a caring situation that a nurse provided basic care to a patient in a coma in a comforting and skillful manner with a beautiful smile and soft words such as "Grandma, please enjoy your meal" every day although she had never received any response from this patient.

However, although this prior qualitative study informed about the characteristics of a good nurse and better nursing, it was limited in terms of the generalizability of findings. To obtain concepts of a good nurse and better nursing that are generally agreed upon by Korean nurses, this study surveyed a large number of nurses and explored these concepts using quantitative evidence. Furthermore, on the basis of the qualitative data of self-reflection in this study, two constructs of a good nurse and better nursing were developed and validated.

Methods

Study Design

This methodological study was designed to develop and validate two instruments for use in Korea. These instruments were (a) a good nurse questionnaire and (b) a better nursing questionnaire.

Ethical Consideration

This study was approved by the institutional review board (No. MC16QISI0067). No individual identification information was collected, and the completed surveys were individually sealed and returned by mail.

Study Procedure and Sample

This study was conducted following the stages of a questionnaire-item development, repeated-construct exploration, and model refinement and validation (Figure 1). The English versions of the instruments were developed using forward–backward translation by bilingual experts.

The questionnaire items were developed based on the interview data of 30 registered nurses (RNs) and tested for content validity on 10 subject experts. The interview data were obtained from a previous study entitled, "A Good Nurse and Better Nursing," in which one of the authors had participated (Um et al., 2017). Preliminary questionnaire items were developed using three steps. First, the interview data were imported to MAXQDA Version 11 (VERBI GmbH, Berlin, Germany), and all meaningful statements were selected, allowing for duplications, which resulted in 475 statements on a good nurse and 285 statements on better nursing. Second, the selected excerpts were restated into general statements applicable across different hospital settings and RNs. For example, a statement "When I did something wrong while taking care of my patient, I let the patients or colleagues know about it" was changed to "A good nurse frankly admits her/his errors and mistakes." As a result, 223 statements on a good nurse and 177 on better nursing were obtained. Third, redundant statements with similar meanings were integrated and removed,

Figure 1
Study process

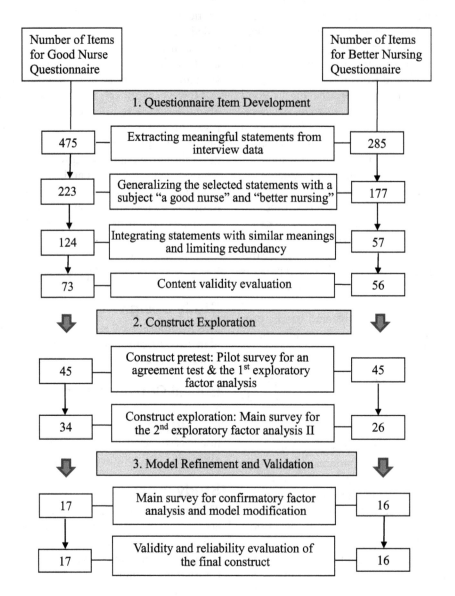

whereas their meanings were clarified using the original data. For example, statements such as "A good nurse accepts even a patient's request that seems unnecessary" and "A good nurse admits and accepts a patient behavior that is annoying and difficult to understand" were combined into one statement of "A good nurse admits and accepts a patient's response that is difficult to understand because (s)he is a patient." At the end of the questionnaire-item development process, there remained 124 statements on a good nurse and 57 on better nursing.

Ten subject experts evaluated the content validity of the questionnaire items using a 4-point scale. The experts were five nursing professors who had studied nursing humanities and five clinical nurses with clinical nursing careers of longer than 5 years each. Items with a content validity index of .80 or higher (Polit & Beck, 2006) were selected for the pilot survey. Four items with a content validity index of .70 were also included in the pilot survey, as they were repeatedly emphasized as critical characteristics of better nursing in the original

interview data. Accordingly, the numbers of survey items for the pilot survey were 73 (58.9%) of 124 statements on a good nurse and 56 (98.2%) of 57 statements on better nursing.

The pilot survey was conducted to pretest the concept and shorten the survey. Perceptions of a good nurse and better nursing were evaluated on a scale ranging from 1 = *not agree at all* to 5 = *strongly agree*. An item was excluded from the first exploratory factor analysis (EFA) if it had less than an average score of 4.0 points. A sample size for factor analysis is at least 100 (Kyriazos, 2018). Thus, 117 of 125 invited RNs (response rate: 93.6%) participated in the pilot survey from four hospitals with 500 or more beds in August 2016. One hundred nine surveys were analyzed after excluding eight unreliable surveys because of most responses being uncompleted or answered without variation.

For the main survey, 1,040 RNs were invited and 950 (91.3% response rate) from 36 hospitals returned the individually sealed paper surveys by mail. These RNs were recruited in two stages. First, 40 hospitals were selected by cluster random sampling from all Korean hospitals grouped by four hospital locations and three hospital sizes (1,000 or more beds, 500–1,000 beds, and less than 500 beds). Second, 1,040 RNs were recruited by convenience sampling from the 40 hospitals.

Nine hundred thirty-seven surveys with reliable responses were selected and randomly assigned using MS Excel software for analysis in the construct exploration stage ($n = 469$) or the refinement and validation stage ($n = 468$). The participants' demographic characteristics, including age, gender, religion, duration of work, type of nursing unit, and work position, were not statistically different at $\alpha = .05$ between the two sets of data.

Data Analysis

SPSS Version 24.0 (IBM, Inc., Armonk, NY, USA) was used for the descriptive statistics analysis and EFA. AMOS 20.0 (IBM, Inc., Armonk, NY, USA) was used for the confirmatory factory analysis (CFA). In the repeated construct exploration stage, items with Pearson's correlation coefficients of either $\geq .80$ or $\leq .30$ were excluded from the factor analysis because of redundancy or low relevancy (Pett et al., 2003). Bartlett's test of sphericity and Kaiser–Meyer–Olkin (KMO) were calculated to evaluate the suitability of the data for EFA. Principal component analysis (PCA) was adopted for factor extraction, and orthogonal rotation (the varimax method) was applied assuming no correlation among factors. A factor loading of $\geq .50$ was accepted. The number of factors was determined if the eigenvalue was greater than 1, percentage of extracted variance was $\geq 5\%$, and cumulative percentage of variance was $\geq 50\%$ (Pett et al., 2003). The reliability of the questionnaire was assessed in terms of internal consistency using Cronbach's α coefficient. As pairwise deletion was adopted, sample sizes differed depending on the variables.

CFA was conducted using the AMOS 20.0 program to refine and validate the factor structure obtained as the result of EFA. Goodness-of-fit indices (GFIs) were adopted to test how well the construct structure from the EFA fits the validation data ($n = 468$). A chi-square test, normed χ^2, root mean square error of approximation (RMSEA), standardized root mean squared residual (SRMR), GFI, and adjusted GFI (AGFI) were used as an absolute fit index, whereas normed fit index (NFI), comparative fit index (CFI), and Tucker–Lewis index (TLI) were used as an incremental index. The EFA factor structure was modified to improve model fit using the modification index (Kang, 2013).

The convergent validity of primitive constructs derived from the EFA results was accepted with standardized factor loading values of $\geq .50$ and average variance extraction (AVE) values of $\geq .50$ (Hair et al., 2010). Construct reliability, also called composite reliability, in CFA was considered acceptable at $\geq .70$ (Hair et al., 2010). Discriminant validity was assessed using the criterion that the confidence interval of the estimated correlation between any two latent constructs

($\pm$ 2 *SEs* from the point estimate) does not include 1 (Haddock & Maio, 2004).

Results

Construct Pretest Stage

In the pilot survey ($N = 109$), most of the participating RNs were female (95.4%, $n = 104$), were an average of 32.72 ± 6.48 years old, self-identified as religious (66.1%, $n = 72$), held a bachelor's degree (52.3%, $n = 57$), worked as a staff nurse (57.8%, $n = 63$), and had an average career duration of 10.26 ± 6.11 years. Before conducting a factor analysis, eight items of "a good nurse" and seven items of "better nursing" were removed because they had a low agreement level (< 4.0).

The KMO values were .90 for both instruments, indicating excellent sampling adequacy, and Bartlett's tests of sphericity were statistically significant ($p < .001$), rejecting the null hypothesis that no relationship exists among the items (Pett et al., 2003). Because all of the items were collapsed into one factor using PCA, a principal axis factoring was used for further item reduction. In the results of factor analysis with orthogonal rotation, items with communality < .50, with factor loadings < .30, or loaded on more than one factor were removed (Mooi, Sarstedt, & Mooi-Reci, 2018). After applying the criteria for factor retention such as the eigenvalue (> 1), percentage of extracted variance ($\geq 5\%$), and cumulative percentage of variance ($\geq 50\%$), 45 items under five factors were retained in the good nurse questionnaire and 45 items under three factors were retained in the better nursing questionnaire.

Construct Exploration Stage

EFA was conducted with the first half of the main survey participants ($n = 469$ RNs). Most of the RNs in this group were female (95.7%, $n = 449$), were an average of 34.77 ± 9.26 years old, self-identified as religious (51.2%, $n = 240$), worked as a staff nurse (81.9%, $n = 384$), and had an average career duration of 11.33 ± 8.36 years. For the instruments, the data were appropriate for factor analysis given that Bartlett's tests of sphericity were statistically significant ($p < .001$) and KMO values were quite high (.97).

Factors were extracted using repetitive PCA with orthogonal rotation, and then the same criteria were used for factor retention. The factor loadings of each item in addition to the eigenvalues of each factor, variance explained, cumulative variance, and Cronbach's α of the good nurse questionnaire are shown in Table 1. The same information about the better nursing questionnaire is presented in Table 2. For the good nurse questionnaire, 34 of the 45 items that loaded on the five factors were extracted, explaining 65.6% of the variance, whereas 26 of the 45 items that loaded on the three factors were identified for better nursing, explaining 67.1% of the variance. No items were cross-loaded or had a factor loading value less than .50.

Table 1

Primitive Construct of the Good Nurse Questionnaire Using Exploratory Factor Analysis and Reliability Analysis

Item	Mean	SD	Factor Loading				
			1	2	3	4	5
A good nurse…							
1. helps fellow nurses keep up with the latest expertise.[a]	4.23	.71	.75	.23	.22	.16	.04
2. focuses on what patients need now by paying careful attention.	4.19	.68	.74	.26	.21	.18	.09
3. respects the expectations and culture of the patient.	4.16	.71	.73	.23	.26	.19	-.03
4. maintains a good relationship with the staffs of other departments based on an understanding of their work.[a]	4.21	.65	.72	.31	.19	.21	.09
5. empathizes with the difficulties of assistance personnel in the hospital and has a warm and respectful attitude.[a]	4.25	.68	.69	.22	.24	.13	.24
6. finds the strengths of fellow nurses and praises them rather than criticizes.[a]	4.17	.70	.69	.21	.16	.16	.14
7. provides all necessary information to patients/guardians as fully as possible even when s/he is busy.	4.24	.68	.69	.26	.22	.10	.17
8. establishes trust with various medical staffs.	4.24	.67	.66	.27	.21	.17	.14
9. reflects on whether nursing care she/he has provided is good enough.	4.17	.68	.66	.33	.13	.18	.24
10. acknowledges that there was a lack of nursing provided to the patient when the patient/guardian complains.	4.07	.71	.65	.10	.10	.15	.39
11. actively approaches nervous patients and helps them calm down.	4.14	.71	.64	.32	.03	.16	.30
12. works with her or his nurse colleagues, helping one another.[a]	4.41	.63	.63	.28	.32	.18	-.03
13. coordinates health examinations and appointments to promote patient comfort.	4.03	.74	.56	.26	.02	.13	.36
14. works fast enough to ensure smooth workflow.[a]	4.27	.66	.31	.74	.21	.26	.12
15. responds quickly to the reports of the patient/family.	4.29	.66	.32	.74	.20	.18	.17
16. thoroughly prepares in advance and constantly checks on the safety of medical treatments.[a]	4.37	.64	.35	.73	.27	.05	.12
17. assesses the patient's critical symptoms in time and informs the doctor, if necessary.	4.47	.61	.28	.71	.30	.09	.09
18. performs proper nursing practices according to my role and work.[a]	4.30	.62	.26	.58	.24	.28	.18
19. is trusted by colleagues because (s)he is devoted to her or his work.	4.24	.66	.35	.58	.30	.33	.05
20. communicates well with other departments and professionals.[a]	4.29	.65	.40	.58	.28	.20	.14
21. gains self-confidence through her or his personal growth experience.	4.13	.73	.37	.58	.14	.37	.17
22. talks to patients in a way they can understand.[a]	4.33	.65	.32	.55	.37	.14	.14
23. cares for patients based on professional ethics.	4.46	.65	.23	.36	.69	.13	.14
24. cares for patients conscientiously and honestly.	4.51	.62	.18	.39	.67	.11	.16
25. listens to patients/guardians carefully and answers their questions sincerely.	4.36	.62	.23	.29	.64	.20	.15
26. does job with a bright and energetic attitude.[a]	4.23	.67	.26	.20	.62	.24	.17
27. believes that s/he can make the most of her or his ability.[a]	4.14	.70	.32	.21	.61	.29	.08
28. is satisfied and happy with working as a nurse.[a]	3.78	.90	.20	.18	.14	.81	.17
29. feels proud and has a sense of achievement after completing a lot of daily work.[a]	4.02	.81	.22	.21	.18	.78	.17
30. feels happy for being helpful to others, even if nobody acknowledges.[a]	3.94	.85	.26	.22	.15	.74	.24
31. thinks the nursing profession is valuable.[a]	4.28	.82	.21	.21	.36	.63	.10
32. has compassion for patients/their families.[a]	3.92	.88	.22	.16	.03	.20	.75
33. feels bad when unable to take care of a patient's request.[a]	4.13	.70	.20	.19	.39	.14	.62
34. shares experiences that can help the patient/guardian.[a]	3.94	.79	.19	.12	.31	.24	.62

(continues)

Table 1

Primitive Construct of the Good Nurse Questionnaire Using Exploratory Factor Analysis and Reliability Analysis, Continued

Item	Mean SD	Factor Loading				
		1	2	3	4	5
Eigenvalue		7.6	5.3	3.7	3.4	2.3
Variance explained (%)		22.4	15.7	10.8	9.9	6.8
Cumulative variance (%)		22.4	38.0	48.9	58.8	65.6
Cronbach's α		.94	.93	.86	.87	.73

[a]Items were retained after confirmatory factor analysis.

Model Refining and Validating Stage

The hypothesized models of the good nurse questionnaire and better nursing questionnaire from the EFA results were tested using CFA on the second half of the main survey participants ($n = 468$ RNs). Most of the participants in this group were female (95.9%, $n = 449$), were an average of 34.49 ± 9.35 years old, self-identified as religious (57.3%, $n = 268$), worked as a staff nurse (83.3%, $n = 390$), and had an average career duration of 11.01 ± 8.46 years.

Good nurse questionnaire

Observational variables of latent construct were examined for reliability and significance using CFA. The model fit indices of the primitive good nurse questionnaire were not satisfactory, as shown in Table 3. Thus, the constructs of the primitive questionnaires from the EFA result were modified using the modification index of CFA. In the modified good nurse model, the number of items was decreased from 34 to 17, and the GFI was improved (normed $\chi^2 = 2.14$, GFI = .95, AGFI = .92, CFI = .97, NFI = .95, TLI = .96, SRMR = .03, and RMSEA = .05). The χ^2 test was significant ($p < .001$), indicating that the sample correlation matrix did not fit the hypothesized model. However, the χ^2 test is particularly sensitive to sample size and is often significant when a large sample is used (Hair et al., 2010). Therefore, examining various fit indices is recommended.

As shown in Table 4, the factor loadings of the 17 items ranged between .57 and .87, indicating statistical significance ($p < .001$). The convergent validity of the final model was acceptable considering that the AVE values ranged from .46 to .63, higher than a criterion of .5, with the exception of one factor that exhibited moderate convergent validity. Moreover, conceptual reliability ranged from .71 to .89, which was higher than the minimum acceptable level of .7, indicating convergent reliability.

To assess discriminant validity, the confidence interval of the estimated correlation between factors was calculated. Whereas factor correlations ranged between .66 (Factor 1 and Factor 5) and .84 (Factor 3 and Factor 4), the confidence interval of the estimated correlations between Factor 3 and Factor 4 ranged from .78 and .90 and did not include 1

(Haddock & Maio, 2004). The five constructs of the final model were considered validly discriminant.

After reviewing the CFA results of a good nurse questionnaire with regard to its use as a tool to measure the virtues of good nurses, the final measurement model consisted of five factors: collaboration (five items), professional competency (four items), self-efficacy (two items), a sense of achievement (three items), and compassion (three items). The Cronbach's alpha for internal consistency was .93, ranging from .70 to .89, depending on a factor of a good nurse. The definition for each factor is provided in Table 5.

Better nursing questionnaire

The model fit indices of the primitive questionnaire of the EFA results for better nursing were not satisfactory, as shown in Table 3, and the model was modified using the CFA. In the modified questionnaire model, the number of items was reduced from 26 to 16, and the GFIs were improved as follows: normed $\chi^2 = 2.06$, GFI = .95, AGFI = .93, CFI = .98, NFI = .97, TLI = .98, SRMR = .03, and RMSEA = .05.

As shown in Table 4, the factor loadings of the 16 items ranged between .75 and .89 ($p < .001$). The AVE values were .61–.74 (> .5), and convergent validity was acceptable. Conceptual reliability ranged between .90 and .93 (> .7), indicating good convergent reliability. Factor correlations ranged between .86 (Factor 2 and Factor 3) and .89 (Factor 1 and Factor 2). The confidence interval for the estimated correlation between Factor 1 and Factor 2 (.83 and .95) did not include 1. Thus, the discriminant validity of the final model was considered acceptable.

After reviewing the CFA results of the better nursing questionnaire, the final measurement model included three factors: person-centered nursing (eight items), proactive nursing (five items), and expertise in nursing (three items). The Cronbach's alpha for internal consistency was .96, ranging from .90 to .93. The definitions of each factor are provided in Table 5.

Discussion

The constructs of a good nurse questionnaire and better nursing questionnaire were validated by conducting exploratory and

Table 2

Primitive Construct of the Better Nursing Questionnaire Using Exploratory Factor Analysis and Reliability Analysis

Item	Mean	SD	Factor Loading		
			1	2	3
Better nursing is to…					
1. create a comfortable atmosphere so that the patient can easily talk about his or her concerns.	4.19	.68	.80	.27	.18
2. allow time for the patient to talk.	4.17	.71	.78	.31	.20
3. understand the patient better by listening attentively to what the patient has to say.	4.12	.71	.77	.31	.09
4. know and practice the importance of holding a patient's hand.[a]	4.16	.73	.74	.36	.16
5. spend time reflecting on and fully understanding herself or himself and thereby better reach out to patients.[a]	4.13	.73	.67	.34	.26
6. try to fulfill the wishes (advance directives) of terminal patients.[a]	4.14	.72	.66	.29	.34
7. facilitate family presence with the dying patient.	4.22	.70	.65	.39	.26
8. take care of patients as her or his own family.[a]	4.14	.78	.64	.38	.33
9. link resources to help patients with economic difficulties.	4.07	.79	.62	.35	.28
10. actively comfort the bereaved family.[a]	4.12	.75	.61	.27	.39
11. respect and consider as fellow human beings patients who are alienated or vulnerable (e.g., homelessness or alcoholism).[a]	4.09	.74	.59	.31	.37
12. feel humble self-awareness about life and death as a human being when witnessing the death of a patient.	4.14	.76	.59	.30	.35
13. treat patients not as objects of work from a disease-oriented perspective but as fellow human beings.[a]	4.10	.74	.56	.36	.29
14. feel glad or healed from taking care of patients.[a]	4.06	.81	.54	.29	.40
15. give attention to the subjective appeals of patients who are in discomfort without relying solely on objective information.	4.27	.71	.32	.74	.15
16. establish, plan, and carry out nursing goals.	4.14	.75	.37	.73	.33
17. approach patients/guardians with a better understanding through diverse experiences.[a]	4.30	.66	.29	.72	.28
18. become an agent for change in terms of fostering a positive relationship with the doctor.[a]	4.10	.75	.39	.72	.18
19. understand each patient's unique situation and find the most appropriate method to communicate and approach.[a]	4.19	.69	.32	.71	.38
20. actively and creatively seek the most appropriate nursing method for the patient.[a]	4.12	.76	.36	.70	.36
21. more actively approach patients who are having difficulties.[a]	4.23	.69	.39	.68	.28
22. approach the patient with an integrated judgment of the patient's situation.	4.21	.71	.31	.68	.40
23. use a nurse as a therapeutic tool.	4.03	.76	.33	.63	.14
24. make professional judgments and try to actively resolve situations.[a]	4.32	.66	.30	.35	.79
25. accurately and quickly respond to emergencies and unexpected situations.[a]	4.35	.68	.32	.28	.77
26. have a certain level of various competences such as responsibility, personality, ethics, and knowledge.[a]	4.26	.69	.30	.35	.74
Eigenvalue			15.0	1.4	1.0
Variance explained (%)			28.8	24.0	14.3
Cumulative variance (%)			28.8	52.8	67.1
Cronbach's α			.95	.94	.89

[a]Items were retained after confirmatory factor analysis.

confirmatory analyses on nationwide survey data of RNs in Korea. In this section, the five constructs of the good nurse questionnaire will be discussed first, followed by a discussion of the features of the better nursing questionnaire. On the basis of the results of this study, a good nurse may be defined as a

professional who performs her or his role well in terms of the essential five virtues of "collaboration, professional competency, self-efficacy, a sense of achievement, and compassion."

The first construct of the good nurse questionnaire, "collaboration," was also recognized as an attribute of a good

Table 3

Model Fit Indices of the Good Nurse Questionnaire and the Better Nursing Questionnaire

Fit Index		Absolute Fit Index							Incremental Fit Index		
		χ^2	p	Normed χ^2	RMSEA	SRMR	GFI	AGFI	NFI	CFI	TLI
Evaluation criteria			> .05	< 3	≤ .05	≤ .08	≥ .9	≥ .9	≥ .9	≥ .9	≥ .9
A good nurse	Original model (34 items)	1701.76 $df = 517$	< .001	3.29	.07	.05	.80	.76	.85	.89	.88
	Modified model (17 items)	232.97 $df = 109$	< .001	2.14	.05	.03	.95	.92	.95	.97	.96
Better nursing	Original model (26 items)	1090.62 $df = 296$	< .001	3.69	.05	.03	.84	.81	.90	.93	.92
	Modified model (16 items)	207.56 $df = 101$	< .001	2.06	.05	.03	.95	.93	.97	.98	.98

Note. RMSEA = root mean square error of approximation; SRMR = standardized root mean squared residual; GFI = goodness of fit index; AGFI = adjusted goodness of fit index; NFI = normed fit index; CFI = comparative fit index; TLI = Tucker–Lewis index.

nurse from the perspective of nurses in a previous study (Catlett & Lovan, 2011; Kim et al., 2019). It may be difficult for patients to be aware of how collaboration among nurses influences their care. The modern code of ethics for nurses emphasizes collaboration with other healthcare professionals based on mutual trust and respect (International Council of Nurses, 2012; Korean Nurses Association, 2013). Collaboration is an ethical responsibility of nurses because quality care and patient safety are possible in today's complex healthcare environments through interdisciplinary care teams working in collaboration with multiple healthcare providers and through nurses creating a bridge between these care teams and patients. Nurses relay patient information to other nurses, doctors, physiotherapists, social workers, dieticians, and other healthcare professionals. Thus, the nursing virtue of collaboration has become even more critical.

The two virtues of "professional competency" and "compassion" on the good nurse questionnaire were frequently identified in previous studies both by nurses (Aydin Er et al., 2017; Catlett & Lovan, 2011; Kim et al., 2019) and by patients (Rchaidia et al., 2009; Van der Elst et al., 2012). There is no question that a good nurse should present appropriate professional knowledge, skills, and attitudes with compassion. Nurses must continuously improve their knowledge and skills as healthcare professionals to adopt new treatments and better technology for the benefit of their patients. At the same time, a good nurse must be able to feel empathy toward patients as well as support and build therapeutic relationships with their patients (Gastmans et al., 1998). A nurse who has excellent nursing knowledge and skills but lacks a compassionate attitude may not be considered to be a good nurse.

Finally, "self-efficacy" and "a sense of achievement" were identified as critical virtues of a good nurse. A good nurse not only believes in his or her own ability with a positive attitude

for patient care but also possesses a strong sense of achievement based on professional pride and satisfaction in his or her nursing practice. These psychological attributes are common characteristics of professionals (Evetts, 2014). Nursing care is a professional response that is customized to a wide array of difficult patient conditions, which may be interpreted quite differently depending on an individual nurse's self-efficacy. In the current healthcare environment, nurses are required to confront and manage diverse challenges. Thus, nurses must possess a high self-efficacy. Furthermore, patients in a Japanese study (Izumi et al., 2006) expressed that they expected a good nurse to have pride in and a passion for nursing work. This study also found that good nurses felt pride and happiness in their nursing work, which related closely to their professionalism. In particular, nurses' professionalism in terms of valuing their work may lead them to remain in their profession and workplace (Çelik & Hisar, 2012; Guerrero et al., 2017). Because of concerns over high rates of professional attrition, sense of achievement has been increasingly considered to be a key virtue in the nursing profession. In conclusion, a good nurse must be able to provide professional care with a compassionate attitude, collaborate with diverse work teams, and present a high level of self-efficacy and sense of achievement.

Three aspects characterize the concept of better nursing, including, in descending order of explained variance, "person-centered nursing" (28.8%), "proactive nursing" (24.0%), and "expertise in nursing" (14.3%). Of nursing practices exhibited by good nurses, better nursing in this study referred to a nurse who performs at a higher level than expected. As anticipated, one of the better-nursing characteristics, "expertise in nursing," facilitates the integration by nurses of professional knowledge and skills into actual practice with a deep understanding of a clinical situation based on their experience. However, this factor explained only 14.3% of the concept.

Table 4

Final Construct of the Good Nurse Questionnaire Using Confirmatory Factor Analysis and Reliability Analysis

Questionnaire/Factor	Item	Mean	SD	λ	SMC	CR	AVE	Cronbach's α
A good nurse								
Factor 1						.89	.62	.89
	4	4.18	0.67	.87	.75			
	6	4.16	0.69	.81	.66			
	5	4.21	0.69	.78	.61			
	12	4.42	0.63	.73	.54			
	1	4.18	0.72	.73	.54			
Factor 2						.85	.59	.79
	16	4.30	0.66	.73	.53			
	18	4.24	0.64	.77	.59			
	22	4.32	0.66	.76	.58			
	20	4.18	0.75	.82	.68			
Factor 3						.71	.55	.71
	27	4.15	0.69	.74	.55			
	26	4.23	0.71	.75	.56			
Factor 4						.83	.63	.83
	29	4.01	0.79	.80	.64			
	30	3.91	0.86	.84	.70			
	28	3.75	0.92	.73	.54			
Factor 5						.71	.46	70
	33	4.12	0.69	.75	.56			
	34	3.94	0.83	.70	.49			
	32	3.93	0.82	.57	.32			
Total								.93
Better nursing								
Factor 1						.93	.61	.93
	14	4.03	0.83	.75	.56			
	13	4.11	0.76	.77	.60			
	11	4.13	0.76	.81	.66			
	6	4.11	0.76	.82	.67			
	10	4.07	0.79	.79	.62			
	8	4.15	0.74	.80	.63			
	4	4.18	0.75	.78	.61			
	5	4.08	0.76	.75	.56			
Factor 2						.91	.66	.91
	20	4.13	0.75	.85	.71			
	19	4.21	0.69	.86	.74			
	18	4.03	0.77	.77	.59			
	21	4.20	0.69	.80	.64			
	17	4.22	0.71	.80	.64			

(continues)

Table 4

Final Construct of the Good Nurse Questionnaire Using Confirmatory Factor Analysis and Reliability Analysis, Continued

Questionnaire/Factor	Item	Mean	SD	λ	SMC	CR	AVE	Cronbach's α
Factor 3						.90	.74	.90
	25	4.33	0.70	.83	.69			
	24	4.30	0.67	.89	.78			
	26	4.23	0.71	.87	.76			
Total								.96

Note. All factor loadings were statistically significant at the $p < .001$ level. λ = standardized factor loading; SMC = square multiple correlation; CR = conceptual reliability; AVE = average variance extraction.

"Person-centered nursing" and "proactive nursing" largely explained the concept of better nursing. In line with "person-centered nursing," nurses are expected to be nonjudgmental and respectful of each patient's life, preserve the personhood of their patients, and feel that they are healed through the therapeutic relationship. Currently in nursing, person-centered care is defined as a holistic approach that provides respectful and individualized care to patients (Morgan & Yoder, 2012). The more that medical treatment depends on high technology to maximize efficiency and accuracy, the more that patients desire to seek humanity in nursing care. Nurses should pursue person-centered care continuously in their own nursing practices without compromising on nursing care quality. Although person-centered care may not be challenging for most patients, it becomes critical for those patients with special needs or complex conditions. Exceptional efforts are required for a nurse to be responsive to and responsible for those patients. Therefore, the concept of person-centered care may not be considered beyond "proactive nursing" in better nursing. "Proactive nursing" means taking an active approach toward patients to address individualized care needs using creative problem-solving abilities and playing a role as an agent for change in the treatment team.

Better nursing practices were highlighted in exemplars cited by Benner (1984). She asserted that these exemplars described excellence and power in nursing, including transformative power, integrative caring, advocacy, healing power, affirmative power, and creative problem solving. Better nursing may require the virtues and excellence of a good nurse. According to Aristotle's virtue ethics, virtue grows mostly from teaching and results from habit. Therefore, being a good nurse is a process that requires teaching, repeated practice, and then habituation in one's work. This study has practical and educational implications. The five essential virtues of a good nurse may be used to guide a prelicensure nursing education program. To train up good nurses, nursing education should cultivate all five of these virtues, which should be taught via classroom and extracurricular activities.

The virtues of a good nurse and the characteristics of better nursing may be used to evaluate nurses and their practice in nursing organizations. Most nursing instruments assess either nursing competencies or caring behaviors separately in relation to a good nurse or better nursing (Park & Kim, 2016). However, being a good nurse and acting better nursing may require both competent practice and caring behavior. Furthermore, nursing professional development must focus

Table 5

Descriptions of the Questionnaires' Dimensions

Questionnaire	Dimension	Description
A good nurse		
Factor 1	Collaboration	Establishing a collaborative relationship with nurses and other personnel
Factor 2	Professional competency	Playing a diverse nurse role based on professional knowledge and skills
Factor 3	Self-efficacy	Believing one's own ability with a positive attitude
Factor 4	A sense of achievement	Having a strong sense of pride and satisfaction in one's nursing care
Factor 5	Compassion	Having empathy to patients and supporting them
Better nursing		
Factor 1	Person-centered nursing	Treating a patient with respect as a whole person, preserving personhood
Factor 2	Proactive nursing	Carrying out proactive roles for caring a patient
Factor 3	Expertise in nursing	Providing care in a fluid and seamless manner

on "what sort of nurse they ought to be," while admitting the importance of learning "what and how to do" for the nursing profession. The concepts of the good nurse questionnaire and better nursing questionnaire may help expose nurses to a good role model for clinical practice in terms of "what sort of nurse they ought to be" as well as "what and how to do." Therefore, the questionnaires may be useful for the evaluation of nurses and their practice in a holistic way and for guiding nurses to reinforce their strengths and improve their weaknesses in terms of being a good nurse and acting better nursing.

The study findings are meaningful given that Korean nurses' understandings of a good nurse and better nursing have never been formally discussed and agreed upon until now. It is timely to have formulated these agreed-upon concepts because of the increasing diversity in the nursing workforce in terms of age, gender, academic background, and previous work experiences. However, the results of this study should be considered in the cultural context of Korean nursing. Because the role and status of nurses vary from country to country, the concept of Korean nurses of "good nurse" and "better nursing" may not be generalizable to other countries. However, on the basis of the findings of previous studies, the characteristics of these two concepts seem to share much in common across countries. If the questionnaires are used in different countries, nursing scholars may compare the related concepts and better understand how different nursing systems and roles influence the concept of a good nurse and better nursing. In addition, these two concepts are changing over time alongside changes in the role of nurses. Therefore, continued study of these concepts is necessary.

Acknowledgments

This research was funded by the Hospital Nurses Association of Korea in 2016. We would like to thank Young Rhan Um and Kyung Ja Song, who conducted the qualitative study titled "A Good Nurse, Better Nursing" and provided significant comments and heartfelt support during the project.

Author Contributions

Study conception and design: MP, EP
Data collection: MP
Data analysis and interpretation: MP, EP
Drafting of the article: MP, EP
Critical revision of the article: MP, EP

References

Aydin Er, R., Sehiralti, M., & Akpinar, A. (2017). Attributes of a good nurse. *Nursing Ethics*, *24*(2), 238–250. https://doi.org/10.1177/0969733015595543

Begley, A. M. (2010). On being a good nurse: Reflections on the past and preparing for the future. *International Journal of Nursing Practice*, *16*(6), 525–532. https://doi.org/10.1111/j.1440-172X.2010.01878.x

Benner, P. (1984). *From novice to expert: Excellence and power in clinical nursing practice*. Addison-Wesley.

Catlett, S., & Lovan, S. R. (2011). Being a good nurse and doing the right thing: A replication study. *Nursing Ethics*, *18*(1), 54–63. https://doi.org/10.1177/0969733010386162

Çelik, S., & Hisar, F. (2012). The influence of the professionalism behaviour of nurses working in health institutions on job satisfaction. *International Journal of Nursing Practice*, *18*(2), 180–187. https://doi.org/10.1111/j.1440-172X.2012.02019.x

Cho, N. O., Hong, Y. S., Han, S. S., & Um, Y. R. (2006). Attributes perceived by cancer patients as a good nurse. *Clinical Nursing Research*, *11*(2), 149–162.

Chou, H. C., Chen, S. Y., Tsai, H. Y., & Chou, H. H. (2007). Treating patients as relatives: Cancer patients' perspectives on the good nurse. *Journal of Evidence-Based Nursing*, *3*(3), 188–194. (Original work published in Chinese)

Evetts, J. (2014). The concept of professionalism: Professional work, professional practice and learning. In S. Billet, C. Harteis, & H. Gruber (Eds.), *International handbook of research in professional and practice-based learning* (pp. XXI, 1383). Springer.

Fry, S. T. (2004). Nursing ethics. In G. Khushf (Ed.), *Handbook of bioethics: Taking stock of the field from a philosophical perspective* (pp. 489–505). Springer Netherlands.

Gallagher, A., Horton, K., Tschudin, V., & Lister, S. (2009). Exploring the views of patients with cancer on what makes a good nurse—A pilot study. *Nursing Times*, *105*(23), 24–27.

Gastmans, C., Dierckx de Casterle, B., & Schotsmans, P. (1998). Nursing considered as moral practice: A philosophical–ethical interpretation of nursing. *Kennedy Institute of Ethics Journal*, *8*(1), 43–69.

Guerrero, S., Chênevert, D., & Kilroy, S. (2017). New graduate nurses' professional commitment: Antecedents and outcomes. *Journal of Nursing Scholarship*, *49*(5), 572–579. https://doi.org/10.1111/jnu.12323

Haddock, G., & Maio, G. R. (2004). *Contemporary perspectives on the psychology of attitudes*. Psychology Press.

Hair, J. F., Black, W. C., Babin, B. J., & Anderson, R. E. (2010). *Multivariate data analysis* (7th ed.). Pearson Prentice Hall.

Han, S., Um, Y., Hong, Y., & Cho, N. (2006). Korean patients' conceptions of a good nurse. *Korean Journal of Medical Ethics Education*, *9*(2), 125–142. (Original work published in Korean)

International Council of Nurses. (2012). *The ICN code of ethics for nurses*. Retrieved from https://www.aynla.org/2012/12/icn-code-of-ethics-for-nurses-2012/

Izumi, S., Konishi, E., Yahiro, M., & Kodama, M. (2006). Japanese patients' descriptions of "the good nurse": Personal involvement and professionalism. *Advances in Nursing Science*, *29*(2), E14–E26.

Kang, H. (2013). Discussions on the suitable interpretation of model fit indices and the strategies to fit model in structural equation modeling. *Journal of the Korean Data Analysis Society, 15*(2), 653–668. (Original work published in Korean)

Kim, G., Jung, E., Cho, M., Han, S. Y., Jang, M., Lee, M., ... Shim, M. S. (2019). Revisiting the meaning of a good nurse. *The Open Nursing Journal, 13*, 75–84. https://doi.org/10.2174/1874434601913010075

Korean Nurses Association. (2013). *The code of ethics for nurses.* KNA. (Original work published in Korean)

Kyriazos, T. A. (2018). Applied psychometrics: Sample size and sample power considerations in factor analysis (EFA, CFA) and SEM in general. *Psychology, 9*, 2207–2230. https://doi.org/10.4236/psych.2018.98126

Mooi, E., Sarstedt, M., & Mooi-Reci, I. (2018). *Market research: The process, data, and methods using Stata.* Springer Singapore.

Morgan, S., & Yoder, L. H. (2012). A concept analysis of person-centered care. *Journal of Holistic Nursing, 30*(1), 6–15. https://doi.org/10.1177/0898010111412189

Park, E. J., & Kim, M. H. (2016). Characteristics of nursing and caring concepts measured in nursing competencies or caring behaviors tools. *Journal of Korean Academy of Nursing Administration, 22*(5), 480–495. https://doi.org/10.11111/jkana.2016.22.5.480

Pett, M. A., Lackey, N. R., & Sullivan, J. J. (2003). *Making sense of factor analysis: The use of factor analysis for instrument development in health care research.* Sage.

Polit, D. F., & Beck, C. T. (2006). The content validity index: Are you sure you know what's being reported? Critique and recommendations. *Research in Nursing & Health, 29*(5), 489–497. https://doi.org/10.1002/nur.20147

Rchaidia, L., Dierckx de Casterlé, B., De Blaeser, L., & Gastmans, C. (2009). Cancer patients' perceptions of the good nurse: A literature review. *Nursing Ethics, 16*(5), 528–542. https://doi.org/10.1177/0969733009106647

Um, Y., Song, K., & Park, M. (2017). *A good nurse, better nursing.* Jongdam Media. (Original work published in Korean)

Van der Elst, E., Dierckx de Casterlé, B., & Gastmans, C. (2012). Elderly patients' and residents' perceptions of 'the good nurse': A literature review. *Journal of Medical Ethics, 38*(2), 93–97. https://doi.org/10.1136/medethics-2011-100046

12

Stress, Workplace Violence and Burnout in Nurses Working in King Abdullah Medical City During Al-Hajj Season

Ahmad RAYAN[1]* • Mo'men SISAN[2] • Omar BAKER[3]

ABSTRACT

Background: The Hajj pilgrimage to Mecca, one of the largest mass gatherings in the world, is associated with various challenges for nurses. One of these challenges is increased levels of workplace violence. Therefore, handling and mitigating workplace violence against nurses during Hajj, when nurses face a higher risk of violence and most experience stress and burnout, is of particular importance.

Purpose: The aims of this study were to identify the types and sources of workplace violence, examine the relationship between burnout in nurses and the variables of stress and workplace violence, and identify from the perspective of nurses measures to effectively handle and mitigate these issues during Hajj season.

Methods: This study used a descriptive correlational design. A convenience sample of 118 nurses completed the Perceived Stress Scale, the Maslach Burnout Inventory, and the modified version of the Joint Programme on Workplace Violence in the Health Sector published by the International Labour Office in Geneva. Data analysis was done using an independent samples t test and Pearson product–moment correlation.

Results: One hundred eighteen nurses completed the study. Over two thirds (65%) were female, and 56% reported experiencing at least one type of violence, of which bullying/mobbing, racial harassment, threats, and physical violence accounted for 61%, 15%, 12%, and 12%, respectively. Nurse managers displayed violent behaviors against 54% of the participants. Participants reported high levels of stress and burnout. A positive relationship was found between stress and emotional exhaustion ($r = .387$, $p < .01$). Providing effective security measures and staff training regarding how to deal with violence at the workplace were the main measures identified to help reduce workplace violence.

Conclusions: Providing effective security measures and tailored intervention programs addressing how to deal with violence in the workplace may enable nurses to handle violent behaviors more effectively.

KEY WORDS:
stress, workplace violence, burnout, Hajj.

Introduction

Hajj is one of the main pillars of Islam. Pilgrimage to the holy place of Mecca in Saudi Arabia takes place once a year during the month of "Thulhijah," which is the last month in the "Hijri" calendar. In 2016, 1.8 million Muslims from all over the world participated in the Hajj (Al Arabiya, 2016). This massive gathering significantly increases the risks for various accident and emergency situations involving the pilgrims. One of the main injuries during Hajj is trauma, which results from factors including walking long distances and motor vehicle accidents in congested areas full of pilgrims and vehicles (Ahmed, Arabi, & Memish, 2006). In addition, the immensely crowded settings increase the risk of transmitting infections such as meningococcal disease and pneumonia (Alsafadi, Goodwin, & Syed, 2011). Dealing with these conditions adds extra burdens on and increases the stress levels of nurses who provide care to Hajj pilgrims.

According to the latest study conducted during the Hajj period, most nurses were found to have limited knowledge and awareness regarding disaster preparedness plans and strategies for managing mass gathering disasters (Alzahrani & Kyratsis, 2017). Subsequently, there is a need to identify nurses' concerns and experiences associated with mass gathering during the Hajj such as workplace violence, stress, and burnout (Alsaqri, 2014; Tsouros & Efstathiou, 2007). In fact, addressing nurses' concerns during Hajj is of special importance and has international significance, as nurses working during the Hajj are of different ethnic and national backgrounds. The current study not only investigates workplace violence, stress, and burnout but also identifies from the perspective of nurses the measures that may help effectively handle and mitigate workplace violence during Hajj season. The findings may be helpful in the development of special intervention programs to control workplace violence in the future.

King Abdullah Medical City in the Holy Capital of Mekkah (KAMC-HC) is one of the largest medical cities in

[1]PhD, Assistant Professor, Psychiatric and Mental Health Nursing, Zarqa University, Jordan • [2]BSN, RN, Oncology Specialist Nurse, King Abdullah Medical City, Mecca, Saudi Arabia • [3]PhD, RN, Associate Professor, College of Nursing, King Saud University, Riyadh, Saudi Arabia.

Saudi Arabia that provides medical care to pilgrims during Hajj season. KAMC-HC has 350 beds covering all specialties and employs nurses of different nationalities. Healthcare manpower at KAMC-HC is not increased during Hajj season. Subsequently, to meet the increased work demands during this period, nurses at KAMC-HC usually work 12 hours a day for at least 15 days or more consecutively. Long shifts and stressful work conditions understandably increase the stress and burnout levels of nurses (Dall'Ora, Griffiths, Ball, Simon, & Aiken, 2015; S. Wu, Zhu, Wang, Wang, & Lan, 2007). Furthermore, during Hajj season, many nurses are reassigned from their normal departments to emergency rooms (ERs), operating rooms, or intensive care units (ICUs). Most standby nurses are not familiar with the daily routine of these critical care units, which may further aggravate their stress levels.

Violence in the workplace is another factor that contributes to stress in nurses and decreases their work productivity (Gates, Gillespie, & Succop, 2011). Violence in the workplace against nurses is a worldwide phenomenon that is largely independent of ethnic/national background (Spector, Zhou, & Che, 2014). However, incidents of violence against nurses typically increase during Hajj because of shortages in nursing staff, language barriers (inability to understand the language of patients who come from all over the world), and shortages of security personnel (Alkorashy & Al Moalad, 2016; Mohamed, 2002). Because of their close contact with patients and their families, nurses face a higher risk of workplace violence than other healthcare professionals (Kwok et al., 2006). It is well documented in the literature that violence in the workplace contributes to work dissatisfaction, decreased productivity, high rates of stress and turnover, and burnout (Gates et al., 2011; Laschinger & Grau, 2012; Stimpfel & Aiken, 2013). To date, limited statistics are available regarding the prevalence of workplace violence against nurses during Hajj season.

A recent study conducted in Saudi Arabia reported that almost 50% of nurses experienced violence at the workplace in 2015 (Alkorashy & Al Moalad, 2016). Alkorashy and Al Moalad (2016) recommended developing specific policies for preventing workplace violence. However, additional preventive measures related to security measures in the workplace and preparing staff to deal effectively with the potential violent incidences during Hajj may be necessary. However, little is known regarding how workplace violence relates to levels of stress and burnout in nurses working during Hajj season, making it difficult to tailor and conduct intervention programs to address this issue and improve working conditions. Therefore, the purpose of this study was to examine the relationship between workplace violence, stress, and burnout in nurses working at KAMC-HC. The related objectives were

- to identify the types and sources of workplace violence toward nurses working at KAMC-HC during Hajj season;
- to identify from the perspective of nurses measures to effectively handle and mitigate workplace violence at

KAMC-HC;
- to assess levels of stress and burnout among nurses working at KAMC-HC during Hajj season; and
- to assess the relationships among workplace violence, stress, and burnout in nurses.

Methods

Data collection was completed using a self-administered questionnaire during the rituals of Al-Hajj from September 1 to 15, 2016. For the purpose of this study, a descriptive, cross-sectional, and correlational design was used. Institutional review board approval was obtained from the KAMC (Approval number 2016/58). Confidentiality was guaranteed for all study participants. Anonymity and autonomy were assured for all participants, and all were free to participate or withdraw from the study at any time without consequence. In addition, participants were briefed about the purpose of the study before data collection. Data were collected by the first author.

Participants

All of the participants in this study were working at KAMC-HC. According to the latest statistics published by the Saudi Arabia Ministry of Health in 2016, the total number of nurses (including midwives) working in Saudi Arabia includes about 180,821 of various nationalities. More than half of these (101,256) work for the Ministry of Health, representing about 57.6% of the nursing workforce. The approximately 900 nurses working at KAMC-HC are nationals of 10 countries, including the Philippines, Jordan, India, Egypt, the United States, Yemen, Lebanon, Malaysia, Pakistan, and Turkistan. The largest percentage (38.3%) are from the Philippines.

On the basis of a G*Power calculation for an independent samples t test with an alpha level of .05, a power of 0.80, and a medium effect size, 102 participants were needed. To obtain more power, the sample size was increased to 120. Inclusion criteria were as follows: being a full-time registered nurse working at KAMC-HC during Al-Hajj season, having over 1 year of experience at KAMC-HC, and working at patient bedsides during Al-Hajj season. Data were not collected from nurses who did not meet the inclusion criteria, including those having less than a year of experience at KAMC-HC, not providing direct care to patients, or not working during Al-Hajj season. Five hundred ninety of KAMC-HC's 900 nurses met the inclusion criteria. A convenience sample of 120 registered nurses working at KAMC-HC was recruited. About 11.2% (66) had been reassigned to work in other departments such as ICU or ER during Hajj season.

Instruments

A demographic questionnaire and three scales, including the modified version of the Joint Programme on Workplace Violence in the Health Sector published by the International

Labour Office, the Perceived Stress Scale (PSS), and Maslach Burnout Inventory (MBI), were included in the questionnaire. A pilot study was conducted on 31 nurses to assess questionnaire validity and reliability. The questionnaire took about 10–15 minutes to complete during the pilot study, and all of the subscales earned a Cronbach's alpha of at least .72.

Demographic Questionnaire

The demographic questionnaire gathered data on age, gender, education level, years of experiences, and marital status.

Questionnaire on the Prevalence, Types, Sources, and Measures Used to Handle Workplace Violence

A survey developed by the "Joint Programme on Workplace Violence in the Health Sector" of the International Labour Office, International Council of Nurses, World Health Organization, and Public Services International (2003) was used in this study. This survey investigates both the types of workplace violence, including psychological violence (threats, bullying/mobbing, and racial harassment) and physical violence, and the sources of violence, including managers, colleagues, and other sources (e.g., visitors, police). Examples of measures taken to handle workplace violence include security measures and restricting public access. In addition, participants had the option to select more than one alternative. Furthermore, participants with no experience of workplace violence were given the chance to select answers concerning the most effective measures to reduce workplace violence based on incidences of violence that they had witnessed. This survey measure has excellent psychometric properties and has been used in countries such as Lebanon, South Africa, Brazil, Portugal, Australia, and Thailand (Di Martino, 2002). In the current study, Cronbach's alpha coefficients for the types, sources, and measures for handling workplace violence were adequate to high, ranging from .76 to .93.

The Perceived Stress Scale

In this study, the 10-item PSS (PSS-10) was used to measure the level of stress of the participants. The PSS is considered one of the most commonly used psychological tools to measure stress perception in individuals (Cohen & Williamson, 1988). It comprises multiple-choice questions that are scored on a 5-point Likert scale (0 = *never* to 4 = *very often*). Items 4, 5, 7, and 8 are reverse scored. The PSS-10 is a reliable scale, and the original total scale has a reported Cronbach's alpha of .78 (Cohen & Williamson, 1988). Recently, the measure has shown evidence of excellent psychometric properties in various populations (Andreou et al., 2011; Chaaya, Osman, Naassan, & Mahfoud, 2010; Reis, Hino, & Añez, 2010). Cronbach's alpha coefficients for the PSS-10 range from .78 to .91 (Cohen, Kamarck, & Mermelstein, 1983; Cohen & Williamson, 1988; Ezzati et al., 2014; S. M. Wu &

Amtmann, 2013). Total scores range from 0 to 40, with 0–7 indicating very low stress, 8–11 indicating low stress, 12–15 indicating average stress, 16–20 indicating high stress, and 21 or over indicating very high stress (Cohen et al., 1983).

Maslach Burnout Inventory

The MBI was used to measure the level of burnout perceived by the participants. The MBI, a 22-item instrument developed by Maslach and Jackson (1981), comprises three subscales. The Emotional Exhaustion (EE) subscale has nine items that address the sense of emotional exhaustion at work, the Personal Accomplishment (PA) subscale has eight items that address the sense of reduced professional competence and decreased positive individual interactions at work, and the Depersonalization (DP) subscale has five items that address the sense of decreased personal involvement with people and emotional disinterest in one's job. The MBI includes frequencies ranging from 0 (never) to 6 (everyday), with low PA scores and high DP and EE scores indicating job burnout. Total EE subscale scores below 17, between 17 and 26, and higher than 26 represent low, moderate, and high levels of job burnout, respectively. Total DP subscale scores below 7, between 7 and 12, and higher than 12 represent low, intermediate, and high levels of burnout, respectively (Maslach, Schaufeli, & Leiter, 2001). Finally, total PA subscale scores below 32, between 32 and 38, and higher than 38 represent high, intermediate, and low levels of burnout, respectively. Maslach and Jackson (1981) reported evidence supporting that the 22-item MBI has both high reliability and validity. The reliability coefficients for the subscales were .89 for EE, .74 for PA, and .77 for DP (Maslach & Jackson, 1981). Furthermore, Iwanicki and Schwab (1981) reported Cronbach's alpha values of .90, .76, and .76 for the EE, DP, and PA subscales, respectively. The scores for each subscale of the MBI should be considered separately and are not suitable for combining into a single total score.

Data Analysis

Data were analyzed using SPSS Version 21 (IBM, Armonk, NY, USA). Descriptive statistics were used to present the sample characteristics, and the independent samples *t* test and Pearson product–moment correlation were used to examine the relationships among workplace violence, stress, and nurse burnout.

Results

Demographic Data

Of the 120 nurses who were invited, 118 nurses completed and returned the study questionnaires, representing a response rate of 98%. The mean age of the participants was 29.14 years. About 65% were female, and most (71%) were married. About 43% worked in close units, and most (91.5%) held a bachelor degree in nursing as their highest level of academic achievement. Mean experience was 7.53

TABLE 1.
Helpful Measures for Handling Workplace Violence From the Perspective of Nurses

Measure	Nurse Mentioned (%)
Security measures (e.g., guards, alarms, portable telephones)	65
Training (e.g., workplace violence, coping strategies, communication skills, conflict resolution, self-defense)	64
Reduced periods of working alone	44
Increased staff numbers	41
Restricted public access	39

(*SD* = 6.8) years. Thirty-seven (31%) had less than 5 years of experience, 64 (55%) had 5–10 years of experience, and 17 (14%) had over 10 years of experience. The largest numbers of participants were from the Philippines (37%), India (28%), and Pakistan (13%), with fewer numbers from other countries, including Jordan, Egypt, Yemen, Lebanon, and Turkistan (22%).

Types and Sources of Workplace Violence Toward Nurses

About 56% of the participants reported experiencing workplace violence during the last 6 months. In terms of types of workplace violence, about 61%, 15%, 12%, and 12% of the participants were exposed to bullying/mobbing, racial harassment, threat, and physical violence, respectively. About 54% of the participants reported experiencing violence from their managers, whereas 32% and 14% reported experiencing violence from colleagues (other nurses) and other sources (e.g., visitors, police), respectively.

Measures Deemed by Nurses as Helpful to Handling Workplace Violence

Table 1 presents the measures recommended by nurses as helpful in handling workplace violence. The most commonly

TABLE 3.
Differences in Stress and Burnout Based on Having Experienced Violence in the Workplace (N = 118)

Variable/Exposed to Any Type of Violence?	Mean	SD	t	p
Stress			3.80	<.001
No	18.24	7.40		
Yes	20.80	6.30		
Emotional exhaustion			1.60	.11
No	29.79	10.69		
Yes	33.53	10.97		
Depersonalization			0.03	.97
No	37.77	9.80		
Yes	37.83	10.33		
Personal accomplishment			1.00	.31
No	9.79	9.54		
Yes	11.92	9.61		

reported included providing effective security measures in the workplace and providing staff training. The least commonly reported measure was restricting public access to workplaces.

Levels of Burnout and Stress

Table 2 presents the levels of stress and burnout, respectively, for each subscale of the MBI. The participants reported high levels of psychological stress, emotional exhaustion, personal accomplishment, and depersonalization, reflecting high overall levels of burnout.

Relationships Among Workplace Violence, Stress, and Burnout

An independent samples *t* test was used to examine if there was a significant difference in stress and burnout based on experiencing violence in the workplace. Expectedly, nurses who were exposed to violence at their place of work reported higher levels of stress and burnout than those who did not. However, stress levels were significantly different only between nurses who were exposed to violence and

TABLE 2.
Levels of Burnout and Stress Among Nurses

Item/Measure Scale	Min	Max	Mean	SD	Indication
Burnout					
Emotional exhaustion	6.00	48.00	31.30	10.93	Scores > 30 indicate high burnout levels
Personal accomplishment	0.00	30.00	10.58	9.58	Scores < 33 indicate high burnout levels
Depersonalization	0.00	48.00	37.92	10.04	Scores > 12 indicate high burnout levels
Stress					
Perceived Stress Scale	1.00	27.00	18.17	8.33	Scores of 16–20 indicate high level of stress

those who were not (Table 3). Pearson product–moment correlation indicated a significantly positive relationship between stress and the EE subscale of MBI ($r = .387$, $p < .01$). However, stress was not significantly correlated with either the PA or DP subscale of MBI ($r = .022$, $p > .05$; $r = .015$, $p > .05$, respectively).

Discussion

The current study investigated the relationships among workplace violence, stress, and burnout in nurses at KAMC-HC during Al-Hajj season 1437 AH. Prevalence of workplace violence, types of violence, and the measures to reduce violence were highlighted. To the best of authors' knowledge, this is the first study to explore the relationships among workplace violence, stress, and nurse burnout during Hajj season. The response rate of 98% is considered favorable given the exploratory nature of this topic. The results indicated that participants who were subject to violence in the workplace experienced higher levels of stress than participants who were not. In addition, a positive relationship was found between stress and the EE subscale of MBI.

Overall, the participants reported very high levels of psychological stress and burnout. In addition, more than half reported having experienced workplace violence in the most recent month. As nursing is a high-pressure profession, high stress levels is an expected outcome, especially during heavy workload periods such as Hajj season. In fact, stress-free environments are rare in the nursing profession. However, some factors such as high workloads and poor working conditions make nurses vulnerable to physical and psychological stress (Geiger-Brown et al., 2012; Trinkoff et al., 2011). Nurse managers should monitor stress levels among their employees, identify stress-contributing factors, and adopt measures to alleviate stress such as providing appropriate work schedules for nurses and improving communications between them (Carr, Kelley, Keaton, & Albrecht, 2011).

In this study, the participants who had been exposed to workplace violence of any type during Hajj season tended to be more stressed than those who had not. Most of the participants were not Arabic speakers, which may affect their levels of stress and burnout, and workplace violence experience. During Hajj season, most nurses are required to work additional hours to compensate for staff shortages while dealing with higher frequencies of emergencies and accidents. According to the literature, mandatory overtime may negatively affect the psychological well-being of nurses because of lack of control (Lobo, Fisher, Ploeg, Peachey, & Akhtar-Danesh, 2013).

Another important finding of this study was that 54% of the participants reported experiencing workplace violence from their managers, which is relatively high when taking into consideration that managers should be a source of support and strength for their nursing staff. In addition, psychological violence was more prevalent than physical violence. Nurse managers should not ignore the huge impact of stress on the functioning of an organization. In addition, these managers should be aware of the relationship between experiencing violence in the workplace and stress among nurses. In fact, both psychological and physical violence in the workplace seriously influence the health and well-being of nurses (Gates et al., 2011).

The participants in this study reported higher levels of burnout compared with a study of multinational nurses working in Saudi Arabia (Al-Turki et al., 2010). Worldwide, comparative studies have shown burnout to be a significant problem inside the world of nursing, with nurses having the highest risk of burnout of any category of healthcare provider (Bernardi, Catania, & Marceca, 2005). The high levels of burnout found in this study may be associated with high levels of stress during Hajj season. In a sample of 1,363 nurses working in hospitals, workload correlated significantly with emotional exhaustion (Greenglass, Burke, & Fiksenbaum, 2001).

Previous research highlighted the importance of developing specific policies for preventing workplace violence (Alkorashy& Al Moalad, 2016). However, providing effective security measures and staff training on how to deal with violence at the workplace were considered by the participants in this study to be the most helpful actions for reducing workplace violence. Thus, these strategies should be given priority consideration when dealing with workplace violence during periods of mass gatherings such as Hajj.

Strengths and Limitations

This study highlighted the contemporary and serious issues faced by nurses of different nationalities working during Hajj season. Because the participants were recruited from one large hospital during a specific period, it may be difficult to generalize the outcomes beyond the limitations of place and situation. However, this study reflects a phenomenon of concern in nursing, as nurses worldwide experience higher workloads during crisis situations. Furthermore, this study explored the relationships among workplace violence, stress, and nurse burnout, which has important implications for nursing practice and research.

Conclusion and Recommendations

This study offers important recommendations for the nursing profession. Preventing workplace violence is more important than providing interventions. In addressing the causes of the problem, it will be necessary to effectively address the related causal factors. Nurses require training to handle violent behaviors effectively. Managers have the primary responsibility to provide adequate staffing and safety measures and to assign sufficient security personnel to critical care areas such as the ER and ICU. Moreover, each hospital should maintain policies addressing violence in the workplace. The policy concerning violence should be appraised on an annual basis (Rayan, Qurneh, Elayyan, & Baker, 2016).

Further research is necessary to further investigate the effectiveness of applying specific strategies to reduce stress levels and burnout and to decrease the incidence of workplace violence. Information concerning circumstances that initiate violent events, burnout, and possible stressors may highlight the results. In addition, it is essential to elicit the predictors and indicators of rising levels of stress or burnout in nurses.

References

Ahmed, Q. A., Arabi, Y. M., & Memish, Z. A. (2006). Health risks at the Hajj. *The Lancet, 367*(9515), 1008–1015. https://doi.org/10.1016/S0140-6736(06)68429-8

Al Arabiya. (2016). *Saudi Arabia says Hajj 2016 receives 1.8 million pilgrims.* Retrieved from http://english.alarabiya.net/en/News/middle-east/2016/09/12/Saudi-Arabia-says-Hajj-2016-receives-1-8-million-pilgrims.html

Alkorashy, H. A., & Al Moalad, F. B. (2016). Workplace violence against nursing staff in a Saudi university hospital. *International Nursing Review, 63*(2), 226–232. https://doi.org/10.1111/inr.12242

Alsafadi, H., Goodwin, W., & Syed, A. (2011). Diabetes care during Hajj. *Clinical Medicine, 11*(3), 218–221. https://doi.org/10.7861/clinmedicine.11-3-218

Alsaqri, S. H. (2014). *A survey of intention to leave, job stress, burnout and job satisfaction among nurses employed in the Ha'il region's hospitals in Saudi Arabia* (Unpublished doctoral thesis). Melbourne, Australia: RMIT University.

Al-Turki, H. A., Al-Turki, R. A., Al-Dardas, H. A., Al-Gazal, M. R., Al-Maghrabi, G. H., Al-Enizi, N. H., & Ghareeb, B. A. (2010). Burnout syndrome among multinational nurses working in Saudi Arabia. *Annals of African Medicine, 9*(4), 226–229. https://doi.org/10.4103/1596-3519.70960

Alzahrani, F., & Kyratsis, Y. (2017). Emergency nurse disaster preparedness during mass gatherings: A cross-sectional survey of emergency nurses' perceptions in hospitals in Mecca, Saudi Arabia. *BMJ Open, 7*(4), e013563. https://doi.org/10.1136/bmjopen-2016-013563

Andreou, E., Alexopoulos, E. C., Lionis, C., Varvogli, L., Gnardellis, C., Chrousos, G. P., & Darviri, C. (2011). Perceived stress scale: Reliability and validity study in Greece. *International Journal of Environmental Research and Public Health, 8*(8), 3287–3298. https://doi.org/10.3390/ijerph8083287

Bernardi, M., Catania, G., & Marceca, F. (2005). The world of nursing burnout. A literature review. *Professioni Infermieristiche, 58*(2), 75–79.

Carr, J., Kelley, B., Keaton, R., & Albrecht, C. (2011). Getting to grips with stress in the workplace: Strategies for promoting a healthier, more productive environment. *Human Resource Management International Digest, 19*(4), 32–38. https://doi.org/10.1108/09670731111140748

Chaaya, M., Osman, H., Naassan, G., & Mahfoud, Z. (2010). Validation of the Arabic version of the Cohen Perceived Stress Scale (PSS-10) among pregnant and postpartum women. *BMC Psychiatry, 10*(1), 111. https://doi.org/10.1186/1471-244X-10-111

Cohen, S., Kamarck, T., & Mermelstein, R. (1983). A global measure of perceived stress. *Journal of Health and Social Behavior, 24*(4), 385–396. https://doi.org/10.2307/2136404

Cohen, S., & Williamson, G. (1988). Perceived stress in a probability sample of the United States. In S. Spacapan & S. Oskamp (Eds.), *The social psychology of health: The Claremont symposium on applied social psychology* (pp. 31–67). Newbury Park, CA: Sage.

Dall'Ora, C., Griffiths, P., Ball, J., Simon, M., & Aiken, L. H. (2015). Association of 12 h shifts and nurses' job satisfaction, burnout and intention to leave: Findings from a cross-sectional study of 12 European countries. *BMJ Open, 5*(9), e008331. https://doi.org/10.1136/bmjopen-2015-008331

Di Martino, V. (2002). *Workplace violence in the health sector—Country case studies (Brazil, Bulgaria, Lebanon, Portugal, South Africa, Thailand and an additional Australian study).* Retrieved from http://www.who.int/violence_injury_prevention/injury/en/WVsynthesisreport.pdf

Ezzati, A., Jiang, J., Katz, M. J., Sliwinski, M. J., Zimmerman, M. E., & Lipton, R. B. (2014). Validation of the Perceived Stress Scale in a community sample of older adults. *International Journal of Geriatric Psychiatry, 29*(6), 645–652. https://doi.org/10.1002/gps.4049

Gates, D. M., Gillespie, G. L., & Succop, P. (2011). Violence against nurses and its impact on stress and productivity. *Nursing Economic$, 29*(2), 59–66.

Geiger-Brown, J., Rogers, V. E., Trinkoff, A. M., Kane, R. L., Bausell, R. B., & Scharf, S. M. (2012). Sleep, sleepiness, fatigue, and performance of 12-hour-shift nurses. *Chronobiology International, 29*(2), 211–219. https://doi.org/10.3109/07420528.2011.645752

Greenglass, E. R., Burke, R. J., & Fiksenbaum, L. (2001). Workload and burnout in nurses. *Journal of Community & Applied Social Psychology, 11*(3), 211–215. https://doi.org/10.1002/casp.614

International Labour Office, International Council of Nurses, World Health Organization, & Public Services International (2003). *Joint programme on workplace violence in the health sector—Workplace violence in the health sector country case studies research instruments survey questionnaire (English).* Retrieved from http://www.who.int/violence_injury_prevention/violence/interpersonal/en/WVquestionnaire.pdf

Iwanicki, E. F., & Schwab, R. L. (1981). A cross validation study of the Maslach Burnout Inventory. *Educational and Psychological Measurement, 41*(4), 1167–1174. https://doi.org/10.1177/001316448104100425

Kwok, R. P., Law, Y. K., Li, K. E., Ng, Y. C., Cheung, M. H., Fung, V. K., … Leung, W. C. (2006). Prevalence of workplace violence against nurses in Hong Kong. *Hong Kong Medical Journal, 12*(1), 6–9.

Laschinger, H. K., & Grau, A. L. (2012). The influence of personal dispositional factors and organizational resources on workplace violence, burnout, and health outcomes in new graduate nurses: A cross-sectional study. *International Journal of Nursing Studies, 49*(3), 282–291. https://doi.org/10.1016/j.ijnurstu.2011.09.004

Lobo, V. M., Fisher, A., Ploeg, J., Peachey, G., & Akhtar-Danesh, N. (2013). A concept analysis of nursing overtime. *Journal of Advanced Nursing, 69*(11), 2401–2412. https://doi.org/10.1111/jan.12117

Maslach, C., & Jackson, S. E. (1981). The measurement of experienced burnout. *Journal of Organizational Behavior, 2*(2), 99–113. https://doi.org/10.1002/job.4030020205

Maslach, C., Schaufeli, W. B., & Leiter, M. P. (2001). Job burnout. *Annual Review of Psychology, 52*(1), 397–422. https://doi.org/10.1146/annurev.psych.52.1.397

Mohamed, A. G. (2002). Work-related assaults on nursing staff in Riyadh, Saudi Arabia. *Journal of Family & Community Medicine, 9*(3), 51–59.

Rayan, A., Qurneh, A., Elayyan, R., & Baker, O. (2016). Developing a policy for workplace violence against nurses and health care professionals in Jordan: A plan of action. *American Journal of Public Health Research, 4*(2), 47–55. https://doi.org/10.12691/ajphr-4-2-2

Reis, R. S., Hino, A. A., & Añez, C. R. (2010). Perceived stress scale: Reliability and validity study in Brazil. *Journal of Health Psychology, 15*(1), 107–114. https://doi.org/10.1177/1359105309346343

Saudi Arabia Ministry of Health. (2016). *Health indicators for the year of 1437H*. Retrieved from http://www.moh.gov.sa/Ministry/Statistics/Indicator/Pages/Indicator-1437.aspx (Original work published in Arabian)

Spector, P. E., Zhou, Z. E., & Che, X. X. (2014). Nurse exposure to physical and nonphysical violence, bullying, and sexual harassment: A quantitative review. *International Journal of Nursing Studies, 51*(1), 72–84. https://doi.org/10.1016/j.ijnurstu.2013.01.010

Stimpfel, A. W., & Aiken, L. H. (2013). Hospital staff nurses' shift length associated with safety and quality of care. *Journal of Nursing Care Quality, 28*(2), 122–129. https://doi.org/10.1097/NCQ.0b013e3182725f09

Trinkoff, A. M., Johantgen, M., Storr, C. L., Gurses, A. P., Liang, Y., & Han, K. (2011). Nurses' work schedule characteristics, nurse staffing, and patient mortality. *Nursing Research, 60*(1), 1–8. https://doi.org/10.1097/NNR.0b013e3181fff15d

Tsouros, A. D., & Efstathiou, P. A. (2007). *Mass gatherings and public health: The experience of the Athens 2004 Olympic games* (1st ed.). Copenhagen, Denmark: WHO Regional Office for Europe.

Wu, S., Zhu, W., Wang, Z., Wang, M., & Lan, Y. (2007). Relationship between burnout and occupational stress among nurses in China. *Journal of Advanced Nursing, 59*(3), 233–239. https://doi.org/10.1111/j.1365-2648.2007.04301.x

Wu, S. M., & Amtmann, D. (2013). Psychometric evaluation of the Perceived Stress Scale in multiple sclerosis. *ISRN Rehabilitation*, 608356. https://doi.org/10.1155/2013/608356

13

The Learning Effectiveness of High-Fidelity Simulation Teaching Among Chinese Nursing Students: A Mixed-Methods Study

Zhen LI[1] • Fei-Fei HUANG[2*] • Shiah-Lian CHEN[3] • Anni WANG[4] • Yufang GUO[5]

ABSTRACT

Background: High-fidelity simulation (HFS) is an interactive and complex experiential learning pedagogy. Given the limited and inconclusive evidence on the effectiveness of HFS in terms of improving student learning outcomes, a more thorough understanding of students' learning experiences and effects of HFS may inform the improvement of nursing training.

Purpose: The aim of this study was to examine the learning effectiveness score of HFS, its influencing factors, and the learning experience of nursing students.

Methods: A convergent parallel mixed-methods research design was adopted. Five hundred thirty-three third-year undergraduate nursing students completed the Simulation Learning Effectiveness Inventory. Semistructured interviews were used to elicit the opinions of 22 participants regarding their participation in the HFS experience.

Results: The quantitative findings showed a moderately high learning effectiveness of HFS among Chinese undergraduate nursing students (121.81 ± 14.93). The learning effectiveness for equipment resources (15.02 ± 2.38), course arrangement (11.18 ± 1.73), and confidence (18.56 ± 3.67) was relatively low. Extroversion and mixed personality ($\beta = 0.14$ and 0.10) and "dislike" or "general like" of the course ($\beta = -0.45$ and -0.33) were found to influence learning effectiveness ($F = 54.79$, $p < .001$, adjusted $R^2 = .29$). In addition, the qualitative findings indicated that the participants felt positively regarding the "debriefing," "clinical abilities," and "problem solving" dimensions of the training.

Conclusions/Implications for Practice: The focus of the education process and curriculum design of HFS activities should be on improving course arrangement, equipment resources, and students' confidence while paying attention to nursing students' personality traits and course preferences.

KEY WORDS:
high-fidelity simulations, nursing, students, mixed-methods design, learning.

Introduction

Emerging health needs and high patient expectations face nurses today, especially those in China, with substantial challenges in delivering high-quality care (Gu et al., 2018).

Because of the deterioration of nurse–patient relationships and the growing attention to patient safety issues, undergraduate nursing students' opportunities to experience direct patient care and clinical practice have been decreasing (Gu et al., 2018; Kim et al., 2016). High-fidelity simulation (HFS) is as ideal substitute for traditional clinical settings, providing nursing students with opportunities to practice decision-making and clinical skills under a wide range of scenarios in a safe, supportive, and realistic clinical environment to meet future nursing challenges without compromising the well-being of patients (Sundler et al., 2015). Thus, HFS has been used widely in nursing education, including in classroom and continuing nursing professional education in clinical practice settings (Kunst et al., 2017).

HFS is an interactive strategy that uses more than computer-based mannequins to show realistic clinical interactions and clinical scenarios (Au et al., 2016). As Jeffries and Rogers (2007) noted, evaluating student learning experiences and outcomes over the phases of HFS is an important component of the teaching process, because it helps instructors assess learning and performance and further improve and refine their teaching strategies (Chen et al., 2015). However, many nurse educators continue to struggle with the problem of how to evaluate the effectiveness of these simulations (Bai et al., 2015; Chu & Chen, 2016).

A substantial body of research findings indicates that HFS may have positive effects on student self-efficacy, learning satisfaction, psychomotor skills, and critical thinking (Aebersold et al., 2018). However, evidence regarding the effect of HFS on student learning efficacy is inconsistent and

[1]BSN, RN, Nursing Manager, Gynaecology and Obstetrics Division, the Affiliated Hospital of Putian University, Putian, People's Republic of China • [2]PhD, RN, Associated Professor, School of Nursing, Fujian Medical University, Fuzhou, People's Republic of China • [3]PhD, RN, Professor, Department of Nursing, National Taichung University of Science and Technology, Taichung, Taiwan, Republic of China • [4]PhD, RN, Lecturer, School of Nursing, Fudan University, Shanghai, People's Republic of China • [5]PhD, RN, Associated Professor, School of Nursing, Shandong University, People's Republic of China

mixed (Yang & Liu, 2016). Nursing educators have highlighted the need to further assess HFS-based teaching strategies and their impact on learning (Blum et al., 2010). Moreover, personal characteristics such level of enthusiasm for the nursing profession, whether a student is a class leader, and personality type may influence the degree to which students engage in their studies (Lin et al., 2018). Further exploration of the factors that influence the learning effectiveness of HFS among Chinese nursing students may help nursing educators better understand their HFS-related learning experience.

HFS is an interactive and complex experiential learning pedagogy (Warren et al., 2016). On the basis of Chen et al. (2015), the learning effectiveness of HFS in this study was defined as the degrees of improvement in clinical ability, confidence in taking care of patients, collaboration with others, and participation in problem-solving activities. Given the limited and inconclusive evidence regarding the effectiveness of HFS, further study is necessary to triangulate the quantitative and qualitative data to provide more comprehensive insight into nursing students' HFS learning experiences and the effectiveness of HFS. Davis et al. (2014) explored the opinions of nursing faculty regarding HFS application using a parallel mixed-methods approach. To our knowledge, the effectiveness of using HFS among nursing students using a mixed-methods approach has not been assessed.

Therefore, the main aims of this study were to examine HFS learning effectiveness and its influencing factors among undergraduate nursing students in China and to explore their perceptions and learning experiences regarding HFS. This study was designed to provide insights that may be applied to the future development and improvement of HFS teaching among nursing students, informing the potential for further integrating HFS into nursing educational curricula.

Methods

Study Design

This sequential parallel mixed-methods research study (Curry et al., 2013) was conducted from June to August 2018. First, self-administered questionnaires were used to assess HFS learning effectiveness in a group of undergraduate nursing students and to collect related sociodemographic and learning characteristics. Then, semistructured interviews were used to explore the opinions of nursing students regarding their HFS learning participation experience. The quantitative and qualitative components of this study were prioritized equally. Ethics approval was obtained from the ethics committee of Fujian Medical University (no. 20170322).

Measurement

The Mandarin Chinese version of the Simulation Learning Effectiveness Inventory (SLEI-SCM; Huang et al., 2019) was adapted from the 31-item, self-report SLEI (Chen et al., 2015). The SLEI-SCM includes three subscales that are used to assess the six domains of HFS learning effectiveness. These domains include course arrangement, equipment resources, debriefing, clinical abilities, problem solving, and confidence. Each item is scored using a Likert-type 5-point scale (1 = *strongly disagree* and 5 = *strongly agree*), and the instrument has a total possible score range of 31–155, with higher scores indicating higher levels of learning effectiveness. The SLEI-SCM has confirmed reliability and validity (Huang et al., 2019), with a Cronbach's α of .95 and a 2-week test–retest reliability of .88.

Demographic information collected from the participants included age, gender, birthplace, whether the student was from a single-child family, whether the student was a class leader, personality type, and whether the student was personally motivated to join the nursing profession. Information on course learning was also collected, including the most impressive experience of HFS learning, the number of role-playing activities participated in, HFS learning preference, and the perceived benefits of HFS learning.

Participants

Five hundred thirty-three third-year undergraduate nursing students were recruited using a nonprobability, convenience, purposive sampling method from a 4-year nursing bachelor program of a medical university in southern China. Students who had completed all 13 HFS classes and were willing to participate were invited to complete the survey, and those who completed the survey were invited to freely and voluntarily share their perceptions of the HFS learning experience. Twenty-two eligible students of various backgrounds (e.g., gender, personality type) were purposively selected to participate in additional, semistructured, individual, in-depth interviews. This sample size met the criteria for theoretical saturation after coding (Speziale & Carpenter, 2007).

The High-Fidelity Simulation Activities

HFS was conducted as a regular part of the curriculum (nursing comprehensive experiment) in a five- and six-semester course of the program undertaken in the simulation nursing laboratory before clinical placement. The HFS course included the use of computerized full-body manikins (METIman Nursing) in a simulated clinical care area, with a viewing room and an adjacent facilitator control room. The purpose of this course was to better cultivate the ability of students to provide nursing care to patients experiencing medical and surgical diseases (e.g., chronic obstructive pulmonary diseases, peptic ulcers, cerebral trauma) and to prepare students for clinical placement.

The HFS course included 13 class sessions, covering common diseases in the fields of medical, surgical, gynecological, and pediatric nursing. During each 2-hour HFS class, students were divided into groups of 16–20 and then further divided into subgroups of three to five for each activity. Generally, three scenarios were performed during each HFS class. Students in each subgroup performed one HFS scenario and were assigned different individual roles, mostly nurses, whereas the students in other subgroups acted as observers. The roles of observer and active participant/nurse were rotated over the course of the entire HFS activity. Three teachers led the course, with one responsible for controlling the computer and simulating the patient's voice during the simulation stage and two serving as facilitators (e.g., doctor, family member).

The simulation class was a 2-hour period that included a 10-minute briefing and preparation and a 50-minute simulation followed by a 60-minute debriefing. The design of the HFS activities was based on the Jeffries simulation model. The HFS class process is shown in Table 1. These simulations require students to complete assigned prereadings that relate to the corresponding scenarios shown on the student learning management platform.

Quantitative Data Collection

Immediately after the end of the last HFS class, two nursing master-degree students distributed the demographic and course-related data form and SLEI-SCM to the participants. Completed surveys were returned anonymously in a secured box. The survey took 10–15 minutes to complete.

Qualitative Data Collection

The qualitative interview guide was developed based on the findings of the quantitative study. In addition, two students were interviewed to further validate the interview script. All of the interviews were held in private at a mutually convenient time for each participant and conducted using the qualitative interview guide. During the interview, the opinions of the interviewees regarding their HFS learning experience were explored in an open and free environment by the interviewers (F. F. H. and A. W.), both of whom hold nursing PhD degrees and are experienced in conducting qualitative studies. Interviews took an average of 40 minutes. The interview responses were transcribed verbatim and translated from Chinese into English, with discrepancies checked by two of the authors. The qualitative interview questions were as follows:

(a) How did your high-fidelity simulation activity experience compare to or differ from the traditional introduction?
(b) What did you gain from the high-fidelity simulation activity?
(c) What were the difficulties or obstacles encountered in the high-fidelity simulation activity?
(d) What are your suggestions for the high-fidelity simulation activity?

Data Analysis

SPSS 16.0 software (SPSS, Inc., Chicago, IL, USA) was used to analyze the quantitative data. Descriptive analysis of the SLEI-SCM scores and the characteristics of participants were reported using means ($\pm$ SD) and frequency distributions.

Multiple stepwise linear regression was performed to identify the predictors of HFS learning effectiveness. The SLEI-SCM

Table 1

The High-Fidelity Simulation Class Process

Stage/Phase	Activity
Before HFS class Online prelearning	Self-directed activity of nursing students.
	A meeting was held by the subject instructors before class to discuss the design of the activity, while a collective lesson preparation was also run among the instructors to ensure the maximization of learning experience and to seek improvement.
Briefing and preparation stage (10 minutes)	(a) Instructors introduced the simulated environment and technology to students. (b) Instructors introduced the HFS learning objectives, activity, amounts of time given, role specifications, and outcome expectancies. (c) Role-players (nursing students) made preparations for the HFS activity and became familiar with the simulated environment.
During HFS class Simulation stage (50 minutes)	(a) Role-players (nursing students) performed preprogrammed HFS scenarios by the use of the think-aloud technique in a simulated clinical care area. (The simulation scenarios were video recorded.) (b) Instructors provided cues, help, and obstacles as necessary in an adjacent facilitator control room. (c) Observers (nursing students) were required to take notes on the clinical presentation, missing data, and reflections in a viewing room.
Verbal debriefing stage (60 minutes)	Students were encouraged to review and discuss the following prompts after the simulation under the guidance of the instructors. When in controversy, the instructors used snippets from the video to guide discussion. (a) Reflecting on what they learned. (b) Analyzing what went right and what went wrong with the simulations. (c) Discussing how to apply knowledge gained to clinical practice. (d) Discussing strengths and weaknesses for future practice and improvement.

Note. HFS = high-fidelity simulation.

score was treated as the dependent variable, and variables showing statistical significance in the *t* test or one-way analyses of variance, including age, nursing students like the HFS learning, and nursing students' personality, were designated as independent variables. Missing data were replaced using mean value substitution, and $p < .05$ was considered to be statistically significant.

The qualitative data were entered into ATLAS.ti software for content analysis (Green & Thorogood, 2004). Two of the researchers read the interview transcripts independently line by line and generated the preliminary coding using an inductive coding approach. Next, the researchers discussed and compared the preliminary coding until consensus was achieved. When discrepancies arose, the original transcripts were reexamined. Finally, the similar codes were summarized to generate the final themes.

In this study, quantitative data analysis was followed by the analysis of qualitative data, with equal weight given to the findings of both analysis methods (NIH Office of Behavioral and Social Sciences, 2018). Finally, both the quantitative and qualitative data were used to interpret the results, and the data on the preparation, process, and learning outcomes of simulation teaching were integrated during interpretation using the Jeffries simulation framework (Jeffries & Rogers, 2007).

Results

Five hundred thirty-three undergraduate nursing students completed the questionnaires, giving a response rate of 96.1%. The mean age of the participants was 21.44 ± 0.87 years. The participants had participated in an average of 4.05 ± 1.72 simulation sessions. The demographic and course-related characteristics of the participants are summarized in Table 2.

Table 2

Participants' Demographics and Course Data

Characteristic	Survey (n = 533)		Interview (n = 22)		Learning Effectiveness Scores		F/t	p
	n	%	n	%	M	SD		
Gender							1.17	.24
Female	463	86.9	20	90.9	123.77	15.95		
Male	70	3.1	2	9.1	121.53	14.78		
Birthplace							−1.05	.30
Urban	365	68.5	8	36.4	121.39	14.56		
Rural	168	31.5	14	63.6	122.85	14.02		
Whether the student was from a single-child family							1.20	.23
Yes	97	18.2	4	18.2	123.45	14.96		
No	436	81.8	18	81.8	121.41	14.86		
Whether the student was a class leader							2.21	.03*
Yes	219	41.1	8	36.4	123.53	14.74		
No	314	58.9	14	63.6	120.62	15.02		
Personal choice to join the nursing profession?							2.18	.03*
Voluntary	235	44.1	13	59.1	123.42	14.36		
Involuntary	298	55.9	9	40.9	120.58	15.28		
Personality type							8.14	< .01*
Extroverted	120	22.5	7	31.8	118.26	13.85		
Introverted	125	23.5	7	31.8	125.85	16.39		
Mixed	288	54.0	8	36.4	121.7	14.39		
Preference of HFS learning							103.36	< .01*
Like	274	51.4	16	72.7	129.01	13.16		
General	241	45.2	2	9.1	115.13	11.56		
Dislike	18	3.4	4	18.2	98.14	20.24		
Gains from HFS learning							1.74	.18
As role-players	366	68.7	15	68.2	122.7	14.35		
As observers	34	6.4	4	18.2	121.17	17.51		
The same as role-players to observers	133	24.9	3	13.6	119.89	15.62		

Note. HFS = high-fidelity simulation.
*$p < .05$.

General Comments on the High-Fidelity Simulation Experience: Both Positive and Negative

The overall learning effectiveness score in this study was 121.81 ± 14.93. Over 70% of the participants reported a high level of satisfaction and positive feelings toward HFS learning, with phrases such as "good, very good"; "interesting,

vivid, practical, funny, exciting"; "it helped linked theory to practice"; and "active learning" frequently expressed.

The participants gave Item 10 ("Discussion with the teacher after class assisted my achieving the learning goals," 4.19 ± 0.70) the highest average score and gave Item 2 ("I understand the objective and evaluation requirements of this course," 3.56 ± 0.73) the lowest average score. The descriptive results of SLEI-SCM are shown in Table 3.

Table 3

Chinese Undergraduate Nursing Students' Response on SLEI-SCM (N = 533)

Factor/Item	Mean	SD
Debrief (score range: 4–20)	16.54	2.29
10. Discussion with the teacher after class assisted my achieving the learning goals.	4.19[a]	0.70
9. The feedback provided by the teacher was immediate and promoted my learning outcome.	4.13[a]	0.71
8. The teacher provided appropriate positive feedback according to the learning situation of students.	4.12	0.73
11. Feedback and discussion of the simulation assisted me in correcting my mistakes and promoting my learning.	4.11	0.72
Clinical ability (score range: 5–25)	20.25	2.89
15. Situational learning enabled me to acquire useful knowledge about clinical practices.	4.12	0.71
14. Situational learning contributed to my mastering the processes of clinical care.	4.11	0.72
12. Situational learning enhanced my understanding of patient problems.	4.08	0.73
16. The contents of situational learning corresponded to my previous learning experience.	4.05	0.71
13. Situational learning promoted my ability to care for patients.	3.90	0.81
Problem solving (score range: 10–50)	40.26	5.35
22. Simulation learning enabled me to identify problems in clinical care that I have not noticed before.	4.16[a]	0.72
30. During the interaction in the situational simulation, I was willing to share workload with other team members.	4.10	0.75
28. Situational simulation practice provided opportunities to practice communicating and cooperating with other members in my team.	4.10	0.73
29. Situational simulation practice enabled me to understand the role that I should play in an interaction with a medical team.	4.07	0.74
25. In participating in simulation learning, I approached solutions to problems through data search.	4.06	0.71
26. In participating in a situational discussion, I identified solutions to problems by understanding argument to topics.	3.98	0.73
27. Simulation courses promoted my problem-solving skills in confronting patient problems.	3.98	0.71
24. Simulation learning enabled me to learn previously unfamiliar learning methods.	3.97	0.76
31. I could discuss patient needs with the medical team by using effective communication skills.	3.94	0.78
23. In participating in simulation learning, I approached new concepts or ideas through observation.	3.91	0.76
Resource (score range: 4–20)	15.02	2.38
5. The equipment and resources for situational exercises contributed to my learning.	3.97	0.70
4. The equipment and resources for situational exercises were sufficient.	3.83	0.80
6. Using the environment and equipment for situational exercises was convenient.	3.65	0.83
7. If I experienced problems or difficulty using the equipment, help was always available.	3.58[b]	0.81
Course (score range: 3–15)	11.18	1.73
3. The activities in this course assisted my achieving the learning goals.	3.84	0.70
1. The course contents were arranged adequately in terms of sequential order and depth, facilitating my learning.	3.78	0.74
2. I understand the objective and evaluation requirements of this course.	3.56[b]	0.73
Confidence (score range: 5–25)	18.56	3.67
17. Situational simulation practice encouraged me to confront future clinical challenges.	3.83	0.83
19. Simulation learning boosted my confidence in handling future clinical problems.	3.74	0.84
18. Situational simulation practice boosted my confidence in my clinical skills.	3.73	0.89
21. Simulation learning contributed to my confidence in future patient care.	3.64	0.86
20. Simulation learning alleviated my anxiety/fear of confronting future clinical patient problems.	3.61[b]	0.90
Total score (range: 31–155)	121.81	14.93

Note. SLEI-CM = Mandarin Chinese version of the Simulation Learning Effectiveness Inventory.
[a] The three greatest score of items. [b] The three lowest score of items.

The qualitative data also revealed the limitations of simulation learning with regard to authenticity and complexity. Most of the participants expressed that the situation was inadequately realistic when using the high-fidelity simulator and that they did not perceive themselves as real clinical nurses during the simulation: "*No, I just had the feeling of performance thinking about what the teacher would ask, and never regarded myself as a real nurse really caring about how to care for a patient. It was a mechanical performance, and I was confused and did not get into it. Our performance cannot reflect reality and focuses more on the practical skills. Even our pre-class review only prioritized the practices. But the teacher paid more attention to how to deal with problems*" (19).

Moreover, the participants expressed that the positive takeaways of the observers were less than those of the actors: "*The observers may not be overly concerned with others sometimes. It was the case that they would watch the performances leisurely and did not do a lot of preparation before class because they did not need to perform*" (6).

Debriefing

Debriefing was the factor that earned the highest average score for perceived simulation learning effectiveness (16.54 ± 2.29). The average scores of the four items under the debriefing factor were each higher than 4, indicating that the debriefing plays a positive role. Similar results emerged in the interviews. Most (80%) of the interviewees perceived the debriefing as fruitful and valuable. They expressed that the debriefing session allowed them to realize their learning strengths and weaknesses and to construct a permanent and vivid body of knowledge. Moreover, the debriefing enabled them to think actively through clinical problems. Half of the interviewees advised that the duration of the debriefing could be longer to promote further discussion of the content.

I like to talk with my teachers and classmates after I have done all the practical training. I really like the process of finding out how to solve problems through such discussions. This kind of process helps me realize when I lack full understanding about the cases. What's more, when I hear the perspectives of the other students who observed (a session) it makes me aware of my deficiencies and strengths in clinical practice. (20)

Although the biggest benefits come from discussions, I prefer scenario performances during which I will think more about the problem and their solutions and the teachers will teach us how to care for patients using clinical thinking. We usually treat nursing practices separately when learning, but HFS is more systematic in that it requires many practices to link it all together, which can be the way to improve our practical skills and gain a better understanding about how to care for patients. Traditional training formats are less flexible. (2)

Abilities

The positive feedback after HFS on the clinical abilities and problem solving of the participants is shown in Table 3. HFS was found to improve clinical nursing care abilities, as the interviewees voiced that the simulation improved their abilities in the realms of observation and analysis, communication, coping, team collaboration, and clinical/critical thinking.

HFS teaching is a comprehensive experience that combines professional theoretical knowledge with practical skills, which will help me improve my clinical thinking and teamwork ability and strengthen our personal knowledge and skills at the same time. (5)

HFS can deepen and consolidate what we have learned and help us apply knowledge into practice. It can also help me find the shortcomings in my practice and then enable me to correct and improve these. What's more, the questions raised by the teachers who played roles as family members or patients are similar to the problems encountered in clinical practice, which can help us improve our clinical practice and communication skills. The HFS really benefits us a lot and has been implemented successfully. (8)

High simulation teaching can cultivate our clinical thinking and train our emergency response abilities, which helps us understand the process of clinical practice more thoroughly and may be a kind of preparation for pre-clinical work. Moreover, it provides us with a clinical atmosphere and training on teamwork. (12)

Resources

The equipment and resources of HFS contributed somewhat to learning effectiveness (15.02 ± 2.38). However, the participants were generally unfamiliar with the simulation equipment. For example, they were unsure of the manikin's capabilities and did not know where to obtain needed supplies or how to use some of the equipment (e.g., patient monitor): "*Some of the equipment used in HFS is different from what we usually use, and so is not very familiar to us, which leads us to panic*" (10) and "*We hope the equipment and models in the laboratory will be thorough. We expect that teachers can show us instructions on how to use the (less familiar) clinical equipment before the HFS activities*" (17).

In addition, the participants stated that they were at a loss and felt anxiety when the teachers set up certain obstacles during the HFS activities and when, during preparation activities, the simulation scenarios unfolded differently than expected: "*Sometimes there exist discrepancies between what you think should take place and what teachers deem should happen in a given scenario*" (21).

Course Arrangement

The scores for the course arrangement factor and its three items indicate that the contribution of course arrangement on learning effectiveness is not consistently positive. In the interview, the participants described that the time given to prepare and gain familiarity with the simulation environment could be longer than currently allowed and include extensions such as providing opportunities to practice in a simulation laboratory. Most of the participants (70%) suggested that the course schedule and allocation of subgroups could be rearranged to better meet students' learning needs and should not be held during the semester immediately before clinical placement. Moreover, the participants expressed hopes of increasing the frequency of simulation-based training within the curriculum to gain greater insight on different clinical issues and knowledge.

> However, the curriculum was always arranged close to the end of the semester. It's too late for some people to prepare. (7)

> I think it's not suitable to arrange students in advance for high simulation. Teachers can assign the scripts of high simulation to the class and can pick students randomly, so that students can cooperate on the spot. As it is, only the pre-arranged actors will think through the case seriously, while the students who are observers seldom think about it. (22)

> I hope HFS can imitate clinical practice better. For example, the teacher can give us the case and practice instructions for the first time, which is reasonable, and the next time we can design them on our own. I still hope that the HFS can be more challenging, containing fewer tips so that we can figure out what to do by ourselves. Even the practice instructions should be prepared on our own in advance. (14)

Confidence

Confidence received the lowest average score of all the simulation learning effectiveness factors (18.56 ± 3.67). The average scores for each of the five items constituting the confidence factor was less than 4. For example, the average score for Item 20, "Simulation learning alleviated my anxiety/fear of confronting future clinical patient problems," was 3.61 ± 0.90. However, the interviewees reported that observing and undertaking practice in simulated scenarios, and receiving feedback and conducting discussions in a supportive environment, allowed them to build confidence to confront future clinical challenges and undertake future patient care. Some also noted that their uncertainty and worry had diminished.

> HFS teaching provided us with an opportunity to practice communicating with future clinical patients, and it could be helpful for us to become familiar with the clinical nursing process. Simulated exercises reduce my fear of facing patients in the future and enhance my abilities to communicate and cooperate with other group members. (2)

> HFS can improve our ability to observe practices, and we will be more relaxed when we face people, which was something we could not deal with ordinarily. (10)

> After HFS practice, I felt more confident in the later clinical internship practice because it wasn't my first time doing it. (1)

The Influencing Factors of Learning Effectiveness

Significant differences in the various independent variables affecting HFS learning effectiveness found in this study are shown in Table 2. These variables include whether the student was a class leader, personal motivation to join the nursing profession, personality type, and HFS learning preference ($p < .05$). On the basis of the results shown in Table 2, these independent variables were included in the regression model.

As shown in Table 4, two influencing factors, namely, enjoyment of HFS learning and having an extroverted/mixed personality type, were found in this study to be predictors of learning effectiveness. These two factors accounted for 29.0% of the total variance ($F = 54.79$, $p < .001$, adjusted $R^2 = .29$) in learning effectiveness scores. In addition, the interview results confirmed the significance of these two factors as predictors.

Discussion

To our best knowledge, this was the first mixed-methods study to provide an overview of simulation learning experiences and effectiveness in undergraduate nursing students. In this study, the qualitative and quantitative data were analyzed and interpreted using the Jeffries simulation framework, which is commonly used to guide the process of designing, implementing, and evaluating simulations in nursing facilities (Jeffries & Rogers, 2007). The findings of both the cross-sectional survey and the interviews revealed that the simulation learning effectiveness levels of the participants were only moderately high and in need of improvement. Furthermore, the findings offer critical insights for developing

Table 4

Independent Predictors of Level of Learning Effectiveness (N = 533)

Predictor	Standardized β	t	p
Constant	0.85	99.57	< .001
Preference of HFS learning			
General	−0.45	−12.03	< .001
Dislike	−0.33	−8.97	< .001
Personality type			
Extroverted	0.14	2.99	< .001
Mixed	0.10	2.14	.030

Note. $F = 54.79$, adjusted $R^2 = .29$, $p < .001$.

new and effective strategies to support and enhance HFS teaching.

As simulation opens door for nursing students to experience today's most complex and challenging clinical cases early in their nursing training, it has the potential to substantively change nursing education. In the sample used in this study, the average SLEI-SCM score was 121.81 ± 14.93, highlighting the positive contributions of HFS. The moderately high simulation learning effectiveness of Chinese nursing students was particularly strong in the dimensions of "debriefing," "clinical abilities," and "problem solving."

The Remarkably High Manifestation of Simulation Learning Effectiveness

Debriefing is not only the "the heart and soul" of the HFS teaching session but also a strong predictor of the efficacy of HFS teaching (Lestander et al., 2016). This finding in this study echoes those of other studies (Jacobs, 2017; Tawalbeh & Tubaishat, 2014; Tuzer et al., 2016) that found evidence in support of the positive effects of video-assisted debriefing educational experiences. In this study, faculty-led supportive, structured debriefing sessions combined with the viewing of recorded video immediately after simulation helped facilitate reflection-on-action and subsequent emotional and cognitive processing in students over time, allowing students to reflect on their responsibilities and actions, realize their mistakes/drawbacks, notice details that may have been overlooked, and learn to apply knowledge gained in different clinical scenarios. Further research is necessary to explore the effects of different debriefing methods (e.g., multimedia debriefing, self-debriefing, and in-simulation instructor-facilitated debriefing) on learning outcomes.

Clinical abilities are the ability and skills necessary for nurses to care for patients with clinical problems (Niu et al., 2014). In line with Kolb's experiential learning theory, HFS teaching provides a learning experience that combines seeing, listening, and touching (Kolb, 1984). Echoing previous findings (Niu et al., 2014; Yuan et al., 2012), we found that HFS activities train the resourceful clinical abilities of participants. The HFS activities allowed the nursing students in this study to integrate theoretical knowledge and a range of skills into practice, including observation, communication, coping, and team collaboration in realistic simulation scenarios. Hence, the participants learned how to identify appropriate ways to solve clinical problems, which establishes a strong basis for future clinical placement. However, questions remain regarding the transferability of competence and knowledge shown in a simulated setting to actual clinical settings, which is an issue that should be studied further using longitudinal/experimental research.

The Relatively Low Manifestation of Simulation Learning Effectiveness

The findings of this study also indicated that nursing students' simulation learning effectiveness with regard to course arrangement and equipment resources was also relatively low. Related problems included inappropriate course time arrangement, inadequate preparation time for HFS activities, and unfamiliarity with the simulation equipment, indicating that the design and conduct of HFS should be improved using several strategies, as subsequently described, to achieve the objectives and effects of HFS courses. First, scenarios for HFS may be selected based on specific course goals, the authenticity and extensibility of scenarios, and the previous learning experience of students. Second, before class, students may be provided adequate preparation time to become familiar with the simulation environment, simulator, and related equipment and resources. It should also be ensured that resources and equipment are adequate, properly functioning, and sufficiently designed to approximate the clinical experience. Third, facilitators may encourage students to freely discuss their HFS experiences and create a supportive and safe environment to enhance their confidence. On the basis of students' learning needs and course goals, teachers should set up the most appropriate and targeted interferences or obstacles during HFS activities. If possible, students may be provided an opportunity to first watch the practices of HFS activities of teachers, which may facilitate a more thorough understanding of the learning goals beforehand and enhance student confidence.

Similar to the findings of Yuan et al. (2012) and Zhang et al. (2014), the positive effect of HFS on the confidence of the participants was mixed. Bandura held the direct experience obtained by an individual during training to be the most influential factor on his or her confidence (Bandura, 1977). The low scores for confidence may be explained by the following reasons based on the interviews and our existing knowledge. First, the participants may have perceived that the METIman was not sufficiently similar to a real human being, so they could not put themselves into a realistic mindset in the scenarios. Second, HFS cannot fully replicate the context of human healthcare because patients' concerns and responses are changeable and complex. Third, the facilitators set up interferences and obstacles during HFS, which may have spurred negative emotions (e.g., anxiety, frustration) in the participants that hindered their learning and performance (Pai, 2016).

It is worth noting that degree of learning effectiveness significantly differed according to HFS learning preferences and participant personality. Compared with introverted students, extroverted and ambiverted students had higher learning effectiveness, possibly because the latter were more likely to challenge and express themselves (Huang et al., 2018) and to actively engage in clinical simulation scenarios and, consequently, achieve better learning efficacy. Echoing the findings of previous studies (Pai, 2016; Zhao & Chen, 2017), HFS-related learning preference was also an important facilitator of HFS learning effectiveness and student engagement.

Implications for Future Practice and Research

The findings of this study have implications for the education process and curriculum design. First, the question of how to improve the positive initiative of nursing students who are either introverted or dislike HFS learning as well as of observers during the course deserves greater attention from nursing educators, especially in large class settings. Teachers may use appropriate strategies to improve positive participation rates and enhance peer learning. For example, during the simulation, observers may be required to complete a stimulated peer assessment tool (Solheim et al., 2017), students may be required to complete a paper about nursing care plans before class, or the instructor may randomly select students to participate in simulated practice in class. Second, future research into this subject should be designed to carefully examine the cost-effectiveness of implementing HFS in nursing programs, including time, space, equipment, and development/maintenance.

Study Limitations

When interpreting the results of this study, several limitations must be considered First, the sample was confined to one region of Mainland China, of which may limit the generalization of the findings to other universities or countries. Second, comparisons of traditional teaching strategies and HFS teaching and a long-term follow-up of simulation learning effectiveness were not explored. To better understand the efficacy and changes of learning effectiveness during the HFS course, experimental and longitudinal study approaches should be considered in future studies.

Conclusion

This mixed-methods study provides an overview of simulation learning effectiveness among Chinese undergraduate nursing students. The participants showed moderately high HFS learning effectiveness, particularly in the dimensions of "debriefing," "clinical abilities," and "problem solving." However, there remains room for improvement, particularly in areas such as equipment resources, course arrangement, and student confidence. Therefore, efforts to improve the educational process and curriculum design of HFS activities should be targeted toward these areas. On the other hand, the personality and course preferences of students should be assessed and considered.

Acknowledgments

The authors wish to sincerely thank all of the participants without whom this study would have not been possible and Miss Jessica Hahne for her assistance in reviewing and editing this article.

Author Contributions

Study conception and design: FFH
Data collection: ZL
Data analysis and interpretation: AW, YG
Drafting of the article: FFH, ZL
Critical revision of the article: SLC

References

Aebersold, M., Voepel-Lewis, T., Cherara, L., Weber, M., Khouri, C., Levine, R., & Tait, A. R. (2018). Interactive anatomy-augmented virtual simulation training. *Clinical Simulation in Nursing, 15*, 34–41. https://doi.org/10.1016/j.ecns.2017.09.008

Au, M. L., Lo, M. S., Cheong, W., Wang, S. C., & Van, I. K. (2016). Nursing students' perception of high-fidelity simulation activity instead of clinical placement: A qualitative study. *Nurse Education Today, 39*, 16–21. https://doi.org/10.1016/j.nedt.2016.01.015

Bai, B., Ke, Y., Li, M., & Zhang, X. (2015). Application progress on high simulation teaching in nursing science. *Chinese Nursing Research, 29*(12), 1416–1419. (Original work published in Chinese)

Bandura, A. (1977). Self-efficacy: Toward a unifying theory of behavioral change. *Psychological Review, 84*(2), 191–215. https://doi.org/10.1037/0033-295X.84.2.191

Blum, C. A., Borglund, S., & Parcells, D. (2010). High-fidelity nursing simulation: Impact on student self-confidence and clinical competence. *International Journal of Nursing Education Scholarship, 7*(1), Article 18. https://doi.org/10.2202/1548-923X.2035

Chen, S.-L., Huang, T.-W., Liao, I.-C., & Liu, C. (2015). Development and validation of the Simulation Learning Effectiveness Inventory. *Journal of Advanced Nursing, 71*(10), 2444–2453. https://doi.org/10.1111/jan.12707

Chu, H., & Chen, Q. (2016). Research status quo of comprehensive evaluation tool of high-fidelity simulation teaching for foreign nursing. *Chinese Nursing Research, 30*(32), 3988–3991. (Original work published in Chinese)

Curry, L. A., Krumholz, H. M., O'Cathain, A., Plano Clark, V. L., Cherlin, E., & Bradley, E. H. (2013). Mixed methods in biomedical and health services research. *Circulation. Cardiovascular Quality and Outcomes, 6*(1), 119–123. https://doi.org/10.1161/CIRCOUTCOMES.112.967885

Davis, A. H., Kimble, L. P., & Gunby, S. S. (2014). Nursing faculty use of high-fidelity human patient simulation in undergraduate nursing education: A mixed-methods study. *The Journal of Nursing Education, 53*(3), 142–150. https://doi.org/10.3928/01484834-20140219-02

Green, J., & Thorogood, N. (2004). *Qualitative methods for health research* (2nd ed.). Sage.

Gu, Y. H., Xiong, L., Bai, J. B., Hu, J., & Tan, X. D. (2018). Chinese version of the clinical learning environment comparison survey: Assessment of reliability and validity. *Nurse Education Today, 71*, 121–128. https://doi.org/10.1016/j.nedt.2018.09.026

Huang, F., Han, X. Y., Chen, S.-L., Guo, Y. F., Wang, A., & Zhang, Q. (2019). Psychometric testing of the Chinese simple version of the Simulation Learning Effectiveness Inventory: Classical theory test and item response theory. *Frontiers in Psychology*, *11*, 32. https://doi.org/10.3389/fpsyg.2020.00032

Huang, F. F., Lin, T., Chen, L. L., & Xie, Y. F. (2018). A survey of the effects and its influencing factors of high-fidelity simulation teaching among undergraduate nursing students. *Chinese Journal of Nursing Education*, *15*(1), 61–65. (Original work published in Chinese)

Jacobs, P. J. (2017). Using high-fidelity simulation and video-assisted debriefing to enhance obstetrical hemorrhage mock code training. *Journal for Nurses in Professional Development*, *33*(5), 234–239. https://doi.org/10.1097/NND.0000000000000387

Jeffries, P. R., & Rogers, K. (2007). Theoretical framework for simulation design. In P. R. Jeffries (Ed.), *Simulation in nursing education: From conceptualization to evaluation*. National League for Nursing.

Kim, J., Park, J. H., & Shin, S. (2016). Effectiveness of simulation-based nursing education depending on fidelity: A meta-analysis. *BMC Medical Education*, *16*, Article No. 152. https://doi.org/10.1186/s12909-016-0672-7

Kolb, D. A. (1984). *Experiential learning: Experience as the source of learning and development*. Prentice Hall.

Kunst, E. L., Mitchell, M., & Johnston, A. N. (2017). Using simulation to improve the capability of undergraduate nursing students in mental health care. *Nurse Education Today*, *50*, 29–35. https://doi.org/10.1016/j.nedt.2016.12.012

Lestander, Ö., Lehto, N., & Engström, Å. (2016). Nursing students' perceptions of learning after high fidelity simulation: Effects of a three-step post-simulation reflection model. *Nurse Education Today*, *40*, 219–224. https://doi.org/10.1016/j.nedt.2016.03.011

Lin, X. D., Lin, Y., Liu, X. Y., Su, W. J., & Nie, R. J. (2018). The status of study engagement and its influencing factors among nursing arts undergraduates. *Chinese Journal of Nursing Education*, *15*(10), 770–774. (Original work published in Chinese)

NIH Office of Behavioral and Social Sciences. (2018). *Best practices for mixed methods research in the health sciences* (2nd ed.). National Institutes of Health.

Niu, G.-F., Sun, J.-P., Wu, X.-H., Yang, Z.-L., & Song, D. (2014). The effect of high-fidelity simulation teaching on the clinical competence of undergraduate nursing students. *Chinese Journal of Nursing Education*, *11*(5), 351–353. (Original work published in Chinese)

Pai, H. C. (2016). An integrated model for the effects of self-reflection and clinical experiential learning on clinical nursing performance in nursing students: A longitudinal study. *Nurse Education Today*, *45*, 156–162. https://doi.org/10.1016/j.nedt.2016.07.011

Solheim, E., Plathe, H. S., & Eide, H. (2017). Nursing students' evaluation of a new feedback and reflection tool for use in high-fidelity simulation—Formative assessment of clinical skills. A descriptive quantitative research design. *Nurse Education in Practice*, *27*, 114–120. https://doi.org/10.1016/j.nepr.2017.08.021

Speziale, H. S., & Carpenter, D. R. (2007). *Qualitative research in nursing: Advancing the humanistic imperative* (4th ed.). Lippincott Williams & Wilkins.

Sundler, A. J., Pettersson, A., & Berglund, M. (2015). Undergraduate nursing students' experiences when examining nursing skills in clinical simulation laboratories with high-fidelity patient simulators: A phenomenological research study. *Nurse Education Today*, *35*(12), 1257–1261. https://doi.org/10.1016/j.nedt.2015.04.008

Tawalbeh, L. I., & Tubaishat, A. (2014). Effect of simulation on knowledge of advanced cardiac life support, knowledge retention, and confidence of nursing students in Jordan. *The Journal of Nursing Education*, *53*(1), 38–44. https://doi.org/10.3928/01484834-20131218-01

Tuzer, H., Dinc, L., & Elcin, M. (2016). The effects of using high-fidelity simulators and standardized patients on the thorax, lung, and cardiac examination skills of undergraduate nursing students. *Nurse Education Today*, *45*, 120–125. https://doi.org/10.1016/j.nedt.2016.07.002

Warren, J. N., Luctkar-Flude, M., Godfrey, C., & Lukewich, J. (2016). A systematic review of the effectiveness of simulation-based education on satisfaction and learning outcomes in nurse practitioner programs. *Nurse Education Today*, *46*, 99–108. https://doi.org/10.1016/j.nedt.2016.08.023

Yang, Y., & Liu, H. P. (2016). Systematic evaluation influence of high-fidelity simulation teaching on clinical competence of nursing students. *Chinese Nursing Research*, *30*(7), 809–814. (Original work published in Chinese)

Yuan, H. B., Williams, B. A., & Fang, J. B. (2012). The contribution of high-fidelity simulation to nursing students' confidence and competence: A systematic review. *International Nursing Review*, *59*(1), 26–33. https://doi.org/10.1111/j.1466-7657.2011.00964.x

Zhang, J., Zheng, P. P., Li, R. R., Liu, Y., Peng, L. B., & Chen, S. Y. (2014). Perception and experience of simulation teaching among undergraduate nursing students: Benefits, process and barriers. *Chinese Journal of Nursing Education*, *11*(4), 276–281. (Original work published in Chinese)

Zhao, W. L., & Chen, H. (2017). Studies on the self-directed learning situation and its influencing factors for nursing students in universities in a province of the western China. *Chongqin Medicine*, *46*(15), 2102–2105. (Original work published in Chinese)

14

The Relationship Between Psychological Resilience and Stress Perception in Nurses in Turkey During the COVID-19 Pandemic

Hatice KARABULAK[1] • Fadime KAYA[2]*

ABSTRACT

Background: In Turkey, nurses are responsible for the treatment and care of patients with coronavirus disease (COVID-19) and for tracing their contacts. Healthcare professionals exposed to COVID-19 face high levels of stress.

Purpose: This study was designed to determine the influence of psychological resilience and several sociodemographic and professional characteristics on stress perception in nurses during the COVID-19 pandemic.

Methods: A cross-sectional design was used in this study, which was conducted between June 16 and 29, 2020. Two hundred one nurses living in Turkey were enrolled as participants. Data were collected using an information form, the Perceived Stress Scale, and the Brief Psychological Strength Scale. This study aligns with the Strengthening the Reporting of Observational Studies in Epidemiology Checklist.

Results: According to the results of the multivariate linear regression analysis, the psychological resilience score of the participants accounted for 25.2% of the variance related to stress perception ($p < .05$). However, several of the demographic and professional characteristics considered in this study were not found to statistically significantly influence stress perception ($p > .05$).

Conclusions/Implications for Practice: The findings support that psychological resilience is significant in explaining perception of stress in nurses in Turkey. Interventions targeting psychological resilience are needed to reduce nurses' stress perceptions.

KEY WORDS:
pandemic, nurse, perceived stress, psychological resilience.

Introduction

Coronavirus is a large family of viruses that causes disease in animals and humans. In humans, coronaviruses are known to be the cause of many diseases such as the common cold form of Middle East Respiratory Syndrome and more serious respiratory infections such as severe acute respiratory syndrome (World Health Organization [WHO], 2020a). The coronavirus discovered in Wuhan, China, in December 2019 (COVID-19) has been identified as an infectious pneumonia agent (WHO, 2020a). This new coronavirus spread rapidly in China and many other countries and caused a pandemic (Bao et al., 2020). The WHO declared this outbreak a pandemic on March 11, 2020 (WHO, 2020b). The numbers of COVID-19 cases and deaths have increased rapidly worldwide since the outbreak began. As of July 11, 2020, the virus had infected 12,286,664 people and killed 555,642 people in 216 countries (WHO, 2020c). No specific treatment or vaccine has been found for COVID-19; the WHO has recommended only protective measures such as staying at home, social distancing, washing hands with soap or disinfectant, and wearing a mask (Wadood et al., 2020). Until an effective antiviral treatment and vaccine for COVID-19 is found, the psychological effects of this disease will be largely neglected. However, pandemics such as this are not only a medical problem, as they tend to affect quality of life and cause social dysfunction in people who contract the disease (Lai et al., 2020).

Considering the rapid transmission of coronavirus, the high numbers of cases and deaths, and the uncertainties in vaccination and treatment, the outbreak created not only the risk of death because of infection but also high levels of psychological pressure (Cao et al., 2020). Stress, which is expressed as emotional tension caused by the disruption of physiological and psychological adaptation as a result of an organism's interaction with the environment in daily life, may cause a person to experience problems in the physical, emotional, behavioral, and mental dimensions and promote the development of chronic diseases (Özel & Karabulut Bay, 2018). Sources of stress during the outbreak include the unpredictability of the condition and the uncertainty regarding when the disease will be brought under control and the severity of related risks (Bao et al., 2020). In addition, those working in clinics during the pandemic were under great pressure and experienced significant physical and psychological tension

[1]MSN, RN, Ministry of Health, Turkey • [2]PhD, RN, Assistant Professor, Faculty of Health Sciences, Department of Mental Health and Psychiatric Nursing, Kafkas University, Kars, Turkey.

because of insufficient medical resources and the large numbers of seriously ill patients in need of help (Mo et al., 2020; Zhang et al., 2020).

Nurses have played an important public health role in the prevention and control of infection during the COVID-19 pandemic (Smith et al., 2020). The infectious nature, relatively high risk of fatality, and lack of proper medical treatment associated with COVID-19 represent risks to the health and safety of nurses. Anxiety about unknown working environments and processes, a lack of work experience with contagious diseases, fear of transmission, heavy workloads, long-term fatigue, treatment-failure-related depression, having children, and worrying about family members have been identified as important sources of psychological stress (Mo et al., 2020; Shen et al., 2020). A study conducted in China on a large sample of mostly nurses investigated the psychological stress created by the COVID-19 outbreak on healthcare workers. The results found that a significant proportion of participants reported symptoms of depression, anxiety, insomnia, and distress. Nurses, women, frontline health workers, and employees in Wuhan, China, reported severer grades than other healthcare workers of all measures of mental health symptoms (Lai et al., 2020).

An official statement by Turkey's Health Minister on April 29, 2020, noted that 7,428 healthcare workers in the country had been diagnosed with COVID-19 (Turkish Medical Association, 2020). In a study conducted in Turkey, healthcare workers stated that they were uncertain about their working conditions and were particularly concerned about getting infected and transmitting the virus to their families (Eriş & İnan, 2020). A study conducted in Turkey to determine the psychological effect of the COVID-19 outbreak on nurses and midwives found that the lives of 54.5% of nurses and midwives had worsened since the outbreak started, 62.4% had difficulties in dealing with the uncertainty during the outbreak, 42.6% desired psychological support, and 11.8% had become estranged from their professions (Aksoy & Koçak, 2020). The American Nurses Association (2011) identified the acute and chronic effects of stress and overwork as one of the most important safety and health problems in nurses. Nurses' perceived stress affects the care and safety quality in their lives as well as in the lives of their patients (Tehranian, 2018). Addressing the feelings of nurses toward COVID-19 may also promote positive outcomes such as increased job satisfaction, decreased stress levels, and reduced intention to quit the profession (Labrague & de Los Santos, 2020). On the basis of the above, it is important to understand the factors that may assist nurses who are actively engaged in combating the COVID-19 outbreak to withstand and cope effectively with professional stress.

Psychological strength (resilience) refers to the ability of a person to recover from difficult life experiences and overcome disasters successfully (Çam & Büyükbayram, 2017). Psychologically strong individuals manage stress better in business life and exhibit a calmer and more correct attitude in conflict and crisis. They do not allow sources of stress to wear them down or reduce their commitment to the organization, so they do not experience job dissatisfaction (Kavi & Karakale, 2018). In nurses, this feature is undoubtedly important for stress perceptions and coping mechanisms in today's working environment.

This study was designed to determine the influence of psychological resilience and several sociodemographic and professional characteristics on the stress perceptions of nurses during the COVID-19 pandemic. Thus, the following research questions were formulated:

- How do the sociodemographic and professional characteristics of nurses affect their perception of stress?
- How does psychological resilience affect the stress perception of nurses?

Methods

Design and Participants

This research, which used a cross-sectional design, was conducted between June 16 and 29, 2020. Two hundred four nurses currently living in Turkey were enrolled as participants. Sample selection was not used. The inclusion criteria included aged 18 years or older, currently a nurse, and providing online informed consent. The exclusion criteria included working as a nonnurse healthcare worker and filling in the questionnaire incompletely or incorrectly. Three of the enrolled participants were excluded from the research because they failed to complete the questionnaire, leaving the data from 201 participants available for analysis.

Measures

The research data were collected using an information form, the Perceived Stress Scale (PSS), and the Brief Psychological Strength Scale (BPSS).

Information form

The information form was prepared by the researchers and consisted of nine questions, including four questions on sociodemographic features (age, gender, marital status, and school graduated), three questions on professional characteristics (institution, department, and length of tenure), and two questions on the COVID-19 pandemic (training in the institution and worries about uncertainties in the control of the COVID-19 outbreak).

Perceived stress scale

The PSS, developed by Cohen et al. in 1983, was adapted into Turkish by Eskin et al. in 2013. The 14-item PSS was designed to measure the degree to which specific situations are perceived as stressful in the respondent's life. Respondents evaluate each PSS item using a 5-point Likert scale ranging from *never* (0) to *very often* (4). Seven of the items contain positive statements and are scored in reverse (Items 4–7, 9, 10, and 13). The total possible PSS score ranges from 0 to 56, with higher scores indicating excessive stress perceptions. The internal consistency coefficient of this scale was assessed as .84 (Eskin et al., 2013), and in this study, the internal consistency coefficient was .86.

Brief psychological strength scale

The BPSS was developed by Smith et al. (2008) to measure psychological resilience and was adapted into Turkish by Doğan (2015). The BPSS is a six-item, self-report measurement tool that uses a 5-point Likert-type scale ranging from *not suitable at all* (1) to *completely suitable* (5). Items 2, 4, and 6 are reverse scored (Doğan, 2015). After the items in the scale are reverse coded and translated, a higher score indicates higher psychological strength. The internal consistency coefficient of the BPSS was previously assessed as .83, and in this study, it was assessed as .78.

Variables

The dependent variable in this study was the PSS total score. The independent variables were the BPSS total score and the demographic, professional, and COVID-19 characteristics of the participants.

Data Collection

The online questionnaire was uploaded and shared on two website platforms (Facebook and WhatsApp). The questionnaire could be completed via computer or smartphone via the website link. The questionnaire also included a section that described the purpose of the study and the anonymity and privacy policies governing participation. The participants completed the questionnaire by connecting to the website, filling in the questionnaire, and pressing the send button.

Data Analysis

The data obtained in the study were analyzed using SPSS Statistics Version 20.0 (IBM Inc., Armonk, NY, USA). The average and standard deviation of continuous variables and the frequency and percentage values of categorical variables were calculated. The PSS total score was obtained for difference statistics. The two-category variables and PSS total mean score difference were evaluated using independent samples *t* tests. One-way analysis of variance was performed using more than two categorical variables and the total mean score difference of the PSS. The relationship between the PSS total score and the BPSS total score was evaluated using the Pearson correlation coefficient. In the last stage, multivariate linear regression analysis was applied to determine the predictor variables. Statistical significance was set at $p < .05$ for all of the variables.

Ethical Considerations

Permission to conduct this research was obtained on June 8, 2020, from the local noninterventional clinical research ethics committee (#81829502.903/48) and from the Republic of Turkey Ministry of Health. Online informed consent was obtained from all of the participants after they had

received an explanation of the purpose and confidentiality policy of this research.

Results

The sociodemographic and professional characteristics of the participants are presented in Table 1. Their average age was 36.21 years (SD = 8.15, range: 21–56 years), and their average tenure was 14.99 years (SD = 9.19; range: 2 months to 38 years). Nearly all (95.5%) of the participants were women, 63.2% were married, 65.7% held a bachelor's degree, 64.2% worked at public or private hospitals, and 56.2% reported providing services that may be considered risky in terms of COVID-19 (i.e., emergency room, surgery, intensive care, and inpatient services). Two thirds (68.7%) reported having received training on COVID-19 at the institution where they worked, and 95% were concerned about the uncertainties involved in effectively controlling the COVID-19 outbreak. The mean BPSS score of the participants was 19.18 (SD = 4.39, range: 6–30).

Table 1
Descriptive Findings (N = 201)

Variable	n	%
Age (years; *M* and *SD*)	36.21	8.15
Gender		
Female	191	95.5
Male	10	5.0
Marital status		
Single	74	36.8
Married	127	63.2
Education		
Health vocational high school	6	3.0
Two-year degree	33	16.4
Bachelor's degree	132	65.7
Master's degree/doctorate	30	14.9
Institution		
University hospital	47	23.4
Public/private hospital	129	64.2
Primary healthcare organization	25	12.4
Department		
Emergency	24	11.9
Intensive care	17	8.5
Surgery	44	21.9
COVID-19 service	28	13.9
Services outside COVID-19	88	43.8
Length of tenure (months; *M* and *SD*)	14.99	9.19
Received training on COVID-19 at work		
Yes	138	68.7
No	63	31.3
Concerned about uncertainties in controlling the COVID-19 outbreak		
Yes	191	95.0
No	10	5.0
Brief Psychological Strength Scale (*M* and *SD*)	19.18	4.39

Table 2

Nurses' Perception of Stress (N = 201)

Perceived Stress Scale	Mean	SD
1. Feeling uncomfortable because something unexpected has happened	2.28	1.12
2. Feeling like you cannot control the important things in your life	2.28	1.12
3. Feeling nervous and stressed	2.58	1.06
4. Feeling unable to overcome daily challenges	1.62	0.99
5. Feeling unable to deal effectively with significant changes in your life	1.71	0.99
6. Feeling insecure in your ability to handle personal problems	1.66	1.11
7. Do not feel like everything is going right	2.13	1.03
8. Realizing that you cannot handle things that need to be done	1.94	1.05
9. Feeling unable to control the difficulties in your life	1.76	0.95
10. Do not feel like you can handle everything	1.81	0.98
11. Being angry about events beyond your control	2.24	1.08
12. Finding yourself thinking about the things you need to achieve	2.45	1.00
13. Feeling unable to control how you use your time	1.82	1.03
14. Feeling that problems have increased too much for you to overcome them	2.05	1.13
Total score	28.47	7.23

The average scores for stress perception scale items and the overall total score for stress perception in the last month are presented in Table 2. The mean PSS score was 28.47 (SD = 7.23), and the four items with the highest mean scores were "Feeling nervous and stressed" (2.58, SD = 1.06), "Finding yourself thinking about the things you must achieve" (2.45, SD = 1.00), "Feeling uncomfortable because something unexpected has happened" (2.28, SD = 1.12), and "Feeling like you cannot control the important things in your life" (2.28, SD = 1.12).

The differences between participants' demographic, occupational, and COVID-19-related characteristics and stress perceptions are shown in Table 3. No statistically significant differences were found between stress perception score and the variables of gender, marital status, educational level, institution, and department. However, the mean stress perception score of those trained on COVID-19 was statistically significantly lower than those who did not receive COVID-19 training ($p < .05$). In addition, the mean stress perception score of those who stated that uncertainties over control of the COVID-19 pandemic increased their concerns was statistically significantly higher than of those who did not ($p < .05$).

The relationships among PSS scores, participant demographics and professional characteristics, and BPSS scores are presented in Table 4. No statistically significant

relationships between age and length of tenure and PSS score were found ($p > .05$). However, a negative and moderately statistically significant relationship between BPSS total score and PSS total score was found ($p < .001$).

The psychological resilience total score was shown to be a significant predictor of perception of stress (R^2 = .25, F = 22.14, $p < .001$), with psychological resilience scores found to account for 25.2% of the variance in stress perception. Thus, perceived stress decreased as psychological resilience increased (Table 5).

However, the statistically significant effect on stress perception was eliminated when the variables of concern (i.e., uncertainties related to COVID-19 training in their institutions and the control of the COVID-19 outbreak) were included in the regression model ($p > .05$).

Discussion

In order to reduce the stress caused by traumatic situations, to increase the coping skills of the person for long and short-term adaptation, and to improve the quality of care in disaster situations, the stress situations of nurses and the affecting factors should be examined (Kılıç & Şimşek, 2018). The aim of this study was to assess the influence of psychological resilience and several demographic and professional characteristics on nurses' perceptions of stress during the COVID-19 pandemic. The results highlight the importance of psychological resilience in protecting the mental health of nurses.

In line with the first research question, the potential relationships between the several demographic and professional characteristics of nurses and their perceived stress scores were evaluated. No statistically significant relationship was found between the perceived stress score and the variable of age, gender, marital status, educational level, institution, department, or length of tenure. These results show that the mean perceived stress score was similar for all of the participants independent of age, gender, marital status, educational level, institution, department, and length of tenure.

The mean PSS score in this study was 28.47 (SD = 7.23), which indicates a moderate level of perceived stress. The total possible range for PSS scores is 0–56, with higher scores indicating higher perceived stress. This scale has no breakpoint (Eskin et al., 2013). The most stressful situations for the participants during the previous 1-month period were described as feeling nervous and stressed, finding themselves thinking about the things they had to achieve, and feeling uncomfortable because something unexpected had happened. During the COVID-19 pandemic in Turkey, the participants expressed perceiving high levels of stress when feeling nervous or stressed, when they felt compelled to succeed, when they experienced an unexpected event, and when they were unable to control important things in their lives. During the COVID-19 pandemic, two thirds of the nurses participating in a study in Austria and more than half of those in Nepal perceived moderate stress levels (Hoedl et al., 2020; Neupane et al., 2020). In a cross-sectional study that aimed to determine the prevalence

Table 3

Differences Between Independent Variables and Stress Perception Scale (N = 201)

Independent Variable	Perceived Stress Scale			
	Mean	SD	t/F	p
Gender				
Female	28.55	7.19	0.70	.482
Male	26.90	8.25		
Marital status				
Single	28.13	7.00	−0.50	.615
Married	28.66	7.38		
Education				
Health vocational high school/2-year degree	29.64	8.93	1.12	.262
Graduate or higher	28.19	6.76		
Institution				
University hospital	27.31	7.25		
Public/private hospital	28.71	7.40	$F = 0.87$	.419
Primary healthcare organization	29.40	6.24		
Department				
Services with COVID-19-positive hospitalization	28.51	7.88	0.09	.928
Services without COVID-19-positive hospitalization	28.42	6.34		
Received training on COVID-19 at work				
Yes	27.47	6.82	−2.94	.004*
No	30.65	7.66		
Concerned about uncertainties in controlling the COVID-19 outbreak				
Yes	28.78	7.08	2.72	.007*
No	22.50	7.84		

Note. t = independent samples t test; F = one-way analysis of variance.
*$p < .05$.

of perceived stress and risk factors among healthcare providers in Ethiopia, the prevalence of perceived stress was found to be very high among healthcare providers, with the highest stress scores found among nurses (Chekole et al., 2020). In a study conducted in Hubei, China, from January to March 2020 to determine the psychological impact and ways of coping with the outbreak (Cai et al., 2020), health workers reported that they were concerned about their families' safety and increased mortality rates. In another study on health workers in China during the COVID-19 outbreak (Xiao et al., 2020), it was determined that the COVID-19 pandemic induced stress in healthcare workers and that

Table 4

Correlation Between Stress Perception Scale and Independent Variables (N = 201)

Independent Variable	Perceived Stress Scale	
	r	p
Age	−.03	.629
Length of tenure	.03	.728
Brief Psychological Strength Scale	−.49	< .001

healthcare workers experienced high rates of anxiety and depression. During pandemics, the burden on health systems and the workload and stress of health professionals increase significantly. These health professionals experience long working hours, aggravated working conditions, increased expectations and anxiety from society, high patient numbers, and elevated risks of becoming sick themselves. All of these factors affect the overall psychosocial functionality and resilience of health workers (Enli Tuncay et al., 2020). The results of this study indicate that the level of stress perceived by nurses is not significantly influenced by sociodemographic and professional variables.

In this study, the variables related to COVID-19 and the effect of psychological resilience on perceived stress in nurses were evaluated using a multivariate simple linear regression model. When the analysis results were examined, the total psychological resilience score was found to significantly predict the participants' perceptions of stress ($p < .05$). According to Graber et al. (2015), psychological resilience is defined as a developmental process in which individuals exposed to potentially traumatic events experience positive psychological adaptation over time. The ability to return to the psychological state that prevailed before a traumatic experience has been defined as psychological resilience. In other words, psychological resilience refers to the mental processes and behaviors that an individual uses

Table 5

Perceived Stress Scale: Simple Linear Regression Model (N = 201)

Independent Variable	Perceived Stress Scale				
	B	95% CI	β	t	p
Constant	41.12	[34.86, 47.38]		12.96	< .001
Total BPSS point	−0.74	[−0.95, −0.53]	−0.45	−6.92	< .001
Trained on COVID-19 at work (0 = no, 1 = yes)	−1.43	[−3.38, 0.52]	−0.09	−1.45	.149
Concerned about uncertainties in controlling the COVID-19 outbreak (0 = no, 1 = yes)	2.62	[−1.53, 6.76]	0.08	1.24	.215

Note. Adjusted R^2 = .24, R^2 = .25, F = 22.14 (p < .001). BPSS = Brief Psychological Strength Scale; CI = confidence interval.

to protect himself or herself from the potential negative effects of stress factors (Devi, 2020). Psychological resilience is also a concept that represents the functions used to adapt to psychopathologies such as depression, anxiety, and posttraumatic stress disorder (Graber et al., 2015). Enli Tuncay et al. (2020) report that rates of psychiatric disorders such as anxiety, depression, posttraumatic stress disorder, and burnout are higher in healthcare professionals than in the general population during a pandemic. Furthermore, the psychosocial aspects of pandemics affect women and nurses more than others (Enli Tuncay et al., 2020). In light of this information, the results of this study highlight the importance of psychological strength in reducing perceived stress in nurses who live and work in Turkey. Thus, assessing the resilience of nurses is important to assess their mental health.

Limitations

This study was affected by several limitations. First, the sample size of this study was small. To improve statistical significance and the generalizability of the results, future studies on this subject should use larger sample sizes. Another limitation was the use of a cross-sectional design, which does not allow causal relationships to be evaluated.

Conclusions

The complex, infectious, and sensitive nature of the COVID-19 outbreak poses significant challenges for healthcare professionals and nurses working on the front lines. To protect and maintain mental health, it is necessary to focus on improving the psychological resilience of nurses and on understanding their perceived stress. This study showed the presence of perceived stress in nurses, whereas psychological resilience was determined as a factor affecting the perception of stress. The results of this study may be used as a reference for community mental health nurses and psychiatric nurses in psychological intervention programs that will be provided during or after the COVID-19 pandemic in Turkey.

Implications for Practice

The results of this study showed that psychological resilience is an important predictor of perceived stress in nurses. Protecting

the mental health of nursing staff is essential for nurses to combat COVID-19 effectively. Community mental health and psychiatric nurses should develop, implement, and evaluate interventions designed to enhance psychological resilience in clinical nurses. Therefore, community mental health and psychiatric nurses should inform nursing managers and clinician nurses about the active mobilization of nurses' social support systems, assist nurses to deal with stress and express their managerial skills and emotions, and organize leisure activities and training to help healthcare professionals reduce stress.

Author Contributions

Study conception and design: HK
Data collection: HK, FK
Data analysis and interpretation: FK
Drafting of the article: HK, FK
Critical revision of the article: HK, FK

References

Aksoy, Y. E., & Koçak, V. (2020). Psychological effects of nurses and midwives due to COVID-19 outbreak: The case of Turkey. *Archives of Psychiatric Nursing, 34*(2), 427–433. https://doi.org/10.1016/j.apnu.2020.07.011 (Original work published in Turkish)

American Nurses Association. (2011). *2011 Health & safety survey— Hazards of the RN work environment.* https://www.nursingworld.org/~48dd70/globalassets/docs/ana/health-safetysurvey_mediabackgrounder_2011.pdf

Bao, Y., Sun, Y., Meng, S., Shi, J., & Lu, L. (2020). 2019-nCoV epidemic: Address mental health care to empower society.

The Lancet, 395(10224), E37–E38. https://doi.org/10.1016/S0140-6736(20)30309-3

Cai, H., Tu, B., Ma, J., Chen, L., Fu, L., Jiang, Y., & Zhuang, Q. (2020). Psychological impact and coping strategies of frontline medical staff in Hunan between January and march 2020 during the outbreak of coronavirus disease 2019 (COVID-19) in Hubei, China. *Medical Science Monitor, 26*, Article e924171. https://doi.org/10.12659/MSM.924171

Çam, O., & Büyükbayram, A. (2017). Nurses' resilience and effective factors. *The Journal of Psychiatric Nursing, 8*(2), 118–126. https://doi.org/10.14744/phd.2017.75436 (Original work published in Turkish)

Cao, W., Fang, Z., Hou, G., Han, M., Xu, X., Dong, J., & Zheng, J. (2020). The psychological impact of the COVID-19 epidemic on college students in China. *Psychiatry Research, 287*, Article 112934. https://doi.org/10.1016/j.psychres.2020.112934

Chekole, Y. A., Yimer, S., Mekuriaw, B., & Mekonnen, S. (2020). Prevalence and risk factors of perceived stress on COVID-19 among health care providers in Dilla town health institutions, Southern Ethiopia: A cross-sectional study. *Research Square*. Advance online publication. https://doi.org/10.21203/rs.3.rs-23476/v1

Devi, S. (2020). Psychological resilience and coping strategies during COVID-19 pandemic lock down. *Journal of Xi'an University of Architecture &Technology, 12*(4), 2925–2933.

Doğan, T. (2015). Adaptation of the Brief Resilience Scale into Turkish: A validity and reliability study. *The Journal of Happiness & Well-Being, 3*(1), 93–102. (Original work published in Turkish)

Enli Tuncay, F., Koyuncu, E., & Özel, Ş. A. (2020). Review of protective and risk factors affecting psychosocial health of healthcare workers in pandemics. *Ankara Medical Journal, 20*(2), 488–504. https://doi.org/10.5505/amj.2020.02418 (Original work published in Turkey)

Eriş, H., & İnan, M. A. (2020). Covid-19 perceptions and attitudes of health workers in Turkey. *Journal of Critical Reviews, 7* (12), 1142–1150. https://doi.org/10.31838/jcr.07.12.200

Eskin, M., Harlak, H., Demirkıran, F., & Dereboy, Ç. (2013). The adaptation of the perceived stress scale into Turkish: A reliability and validity analysis. *New/Yeni Symposium Journal, 51*(3), 132–140. (Original work published in Turkish)

Graber, R., Pichon, F., & Carabine, E. (2015). *Psychological resilience: State of knowledge and future research agendas* (working paper). Overseas Development Institute. https://www.odi.org/publications/9596-psychological-resilience-state-knowledge-future-research-agendas

Hoedl, M., Bauer, S., & Eglseer, D. (2020). Influence of nursing staff working hours on the stress level during the COVID-19 pandemic: A cross-sectional online survey. *MedRxiv*, 1-18. https://doi.org/10.1101/2020.08.12.20173385

Kavi, E., & Karakale, B. (2018). Psychological resilience related to labor psychology. *HAK-İŞ International Journal of Labour and Society, 7*(7), 55–77. https://doi.org/10.31199/hakisderg.391826 (Original work published in Turkish)

Kılıç, N., & Şimşek, N. (2018). Psychological first aid and nursing. *Journal of Psychiatric Nursing, 9*(3), 212–218. https://doi.org/10.14744/phd.2017.76376 (Original work published in Turkey)

Labrague, L. J., & de Los Santos, J. (2020). Fear of COVID-19, psychological distress, work satisfaction and turnover intention among frontline nurses. *Journal of Nursing Management, 29*(3), 395–403. https://doi.org/10.21203/rs.3.rs-35366/v1

Lai, J., Ma, S., Wang, Y., Cai, Z., Hu, J., Wei, N., Wu, J., Du, H.,

Chen, T., Li, R., Tan, H., Kang, H., Yao, L., Huang, M., Wang, H., Wang, G., Liu, Z., & Hu, S. (2020). Factors associated with mental health outcomes among health care workers exposed to coronavirus disease. *JAMA Network Open, 3*(3), Article e203976. https://doi.org/10.1001/jamanetworkopen.2020.3976

Mo, Y., Deng, L., Zhang, L., Lang, Q., Liao, C., Wang, N., Qin, M., & Huang, H. (2020). Work stress among Chinese nurses to support Wuhan in fighting against COVID-19 epidemic. *Journal of Nursing Management, 28*, 1002–1009. https://doi.org/10.1111/jonm.13014

Neupane, M. S., Angadi, S., Joshi, A., & Neupane, H. C. (2020). Stress and anxiety among nurses working in tertiary care hospitals in Nepal during COVID-19 pandemic. *Journal of Chitwan Medical College, 10*(3), 8–11. https://doi.org/10.3126/jcmc.v10i3.32001

Özel, Y., & Karabulut Bay, A. (2018). Daily living and stress management. *Turkish Journal of Health Sciences and Research, 1*(1), 48–56. (Original work published in Turkish)

Shen, X., Zou, X., Zhong, X., Yan, J., & Li, L. (2020). Psychological stress of ICU nurses in the time of COVID-19. *Critical Care, 24*, – Article No. 200. https://doi.org/10.1186/s13054-020-02926-2

Smith, B. W., Dalen, J., Wiggins, K., Tooley, E., Christopher, P., & Bernard, J. (2008). The brief resilience scale: Assessing the ability to bounce back. *International Journal of Behavioral Medicine, 15*(3), 194–200. https://doi.org/10.1080/10705500802222972

Smith, G. D., Ng, F., & Li, W. H. C. (2020). COVID-19: Emerging compassion, courage and resilience in the face of misinformation and adversity. *Journal of Clinical Nursing, 29*(9–10), 1425–1428. https://doi.org/10.1111%2Fjocn.15231

Tehranian, A. (2018). *Compassion and perceived stress in registered nurses: Impact on patient-safety culture* (Unpublished doctoral dissertation). The Chicago School of Professional Psychology.

Turkish Medical Association. (2020). *If the rights of healthcare workers who get sick from COVID-19 cannot be protected, it means that no one can claim rights.* https://www.ttb.org.tr/kollar/COVID19/haber_goster.php?Guid=eb366d92-8ad5-11ea-911b-f85bdc3fa683 (Original work published in Turkish)

Wadood, A., Mamun, A., Rafi, A., Islam, K., Mohd, S., Lee, L. L., & Hossain, G. (2020). Knowledge, attitude, practice and perception regarding COVID-19 among students in Bangladesh: Survey in Rajshahi University. *MedRxiv*. Advance online publication. https://doi.org/10.1101/2020.04.21.20074757

World Health Organization. (2020a). *Coronavirus disease (COVID-19).* https://www.who.int/emergencies/diseases/novel-coronavirus-2019/question-and-answers-hub/q-a-detail/q-a-coronaviruses

World Health Organization. (2020b). *Coronavirus disease 2019 (COVID-19) Situation Report-51.* https://apps.who.int/iris/handle/10665/331475

World Health Organization. (2020c). *Coronavirus disease (COVID-19) outbreak situation.* https://www.who.int/emergencies/diseases/novel-coronavirus-2019

Xiao, X., Zhu, X., Fu, S., Hu, Y., Li, X., & Xiao, J. (2020). Psychological impact of healthcare workers in China during COVID-19 pneumonia epidemic: A multi-center cross-sectional survey investigation. *Journal of Affective Disorders, 274*, 405–410. https://doi.org/10.1016/j.jad.2020.05.081

Zhang, H. J., Yin, L., Peng, Y., Chen, Q., Lv, C., Juan, L., Fan, L., Tong, T., Liu, R., Zhao, L., Liang, T., & Tian, S. (2020). A qualitative study on the inner experience of first-line nurses in the clinical fight against COVID-19. *Research Square*. Advance online publication. https://doi.org/10.21203/rs.3.rs-33438/v1

15

The Relationship Between Critical Thinking Skills and Learning Styles and Academic Achievement of Nursing Students

Fatemeh SHIRAZI[1] • Shiva HEIDARI[2]*

ABSTRACT

Background: Academic achievement is one of the most important indicators in evaluating education. Various factors are known to affect the academic achievement of students.

Purpose: This study was performed to assess the relationship between critical thinking skills and learning styles and the academic achievement of nursing students.

Methods: In this cross-sectional study, 139 sophomores to senior-year nursing students were selected using a simple random sampling method. The data were gathered using a three-part questionnaire that included a demographic questionnaire, the Kolb's Learning Style Standard Questionnaire, and the California Critical Thinking Skills Questionnaire. The previous semester's grade point average of the students was considered as a measure of academic achievement. The data were analyzed using descriptive and analytical statistics in SPSS 20.

Results: The mean score for critical thinking skills was 6.75 ± 2.16, and the highest and lowest scores among the critical thinking subscales related to the evaluation and analysis subscales, respectively. No relationship between critical thinking and academic achievement was identified. "Diverging" was the most common learning style. The highest mean level of academic achievement was earned by those students who adopted the "accommodating" style of learning. A significant relationship was found between learning style and academic achievement ($p < .001$).

Conclusions: According to the findings, the critical thinking skills score of students was unacceptably low. Therefore, it is essential to pay more attention to improving critical thinking in academic lesson planning. As a significant relationship was found between learning style and academic achievement, it is suggested that instructors consider the dominant style of each class in lesson planning and use proper teaching methods that take into consideration the dominant style.

KEY WORDS:
academic achievement, critical thinking skills, learning styles, nursing student.

academic failure may cause a decrease in academic accomplishment and an increase in the costs of education (Jayanthi, Balakrishnan, Ching, Latiff, & Nasirudeen, 2014). Academic achievement, the level to which students attain predetermined educational goals, depends on family and individual, socioeconomic, education, training, and psychological factors (Farooq, Chaudhry, Shafiq, & Berhanu, 2011). Assessing these factors and determining the contribution of each to academic achievement are critical to developing strategies for identifying the factors that contribute to academic success and failure and help educational planners focus on promoting the positive factors and reducing the impact of negative factors (Gordon, Williams, Hudson, & Stewart, 2010). Critical thinking is one of the contributing factors in academic achievement as well as an essential component in clinical decision making, nursing practice, and education (Fero et al., 2010).

There are many reasons for nurses to learn critical thinking skills. The first reason is that thinking is the key component in problem solving, and nurses without these proficiencies become part of the problem. In addition, nurses should be capable of making major decisions independently and quickly in critical situations. Critical thinking skills enable them to identify essential data and distinguish between problems that require urgent intervention and those that are not life-threatening. Thus, nurses should be able to reflect on their actions and consider the possible consequences of each action to make precise and proper decisions (Eslami & Maarefi, 2010).

Various investigations have suggested that it is necessary to design educational strategies that are based on student learning style to improve students' critical thinking. In addition to critical thinking, the learning styles of students are an important factor that plays a fundamental role in the process

[1]PhD, Assistant Professor, Department of Nursing, School of Nursing and Midwifery, Shiraz University of Medical Sciences, Shiraz, Iran • [2]MSN, Instructor, Department of Nursing, Urmia Branch, Islamic Azad University, Urmia, Iran.

Introduction

Academic achievement is crucial to the future success of students, and lack of attention to this basic issue and subsequent

of problem solving and learning. Learning style describes the method used to process information, which differs from person to person. Identifying the methods that students use to process information and their learning styles allows educators to assist them to advance toward the higher goals of training and achieve broader critical thinking and problem-solving skills (Lau & Yuen, 2010). Perhaps, the best definition of learning styles was provided by Kolb, who defined learning styles as an individual's method of emphasizing certain learning abilities over other abilities. Kolb's experiential learning theory is the result of the combination of three templates from the experiential learning process, including Lewin's practical and laboratory model, Dewey's learning model, and Piaget's pattern of learning and cognitive development. Kolb believed learning to be the result of resolving the conflicts among these three models (Kolb & Kolb, 2005). Many studies have investigated the relationships between learning styles and other variables. The academic achievement of learners is one of the key variables to be studied with regard to its relationship with learning style (Zainol Abidin, Rezaee, Abdullah, & Singh, 2011). Most of these studies have shown thinking to be the combination of knowledge, skills, and attitudes. This combination empowers thoughtful persons to become wiser and more competent in different sciences and technologies and, consequently, gives them momentum along the path to success (Can, 2009). The study of Aripin, Mahmood, Rohaizad, Yeop, and Anuar (2008) showed that paying attention to students' learning styles and matching these with a learning framework significantly improved students' academic performance, whereas a mismatch between learning styles and curriculum reduced performance levels. Other studies that surveyed the relationship between critical thinking and its subdomains and different learning styles obtained different results (Ghazivakili et al., 2014; Noohi, Salahi, & Sabzevari, 2014).

The review of studies highlighted conflicting results in the relationship between critical thinking, learning styles, and academic achievement. Some studies have emphasized a positive relationship (Ashoori, 2014; Ghazivakili et al., 2014), whereas others have found a negative relationship (Aghaei, Souri, & Ghanbari, 2012) or an absence of a significant relationship. These conflicting results may be caused by differences among individual student characteristics and their educational culture (Abdollahi Adli Ansar, FathiAzar, & Abdollahi, 2015). On the basis of these differences in results and the diversity of students and educational systems in different academic contexts, this study was designed to determine the relationship between critical thinking skills and learning styles and the academic achievement of nursing students studying at Urmia Islamic Azad University.

Methods

In this cross-sectional study, 139 nursing students between their sophomore and senior years were selected randomly out of 360 nursing students studying at Islamic Azad University in Urmia, Iran. The students were divided into three groups according to their years of education, and each group was random sampled using a table of random numbers. The researcher delivered the questionnaires and consent forms to the selected students. After explaining how to answer the questions, the completed questionnaires were collected 2 days later. Data collection lasted from October to December 2015.

This study was approved by the research council and the ethics committee of the Urmia branch of Islamic Azad University, Urmia, Iran (Code: 27827). A three-part questionnaire was used for data collection. The first part of the questionnaire assessed demographic information such as age, marital status, and educational level. Besides that, the grade point average (GPA) of each student for the previous semester was recorded as a measure of academic achievement. The second part of the questionnaire was California Standardized Critical Thinking Skills Test, Form B, published by Facione and Facione in 1994. This test contains 34 multiple (4–5)-choice questions with one correct answer each. These questions address the five domains of the cognitive skills of critical thinking (deductive, inductive, assessment, analysis, and inference). One score is assigned for each correct answer, and the total test score is obtained by summing the number of correct answers. The minimum and maximum possible scores are 0 and 34, respectively. The midpoint score of the scale is 15.98, indicating that lower scores represent relatively weak critical thinking and higher scores represent relatively strong critical thinking. The reliability of this questionnaire was reported as .86 by Hariri (Hariri & Bagherinejad, 2012). In this study, the reliability of the test was checked using test–retest, with an earned score of .79.

The third part of the questionnaire was Kolb's Learning Styles Inventory, which includes 12 sentences. Each sentence includes four parts that respectively measure reflective observation, concrete experience, active experimentation, and abstract conceptualization. The four scores obtained from the sum of these four parts in the 12 questions of the questionnaire indicate the four styles of learning. Two scores are obtained from two-by-two subtraction of these styles, that is, the subtraction of abstract conceptualization from concrete experience and active experimentation from reflective observation. These two scores are placed on the axis, which constitutes the four quarters of a square, identified by the four learning styles as diverging, converging, assimilating, and accommodating (Kolb & Kolb, 2005). Emamipour reported the alpha coefficients of abstract conceptualization, concrete experience, active experimentation, and reflective observation as .49, .51, .47, and .53, respectively (Emamipour & Shams Esfandabad, 2007).

After collecting the completed questionnaires, the data were analyzed using SPSS software Version 20 with descriptive and analytical statistical tests such as Student t test, one-way analysis of variance, chi-square, and correlation test.

Results

The data analysis showed that all of the participants were female, with a mean age of 21.88 ± 2.09 years and an age

TABLE 1.

Demographic Characteristics of Participants (N = 139)

Variable	n	%
Age (years; M and SD)	21.88	2.09
19–23	112	80.6
24–29	21	15.1
Not declared	6	4.3
Marital status		
Single	119	85.6
Married	18	13.0
Widowed/divorced	2	1.4
Educational level		
Sophomore (second year)	48	34.2
Junior (third year)	46	33.4
Senior (fourth year)	45	32.4

TABLE 3.

Relationship Between Learning Style and Demographic Variables and Academic Achievement

Variable	Learning Style	
	χ^2/F	p
Age	0.95	.81
Marital status	64.73	< .001
Educational level	6.03	.73
Grade point average	$F = 6.96$	< .001

range of 19–29 years. Most (85.6%) were single (Table 1). The mean GPA of the students was 15.78 ± 1.35, ranging from 12 to 18.79.

The mean score of critical thinking was 6.75 ± 2.16, and the highest and lowest mean critical thinking skill subdomain scores were for evaluation skill (6.75 ± 2.16) and analysis skill (1.58 ± 1.85), respectively. No significant relationship between critical thinking and academic achievement was found. Moreover, the critical thinking subdomains were not significantly related to academic achievement. In addition, no significant relationship was found between the total score and the subscales of critical thinking and marital status, age, or educational level. However, a significant relationship was found between the total score of critical thinking and educational level. Therefore, the senior students in this study earned a higher mean score for critical thinking than their lower-grade peers ($p = .04$; Table 2).

Most participants (55.4%) used a "diverging" learning style, whereas 0.7% used a "converging" style. There was a significant relationship between learning styles and academic achievement, with academic achievement (represented by GPA) highest in the accommodating learning style subgroup followed by the diverging, converging, and assimilating learning-style subgroups.

Whereas no significant relationship was found between learning style and either age or educational level, a significant relationship was found between learning style and marital status (Table 3).

Using one-way analysis of variance, the relationship between learning style and critical thinking skills and also the comparison of the mean score for each skill in four styles are reported in Table 4. The findings showed no statistically significant relationship between learning style and critical thinking or its subscales (Table 4).

Finally, a significant relationship was found between academic achievement and educational level, which meant that senior students had the highest level of academic achievement ($p = .01$). However, academic achievement had no

TABLE 2.

The Relationship Between Critical Thinking Styles and Demographic Variables and Academic Achievement

Variable	Age		Marital Status		Educational Level		GPA[a]	
	r	p	F^b	p	F	p	r	p
Assessment	.02	.86	2.02	.13	1.27	.28	−.01	.87
Analysis	−.20	.07	0.65	.52	0.11	.89	.02	.81
Inference	−.12	.20	1.07	.34	0.20	.81	.06	.60
Inductive reasoning	−.06	.57	1.28	.28	0.97	.38	.002	.98
Deductive reasoning	−.12	.23	1.49	.23	0.18	.83	−.06	.57
Total critical thinking score	−.15	.18	2.15	.12	0.54	.04	.05	.74

Note. GPA = grade point average.
[a]An indicator of academic achievement. [b]Analysis of variance.

TABLE 4.
Relationship Between Critical Thinking Skills and Learning Style

Critical Thinking	Learning Style								
	Divergent		Convergent		Accommodator		Assimilator		
	Mean	SD	Mean	SD	Mean	SD	Mean	SD	p
Assessment	3.51	1.46	2.00	0	2.50	1.29	3.30	1.74	.41
Analysis	1.73	1.27	2.00	0	2.66	0.57	1.31	0.90	.13
Inference	1.82	1.26	1.00	0	2.66	0.57	1.89	0.93	.56
Inductive reasoning	3.25	1.37	2.00	0	3.25	1.50	3.17	1.46	.93
Deductive reasoning	3.09	1.59	1.00	0	3.00	1.00	2.65	1.71	.51
Total critical thinking	6.94	2.36	5.00	0	6.50	0.70	6.52	2.01	.70

significant relationship with other variables such as age and marital status (Table 5).

Discussion

This study found no significant relationship between any of the demographic variables such as age and marital status and academic achievement. However, years of education were associated positively with academic achievement. This finding is consistent with that of Edraki, Rambod, and Abdoli (2011). Fewer courses in higher academic grades, familiarization with the university atmosphere, and the stronger emphasis on clinical courses during the years of education may help students to effectively increase their GPA and improve their academic achievements.

The mean score for critical thinking in this study was 6.75 ± 2.16. Similar to the results of this study, Taghavi Larijani, Mardani Hmouleh, Rezaei, Ghadiriyan, and Rashidi (2014) reported a mean score for critical thinking of 9.33 ±

TABLE 5.
Relationship Between Demographic Variables and Academic Achievement

Variable	Grade Point Average			
	M	SD	t/F	p
Age (years)			t = 5.70	.76
19–23	15.80	1.25		
24–29	15.66	1.83		
Marital status			1.24	.29
Single	15.73	1.30		
Married	16.23	1.68		
Widowed/Divorced	14.84	1.18		
Educational level			3.88	.01
Sophomore (second year)	15.36	1.20		
Junior (third year)	15.52	1.47		
Senior (fourth year)	16.34	1.09		

3.33. In addition, a study conducted in the United States found that most students earned relatively low scores for critical thinking (Shinnick & Woo, 2013). On the contrary, a 2010 study in Norway found that participants earned good scores for critical thinking (Wangensteen, Johansson, Björkström, & Nordström, 2010). Researchers believe that the multiple, intertwining factors involved in decreasing critical thinking scores include educational failure, focusing on rote memorization, presenting concepts in manners that do not require deep questioning/consideration, emphasis on multiple-choice examinations, lack of appropriate mental or psychological security for questioning and answering between the students and instructors, and poor development of critical thinking abilities (Hosseini, 2009). The low critical thinking score of the students in this research as well as in other studies conducted in Iran compared with the scores of students in other countries suggests that current education methods in Iran do not effectively strengthen the critical thinking of students and thus should be revised (Azodi, Jahanpoor, & Sharif, 2010).

In addition, in this study, the maximum and minimum subdomain scores for critical thinking were for assessment and analysis, respectively. Similarly, Ghazivakili et al. found that the minimum score for critical thinking was in the dimension of analysis (Ghazivakili et al., 2014). On the basis of the findings of this study, no significant relationship was observed between the critical thinking and the academic achievement of the students, which is consistent with the results of Azodi et al. (2010). Furthermore, the findings of Ghazivakili et al. suggested a relationship between critical thinking skills and the previous semester's GPA as a criterion for determining academic achievement. In the study of Ghazivakili et al., the mean GPA score of the students was increased by increasing the understanding skill of critical thinking (Ghazivakili et al., 2014).

This study did not show any relationship between critical thinking and either age or marital status. However, Azodi et al.'s study showed a positive relationship between age and critical thinking (Azodi et al., 2010). Age is an important demographic variable that is often correlated with critical thinking. This relationship is based on the assumption that critical thinking improves with age (Babamohammadi, Esmaeilpour, Negarande, & Dehghan Nayeri, 2011).

The relationship between the total score for critical thinking and educational level was significant. Thus, the total score for critical thinking increased with the number of years of enrollment. However, no relationship was observed between the subdomains of critical thinking and educational level, which is consistent with the findings of Noohi et al. (2014).

The results showed that diverging, assimilating, accommodating, and converging were, respectively, the most-to-least used learning styles of the participants in this study. This ranking of students' learning styles differs from those of other studies that were conducted domestically and outside Iran. Most participants adopted the assimilating learning style in the research of Tulbure (2012), whereas Orhun (2012) found that most participants preferred the converging learning style. This variation may reflect differences in educational settings and/or educational methods.

It seems that the diverging learning style is more appropriate for the field of nursing due to the nature of the field and the career prospects of nursing and midwifery students (Ahanchian, Mohamadzadeghasr, Garavand, & Hosseini, 2012). This learning style encourages students to be holistic and sociable; to use their ingenuity and thoughts in social situations and communication, especially with patients; and to be creative learners. These students develop and implement creative, workable, and effective solutions when dealing with complex patient issues and instill strong problem-solving capabilities. Thus, it is better to select those students who have diverging and accommodating learning styles for the field of nursing (Mohammadi, Sayehmiri, Tavan, & Mohammadi, 2013).

In determining the relationship between learning style and academic achievement, the results showed a significant relationship between these two variables. Thus, the highest average of academic achievement was earned, in rank order, by students who used accommodating, diverging, converging, and assimilating learning styles. A relationship between learning styles and academic achievement has also been suggested by Ahadi, Abedsaidi, Arshadi, and Ghorbani (2010) and Ghazivakili et al. (2014), but not by Farmanbar, Hosseinzadeh, Asadpoor, and Yeganeh (2013). The accommodating learning style is created from the combination of active experimentation and concrete experience. Users of this style learn and enjoy through practical work, work on projects, and engage in new tasks and controversial experiences. Preferred methods for accommodators include role playing and computer simulations. Accommodators have a tendency to engage in experimental work and to use various methods to achieve a goal (Pazargadi & Tahmasebi, 2010).

From the perspective of Kolb, learning style is a combination of cognitive, affective, and psychological properties. People advance their knowledge based on their learning style that has a significant role in their academic achievement. People have their own style of learning. Therefore, if the learning strategies of an individual match his or her learning style, performance is expected to improve (Panahi, Kazemi, & Rezaie, 2012).

Comprehending the learning styles of students is crucial for teachers, because each learning style requires the provision of appropriate educational materials (Gurpinar, Alimoglu, Mamakli, & Aktekin, 2010). The alignment of instructors' teaching styles to students' learning styles results in improved student understanding (Mlambo, 2011).

In surveying the relationship between critical thinking and learning styles, the critical thinking score was not statistically different among the four learning-style groups. Nevertheless, the results showed that the mean scores for critical thinking skill were found, from highest to lowest, in the diverging, assimilating, accommodating, and converging learning-style groups. In terms of the subscales, the highest average score was "assessment" in the diverging style group. The results of Noohi et al. also showed a higher score for critical thinking among converging people than among assimilating, accommodating, and diverging people (Noohi et al., 2014). Unlike the finding of this study, Ghazivakili et al. found that the total score of critical thinking differed among the four learning-style groups and that two of the subscales of critical thinking (evaluation and inductive reasoning) were positively related to learning styles (Ghazivakili et al., 2014).

Whereas no significant relationship was observed between learning style and either age or educational level in this study, significant relationships were found in the study of Ghazivakili et al. (2014). Furthermore, whereas both this study and Ahadi et al.'s (2010) study found a positive relationship between marital status and learning styles, Ghazivakili et al. reported no relationship with these two variables.

Conclusions

The findings show that the mean scores of critical thinking skills and its subdomains were low among the nursing students who were surveyed for this study. Some strategies that may be used to improve critical thinking in this population include frequent use of individual and group active learning strategies, empowering instructors to prepare tests that target high levels of cognitive domain and present probing questions, encouraging students and instructors to participate in problem analysis and discussions, providing different ideas and opinions, and promoting self-directed learning (Shirazi, Sharif, Molazem, & Alborzi, 2016). It is hoped that the findings of this research attract the attention of instructors and managers regarding the importance of critical thinking evaluation in students. In addition, obtaining information about the dominant learning styles of students may encourage and enable nursing instructors to create appropriate learning environments and prepare the areas for academic achievement of the students. Learning outcomes improve when training matches the learning styles of the students.

Acknowledgments

The authors wish to thank the Research Department of Islamic Azad University, Urmia Branch, and all of the students who participated in this study. In addition, the authors wish to thank the Research Consultation Center at the Shiraz University of Medical Sciences for their invaluable assistance in editing this article.

References

Abdollahi Adli Ansar, V., FathiAzar, A., & Abdollahi, N. (2015). The relationship of critical thinking with creativity, self-efficacy beliefs and academic performance of teacher–students. *Journal of Research in School and Virtual Learning, 2*(7), 41–52. (Original work published in Persian)

Aghaei, N., Souri, R., & Ghanbari, S. (2012). Comparison of the relationship between critical thinking and academic achievement among physical education students and students in other fields of study in Bu Ali Sina University, Hamedan. *Management of Sport and Movement Sciences, 2*(4), 35–45. (Original work published in Persian)

Ahadi, F., Abedsaidi, J., Arshadi, F., & Ghorbani, R. (2010). Learning styles of nursing and allied health students in Semnan University of Medical Sciences. *Koomesh, 11*(2), 141–146. (Original work published in Persian)

Ahanchian, M., Mohamadzadeghasr, A., Garavand, H., & Hosseini, A. (2012). Prevalent learning styles among nursing and midwifery students and its association with functionality of thinking styles and academic achievement a study in Mashhad School of Nursing and Midwifery. *Iranian Journal of Medical Education, 12*(8), 577–588. (Original work published in Persian)

Aripin, R., Mahmood, Z., Rohaizad, R., Yeop, U., & Anuar, M. (2008). *Student learning styles and academic performance.* Paper presented at the Proceedings of the 22nd Annual SAS Malaysia Forum, Malaysia.

Ashoori, J. (2014). Relationship between self-efficacy, critical thinking, thinking styles and emotional intelligence with academic achievement in nursing students. *Scientific Journal of Hamadan Nursing & Midwifery Faculty, 22*(3), 15–23. (Original work published in Persian)

Azodi, P., Jahanpoor, F., & Sharif, F. (2010). Critical thinking skills of students in Bushehr University of Medical Sciences. *Interdisciplinary Journal of Virtual Learning in Medical Sciences, 1*(2), 10–16. (Original work published in Persian)

Babamohammadi, H., Esmaeilpour, M., Negarande, R., & Dehghan Nayeri, N. (2011). Comparison of critical thinking skills in nursing students of Semnan and Tehran Universities of Medical Sciences. *Journal of Rafsanjan University of Medical Sciences, 10*(1, Suppl.), 67–78. (Original work published in Persian)

Can, Ş. (2009). The effects of science student teachers' academic achievements, their grade levels, gender and type of education they are exposed to on their 4mat learning styles (Case of Muğla University, Turkey). *Procedia-Social and Behavioral Sciences, 1*(1), 1853–1857. https://doi.org/10.1016/j.sbspro.2009.01.327

Edraki, M., Rambod, M., & Abdoli, R. (2011). The relationship between nursing students' educational satisfaction and their academic success. *Iranian Journal of Medical Education, 11*(1), 32–39. (Original work published in Persian)

Emamipour, S., & Shams Esfandabad, H. (2007). *Learning and cognitive styles: Theories and tests* (pp. 453–472). Tehran, Iran: Samt Publisher. (Original work published in Persian)

Eslami, A. R., & Maarefi, F. (2010). A comparison of the critical thinking ability in the first and last term baccalaureate students of nursing and clinical nurses of Jahrom University of Medical Sciences in 2007. *Journal of Jahrom University of Medical Sciences, 8*(1), 37–45. (Original work published in Persian)

Facione, P. A., & Facione, N. (1994). *The California Critical Thinking Skills Test: Test manual.* Millbrae, CA: California Academic Press.

Farmanbar, R., Hosseinzadeh, T., Asadpoor, M., & Yeganeh, M. (2013). Association between nursing and midwifery students' learning styles and their academic achievements, based on Kolb's model. *Journal of Guilan University of Medical Sciences, 22*(86), 60–68. (Original work published in Persian)

Farooq, M. S., Chaudhry, A. H., Shafiq, M., & Berhanu, G. (2011). Factors affecting students' quality of academic performance: A case of secondary school level. *Journal of Quality and Technology Management, 7*(2), 1–14.

Fero, L. J., O'Donnell, J. M., Zullo, T. G., Dabbs, A. D., Kitutu, J., Samosky, J. T., & Hoffman, L. A. (2010). Critical thinking skills in nursing students: Comparison of simulation-based performance with metrics. *Journal of Advanced Nursing, 66*(10), 2182–2193. https://doi.org/10.1111/j.1365-2648.2010.05385.x

Ghazivakili, Z., Norouzi Nia, R., Panahi, F., Karimi, M., Gholsorkh, H., & Ahmadi, Z. (2014). The role of critical thinking skills and learning styles of university students in their academic performance. *Journal of Advances in Medical Education & Professionalism, 2*(3), 95–102.

Gordon, C. D., Williams, S. K. P., Hudson, G. A., & Stewart, J. (2010). Factors associated with academic performance of physical therapy students. *West Indian Medical Journal, 59*(2), 203–208.

Gurpinar, E., Alimoglu, M. K., Mamakli, S., & Aktekin, M. (2010). Can learning style predict student satisfaction with different instruction methods and academic achievement in medical education? *Advances in Physiology Education, 34*(4), 192–196. https://doi.org/10.1152/advan.00075.2010

Hariri, N., & Bagherinejad, Z. (2012). Evaluation of critical thinking skills in students of health faculty, Mazandaran University of Medical Sciences. *Journal of Mazandaran University of Medical Sciences, 21*(1), 166–173. (Original work published in Persian)

Hosseini, Z. (2009). Cooperative learning and critical thinking. *Developmental Psychology (Journal of Iranian Psychologists), 5*(19), 199–208. (Original work published in Persian)

Jayanthi, S. V., Balakrishnan, S., Ching, A. L. S., Latiff, N. A. A., & Nasirudeen, A. M. A. (2014). Factors contributing to academic performance of students in a tertiary institution in Singapore. *American Journal of Educational Research, 2*(9), 752–758. https://doi.org/10.12691/education-2-9-8

Kolb, A. Y., & Kolb, D. A. (2005). *The Kolb learning style inventory—Version 3.1 2005 technical specifications.* Boston, MA: Hay Resources Direct.

Lau, W. W. F., & Yuen, A. H. K. (2010). Gender differences in learning styles: Nurturing a gender and style sensitive computer science classroom. *Australasian Journal of Educational Technology, 26*(7), 1090–1103. https://doi.org/10.14742/ajet.1036

Mlambo, V. (2011). An analysis of some factors affecting student academic performance in an introductory biochemistry course at the University of the West Indies. *Caribbean Teaching Scholar, 1*(2), 79–92.

Mohammadi, I., Sayehmiri, C., Tavan, H., & Mohammadi, E. (2013). Learning styles of Iranian nursing students based on Kolb's theory: A systematic review and meta-analysis study. *Iranian Journal of Medical Education, 13*(9), 741–752. (Original work published in Persian)

Noohi, E., Salahi, S., & Sabzevari, S. (2014). Association of critical thinking with learning styles in nursing students of school of nursing and midwifery, Iran. *Journal of Strides in Development of Medical Education, 11*(2), 179–186. (Original work published in Persian)

Orhun, N. (2012). The relationship between learning styles and achievement in calculus course for engineering students. *Procedia-Social and Behavioral Sciences, 47*, 638–642. https://doi.org/10.1016/j.sbspro.2012.06.710

Panahi, R., Kazemi, S., & Rezaie, A. (2012). The relationship between learning styles and academic achievement: The role of gender and academic discipline. *Developmental Psychology (Journal of Iranian Psychologists), 8*(30), 189–196. (Original work published in Persian)

Pazargadi, M., & Tahmasebi, S. (2010). Learning styles and their application in nursing. *Iranian Journal of Educational Strategies, 3*(2), 73–76. (Original work published in Persian)

Shinnick, M. A., & Woo, M. A. (2013). The effect of human patient simulation on critical thinking and its predictors in prelicensure nursing students. *Nurse Education Today, 33*(9), 1062–1067. https://doi.org/10.1016/j.nedt.2012.04.004

Shirazi, F., Sharif, F., Molazem, Z., & Alborzi, M. (2016). Dynamics of self-directed learning in M.Sc. nursing students: A qualitative research. *Journal of Advances in Medical Education & Professionalism, 5*(1), 33–41.

Taghavi Larijani, T., Mardani Hmouleh, M., Rezaei, N., Ghadiriyan, F., & Rashidi, A. (2014). Relationship between assertiveness and critical thinking in nursing students. *Journal of Nursing Education, 3*(1), 32–40. (Original work published in Persian)

Tulbure, C. (2012). Learning styles, teaching strategies and academic achievement in higher education: A cross-sectional investigation. *Procedia-Social and Behavioral Sciences, 33*, 398–402. https://doi.org/10.1016/j.sbspro.2012.01.151

Wangensteen, S., Johansson, I. S., Björkström, M. E., & Nordström, G. (2010). Critical thinking dispositions among newly graduated nurses. *Journal of Advanced Nursing, 66*(10), 2170–2181. https://doi.org/10.1111/j.1365-2648.2010.05282.x

Zainol Abidin, M. J., Rezaee, A. A., Abdullah, H. N., & Singh, K. K. B. (2011). Learning styles and overall academic achievement in a specific educational system. *International Journal of Humanities and Social Science, 1*(10), 143–152.

16

Using Reflective Teaching Program to Explore Health-Promoting Behaviors in Nursing Students

Yi-Ya CHANG[1] • Miao-Chuan CHEN[2]*

ABSTRACT

Background: The attitudes of nurses toward health promotion affect patients. However, current classroom teaching does not provide nursing students with actual experiences. An experiential and reflective teaching design will help nursing students practice actual health behaviors and record their feelings. This will help nursing students better understand the difficulties and feelings experienced by nurses when encouraging patients to make behavioral changes in clinical settings.

Purpose: This study aimed to explore the experiences and factors affecting health-promoting learning with reflective teaching in nursing students.

Methods: This explorative study integrated the "reflective assessment, engagement, and action-reflection" strategy of reflective teaching into the standard health-promotion teaching curriculum to understand the experiences of nursing students when executing health-promoting behaviors. Fifty-seven second-year nursing students from a university in northern Taiwan participated in this course, which was conducted between September 2017 and January 2018. The data were collected from the contents of the reflective journals written by the nursing students and analyzed using thematic analysis.

Results: The three health-promoting behaviors performed by most of the students were regular exercise, balanced and healthy diet, and adequate daily water intake. The feelings experienced by the nursing students during the execution of health-promoting behaviors included easier said than done, compromise and adjustment, and continuation of health behaviors. Accommodation, peer encouragement, and support were important, facilitating factors of health-promoting behaviors in this study.

Conclusions/Implications for Practice: The results of this study may serve as a reference for nursing lecturers when employing reflective teaching in the classroom. Reflective teaching designs for actual experiences help nursing students experience the crucial factors and benefits of executing health-promoting behaviors.

KEY WORDS:
nursing students, health promotion, reflective journal, reflective teaching.

Introduction

Nurses are healthcare professionals. One of their major tasks is to provide health education to patients that helps the latter pursue healthier lifestyles. However, nurses often find that, although they provide health education to patients, patients are not always able to make behavioral changes. Moreover, nurses lack the deep understanding of the problems and difficulties faced by their patients necessary to tailor behavioral change suggestions to individual patient needs. Therefore, the patient's problem may still persist.

Classroom teaching typically provides only knowledge related to health-promoting behaviors and not actual experience with practicing behaviors. However, one responsibility of nurses is to teach patients to practice healthy behaviors. If nurses do not understand how to practice health-promoting behaviors themselves, how can they teach their patients? This gap continues to exist between nurses and patients. Therefore, actual practice will help nurses understand the challenges encountered in achieving success. Thus, early implementation of the relevant scenarios of health-promoting behaviors in the nursing curriculum may help nursing students improve their problem-solving abilities and empathize with the difficulties faced by patients who are unable to make behavioral changes.

Recently, conventional "spoon-feeding" teaching has started to undergo changes, with various types of flipped teaching methods under active development. A number of innovative teaching methods have already been employed in different courses for students of various ages. A Chinese literature teacher in Taiwan developed the "flipping-literature class"

[1]PhD, RN, Assistant Professor, Department of Nursing and Clinical Competency Center, Chang Gung University of Science and Technology, and Assistant Research Fellow, Chang Gung Medical Foundation, Taiwan, ROC • [2]PhD, RN, Associate Professor, Department of Nursing, Chang Gung University of Science and Technology, Taiwan, ROC.

method to reverse the traditional one-way learning environment by allowing students to self-learn, reflect, and express themselves during instruction (Chang, 2016). The flipped teaching classroom created by Professor Yeh used the "By the Student" teaching method and promoted using Facebook and Google Form as learning platforms (Yeh, 2015). Under flipped teaching, nursing lecturers have begun employing scenario-based learning to increase self-confidence, professional capabilities, teamwork, and communication abilities in their nursing students (Huang, Hsieh, & Hsu, 2014; Kim & Jang, 2017; Kunst, Mitchell, & Johnston, 2017). These experiences have encouraged scholars to incorporate different teaching methods into the nursing curriculum.

Some studies found that reflective teaching may increase the communication, caring, and critical thinking abilities of students (Chen, 2010; Lo, Chang, & Chen, 2014). One study found that the methods that affected nursing students' reflective abilities were, from higher to lower importance: reflective journals, classroom discussions, and book reviews (Lo et al., 2014). Writing reflective journals has been found to affect the knowledge, attitudes, and behavior of nursing students positively (Ross, Mahal, Chinnapen, Kolar, & Woodman, 2014). Therefore, reflective learning interventions should be introduced into the nursing curriculum as early as possible to ensure the nurses are equipped with problem-solving and caring abilities. In this study, a nursing curriculum was designed that employed a reflective teaching intervention approach. In this curriculum, the nursing students execute health-promoting behaviors, which conform to the "learning-by-doing" philosophy advocated by John Dewey. However, reflection is an intrinsic process that is difficult to assess (Chen, Lai, Chang, Hsu, & Pai, 2016). To understand the experience of nursing students in achieving behavioral change, this study employed a reflective teaching program wherein nursing students wrote reflective journal entries during the health-promoting behaviors' implementation process.

Methods

Design

This was an explorative study that used qualitative data analysis. The "reflective assessment, engagement, and action-reflection" teaching strategy was employed to conduct reflective teaching in health promotion courses. Classroom discussions and reflective journals were used to encourage students to introspect their unhealthy behaviors in this study. The reflection journal entries of the students that corresponded to the execution of health-promoting behaviors were analyzed. The course was conducted, and the data were collected between September 2017 and January 2018.

Teaching Strategy

A reflective teaching program was designed and "reflective assessment, engagement, and action reflection" was employed in a course for students. In the first 9 weeks of the course,

classroom teaching was performed to equip students with health-promotion-related knowledge and skills, thereby enabling students to identify their personal health challenges. The principles of behavioral changes or health promotion action strategies were used to develop a 4-week health promotion plan.

In teaching strategy, "reflective assessment" refers to stimulating the willingness and motivation of students to make the changes necessary to eliminate unhealthy behaviors. The relationship between unhealthy behaviors and disease was explained to the students, and an assessment was conducted to analyze the unhealthy behaviors that the students practiced in their everyday lives. In addition, in the "reflective assessment" stage, the instructor guided nursing students to discuss their unhealthy behaviors and strategies for changing these behaviors. After the discussions, nursing students decided to perform their health-promoting behavior and plan.

In the "engagement" stage, the students learned to self-assess health-promoting behaviors that conformed to the health principles and to design health-promoting behaviors that are tailored to their personal needs. In the "action-reflection" stage, the students recorded in their reflective journal over a period of 4 weeks what health-promoting behaviors they had executed using pictures and/or text, their feelings regarding executing the health promotion action plans, and the reasons for their success or the difficulties they experienced in achieving their goals.

The teaching strategy of "reflective assessment, engagement, and action-reflection" helped assess (a) "What kinds of health problems and unhealthy behaviors do the nursing students have?", (b) "What kinds of health-promoting behaviors and planning did the nursing students pursue?", and (c) "What are the positive and negative factors that influenced the execution of health-promoting behaviors?"

Participants

Fifty-seven second-year nursing students (16 men and 41 women) at a university in northern Taiwan participated in the "health promotion" course used in this study.

Data Collection

Data were collected from the reflective journals written by the 57 participants over a period of 4 weeks, during which time they were executing health-promoting behaviors. One reflective journal entry was written per week. Thus, each participant wrote four journal entries in total. These reflective journals were submitted online, and each journal was numbered and stored in the flash drive that was accessed for this project.

Data Analysis

This study employed the six steps of the thematic analysis method of Braun and Clarke (2006) in data analysis. The six steps were as follows: (a) data familiarization: the reflective journals were repeatedly read, and the thoughts on meaningful data were jotted down; (b) generating initial codes:

after reading the content of the reflective journals, meaningful content was coded; (c) searching themes: related and similar codes were analyzed and grouped together to form potential themes; (d) reviewing themes: the themes were repeatedly read, and the relevance of their context was confirmed; (e) defining and naming themes: the nature of each theme was examined, and the data described by each theme were confirmed; and (f) writing the report.

In addition, a Fisher's exact test was used to analyze the effect of gender on the observed health-promoting behaviors.

Rigor

Rigor in this study was maintained by adhering to credibility, dependability, transferability, and confirmability (Lincoln & Guba, 1985). In terms of credibility, the data in this study originated from the reflective journals, which were written by the 57 participants. The contents of these reflective journals reflected the personal experiences of the participants in making health-promoting behaviors, and the data were highly credible. In terms of dependability, data coding and theme formulation were conducted by the first author by repeatedly reading the reflective journals and discussing the content with the second author. When there were differences in opinion between the two authors, the relevant reflective journal entries were reread to clarify the context and achieve consistency. In terms of transferability, the researchers dispassionately analyzed the experiences of the participants and avoided adding subjective viewpoints to ensure that the rich study results were inferred from real-life scenarios. In addition, the researchers reflected on the effects of their subjective values on the study during the study process to avoid generating bias during interpretation and to achieve confirmability.

Ethical Considerations

Before implementation, this research proposal was approved by the research ethics committee of a medical center (Reference No. 201701256B0) and by related departments in the university. To protect the rights of the nursing students and ensure the security of the data, numbers were used in place of participant names during data analysis.

Results

Regular exercise was the health-promoting behavior most often cited by the participants (22 students), followed, in descending order, by a balanced and healthy diet (15) and adequate daily water intake (10). In addition, five participants cited getting enough sleep, and five cited reducing the time they spent online. The female participants cited a balanced and healthy diet twice as frequently as their male peers. No significant gender difference was found for any of the health-promoting behaviors (Table 1).

Emerging Themes

Six subthemes and three main themes emerged from the participants' reflective journals, as shown in Table 2. The main

TABLE 1.

Comparison of Health-Promoting Behaviors Between Male and Female Participants (N = 57)

Item	Male (n = 16) n	%	Female (n = 41) n	%	χ^2	p
Health-promoting behaviors					1.94	.79
Regular exercise	6	37.5	16	39.02		
Balanced and healthy diet	2	12.5	10	24.39		
Adequate daily water intake	4	25.0	9	21.95		
Get enough sleep	2	12.5	3	7.32		
Reduce Internet use	2	12.5	3	7.32		

themes included easier said than done, compromise and adjustment, and continuation of health behaviors.

Executing the health behavior self-assessment and writing reflective journals when executing health-promoting behaviors over the 4-week period provided an opportunity for the participants to change their unhealthy behaviors. However, this was easier said than done, as the participants learned that behavioral change is difficult. They readjusted their expectations, pursued compromise, and made adjustments to make progressive changes. Moreover, they looked to technological aids and peer encouragement to find the strength to continue the process of behavioral change. Thus, the participants may think of continuing their health behaviors when they experience slight physical changes and a sense of achievement in achieving their goals.

Theme 1: Easier Said Than Done

After the participants completed an analysis of their lifestyle, they identified certain aspects that required changes, thereby setting goals. However, when they started making behavioral changes, they found that making these changes was "easier said than done." Therefore, they experienced feelings of "easy to know but difficult to practice," which embodied the opportunity to achieve actual change.

Opportunity for change

The teachers guided the participants to reflect on their lifestyle in the classroom and requested that they establish a health behavior for 4 weeks as an assignment for this course. Therefore, the participants shared that they had an opportunity to make behavioral changes because of this class assignment.

Student no. 43 mentioned: "This assignment is a great motivation and gives me a goal to continue exercising." Other participants mentioned that:

"I have often thought of slimming down. Now, I experience stress from the assignment, wherein written reflective

TABLE 2.
Emerged Themes and Subthemes

Theme	Subtheme
Easier said than done	(a) Opportunity for change
	(b) Everything is difficult in the beginning
Compromise and adjustment	(a) Progressive changes
	(b) Identification of the strength to persist
Continuation of health behaviors	(a) Experience physical changes
	(b) Achieving a sense of accomplishment

journals provide me with greater motivation to exercise.... This assignment provided me with an impetus to convert thought to action" (Nursing Student no. 14) and *"With this assignment, I have a goal to execute an exercise plan. Completing this assignment enabled me to cultivate good exercise habits. My reasons for not exercising in the past now appear as excuses."* (Nursing Student no. 44)

Everything is difficult in the beginning

After the participants set their goals for behavioral changes, they discovered as they began to invest related efforts that achieving these goals would not be easy. Therefore, they realized that it was not easy to make behavioral changes and felt that everything was difficult in the beginning.

Nursing Student no. 14 wrote in the reflective journal on regular exercise that *"I thought it could be achieved very easily, but I never thought that it would be quite tiring at the beginning."*

Nursing Student no. 30 mentioned: *"It was really agony at the start to drink so much water every day."*

In working to eat a balanced and healthy diet, Nursing Student no. 12 mentioned that *"I forgot about this goal or did not follow the necessary habits for this goal during the first week, resulting in my not being able to achieve the set goal."*

One participant wrote: *"I initially thought it would be easy. But in reality, I found that it is really difficult to exercise continuously and that this assignment is tougher than I thought."* (Nursing Student no. 38)

Theme 2: Compromise and Adjustment

After Week 1 of the behavioral change program, the participants began to reflect on whether the behavioral change goals they had set were overly high or ideal. Thus, they either adjusted their goals for the second week or devised new ways to help them achieve their set behavioral changes. During this adjustment and adaptation to behavioral changes, the participants employed a number of methods to help them make these changes, including progressive changes and identification of strength to persist.

Progressive changes

After the first week, the participants began to believe that achieving behavioral change would not be easy. Therefore, they adopted a series of progressive goals that they hoped would help them achieve their behavioral change goals, albeit more gradually. In the reflective journals, the participants shared how they made behavioral changes. Nursing Student no. 30 mentioned *"using progressive methods so that I can slowly get used to it is an effective method."* Nursing Student no. 8 wrote: *"It is troublesome to carry a water bottle when going out and that water is tasteless. In the beginning, I forgot to carry a water bottle with me because I rushed out in the morning. I developed the habit of drinking water with a water bottle during the third week."*

Other participants shared: *"I did not set a high goal at the start because I hoped I could achieve the goal. I will increase my goal after I gradually get used to it."* (Nursing Student no. 36)

Identification of the strength to persist

To achieve the goal of cultivating health behaviors, the participants started to search for the strength to persist from sources such as technological products and peer encouragement and support. All of the participants lived in the university dormitory, and all owned and frequently used mobile phones or smartphones. They used various functions on their smartphones to generate regular reminders of the need to achieve behavioral change. Some used their smartphone's camera function to record the food they ate daily for each meal and used the alarm clock function to self-notify when it was time to drink water. Nursing Student no. 14 even used a mobile phone app to record the distance and calories consumed through walking and cycling each day. Five participants used an app to control the time they spent online on their smartphone. Other participants mentioned that *"I initially did not record my dietary habits. However, I started recording my lunch for this assignment. Looking at the daily records (using pictures), I started to realize that my diet is not balanced."* (Nursing Student no. 5) and *"I set a timer to remind myself to drink water, and immediately drank water when the alarm rang. My laziness gradually decreased and my self-confidence and sense of achievement increased."* (Nursing Student no. 6). One participant shared that *"I do not drink a lot of water because other beverages taste better than water, and there are various new types of drinks sold in the supermarket. Adding lemon slices or honey to the water to add some flavor helped make me like drinking water."* (Nursing Student no. 20)

In addition, the participants shared that part of the incentive to make behavioral changes was the encouragement and support from peers. Nursing Student no. 29 mentioned: *"Exercising together with my partners provides me with more impetus to exercise."* Nursing Student no. 13 shared that *"I feel that looking for an exercise partner is a good idea, as you can encourage each other."*

Theme 3: Continuation of Health Behaviors

After the participants had experienced an implementation process that was initially difficult and identified effective self-help methods, they slowly experienced the benefits of their changed health behaviors and improved physical condition (many mentioned improvements in constipation and skin conditions). In the third and fourth week, the participants wrote in their reflective journals about the joy of successfully accomplishing their goals and their resulting sense of achievement. They also expressed hope regarding their ability to continue this health behavior.

Experience physical changes

After making positive changes to their health behaviors, many of the participants perceived improvements in their physical condition, as described in the following:

"It has only been one month between when I began, when I didn't feel acclimated, and now, when I feel it is natural. My body's metabolism has shown improvements. In the past, I often experienced constipation, but now I have normal bowel movements." (Nursing Student no. 27)

"It is difficult to drink a lot of water daily but there are many benefits. I do not experience constipation and my pores have shrunk, enabling me to have more energy." (Nursing Student no. 30)

"I am slowly starting to like the feeling of a slow jog. This is because my sleep quality has improved after I started exercising, and I do not experience insomnia late at night or watch movies at night like I often did in the past. Exercise has really improved my work and rest habits." (Nursing Student no. 37)

Achieving a sense of accomplishment

The participants recorded their reflective journal entries every week and analyzed whether they had achieved their behavioral change goals. When preset goals were achieved, they shared their related joy, which reflected their sense of achievement. The reflective journal entry of Nursing Student no. 44 on carrying out regular exercises mentioned: *"I enjoy these changes. In the future, even if I am busy and tired, I will continue my exercise habits."*
Some of the participants shared:

I had always thought of changing my habits and myself. However, every time I only talked about it but did not act. This time, I really persisted for a period. I realized I could actually do it. So, it depends on whether I want to carry out a behavior or not! This activity enabled me to drastically change my lifestyle habits and become healthier. (Nursing Student no. 15)

When I have consumed the targeted amount of water, I experience a sense of achievement and realize that this change will persist as long as I have the perseverance! (Nursing Student no. 6)

Maybe I was not used to it at first. However, after I got used to it, I realized that it was not so difficult. I feel that even if there is no need to do such assignments in the future, I will continue to exercise. (Nursing Student no. 14)

Discussion

This study found that the top three health-promoting behaviors performed by the participants were regular exercise, balanced and healthy diet, and adequate daily water intake. These three behaviors highlight the concerns of nursing students about unhealthy behaviors and their desired responses in terms of health-promoting behaviors. The choice of exercise and diet as the most desired health-promoting behaviors echoes Tang, Su, and Huang (2015), who found the top three worse health-promoting behaviors among university students to be health responsibility, exercise, and nutrition. The similarity in findings may reflect the similar backgrounds, and thus problems, of students in both studies. Moreover, Chang, Liao, and Shia (2014) found that 52.4% of university students in Taiwan do not exercise. Hung and Chiu (2011) found that the lifestyle of university students still has room for improvement in terms of developing healthy behaviors and regular exercise. These studies show that university students need to perform health-promoting behaviors such as exercising regularly and eating a balanced diet. Therefore, the performance by the participants in this study of health-promoting behaviors such as regular exercise and healthy and balanced diet was consistent with the findings of previous studies that inadequate exercise and poor diet are major health behavior problems among university students. Furthermore, the results of this study found that female students were twice as likely as male students to consume a balanced and healthy diet, suggesting that female students are more concerned about diet-related body weight problems. This finding is similar to previous studies that found adolescent girls to be more concerned than adolescent boys about their appearance and size (Ganesan, Ravishankar, & Ramalingam, 2018; Šmídová, Švancara, Andrýsková, & Šimůnek, 2018).

The choice of some participants in this study to focus on drinking an adequate amount of water each day highlights an issue that has not been explored in previous studies. The reflective journal of Nursing Student no. 6 notes that he or she does not have a habit of drinking water or carrying a water bottle and often drinks beverages instead of plain water. Nursing Student no. 8 wrote that he or she feels it troublesome to carry a water bottle when going out and that water is tasteless. Many drinks shops are located outside the university that sell beverages at prices comparable with bottled water. Therefore, he or she (Nursing Student no. 8) chose to purchase beverages. Nursing Student no. 20 stated that the reason why he or she does not drink a lot of water is because other beverages taste better than water and because there were new types of drinks sold in the supermarket. In addition, it was easier to purchase these beverages than water. Therefore, the participants in this study frequently purchase beverages to drink. The descriptions provided by the participants explain why students do not drink water and prefer other beverages. Currently, there are many types of tea beverages sold in Taiwan, encouraging people to choose these instead of water and to discount the importance of drinking water. Drinking beverages habitually increases the risks of health problems because of the sugar and other ingredients in these drinks. Therefore, future studies should further explore the knowledge and behavior of university students related to water consumption.

A previous study found a 20.3% prevalence of Internet "addiction" among university students in Taiwan (Yang, 2014). A prevalent desire among the participants to reduce Internet usage and to get enough sleep was one of the findings of this study. Previous correlation studies have focused on the issue of Internet addition among university students (Akın, 2012; Chou et al., 2017; Jiang, Zhu, Ye, & Lin, 2012; Mazhari, 2012; Yao, He, Ko, & Pang, 2014). Thus, it is apparent that Internet addiction is a problem in university settings. More intervention studies on Internet addition are needed in the future. Furthermore, the phenomena of sleeping late and heavy Internet use on mobile phones are related to one another. Both phenomena are common today, justifying greater researcher attention.

This study found that the participants were aware of what changes in personal behaviors were needed and that the course assignment enabled them to achieve their health behavior goals and develop real experiences. Therefore, the participants felt that this assignment provided an opportunity to make positive health-related changes in behavior. The results of this study were similar to those of a Canadian study in which students in a course attempted to make health-related behavior changes and write a reflective report, with investigators finding that the students could facilitate the change process (Lee, Yanicki, & Solowoniuk, 2011). Although effecting self-change is difficult, using courses to provide students with opportunities to make health-promoting behavior changes is feasible. Thus, it is recommended that relevant courses be designed for nursing students to help them make changes to their own health-promotion behaviors and to gain experience from learning by doing. In addition, the participants in this study experienced difficulties when they began performing their desired health-promoting behaviors. They found that these behaviors were conceptually easy but difficult to put into practice, a finding that is similar to another study that found that university students possessed knowledge regarding oral hygiene but found this knowledge difficult to put it into practice (Chenh, Yang, Hone, & Shieh, 2002).

During the compromise and adjustment process involved in improving health-promoting behaviors, the participants utilized their problem-solving abilities to achieve their behavior goals. The participants used app functions on their smartphones to assist in making health-promoting behaviors. Therefore, using smartphone functions to facilitate health-promoting behaviors was a characteristic of this group of participants. Furthermore, because the participants ranged in age from 19 to 21 years, most lived in the university dormitory, where interactions with peers are typically a regular facet of daily life. The reflective journal entries indicated that the participants carried out health-promoting behaviors cooperatively with their classmates. Therefore, peer encouragement and support were important factors for implementing health-promoting behaviors. These results are similar to those of other studies that found accommodation to be a factor affecting health-promoting behaviors in university students (Bakouei, Seyedi-Andi, Bakhtiari, & Khafri, 2018; Hung & Chiu, 2011).

In participating in the 4-week health behavior change assignment, the participants gradually realized that they were capable of making these changes on their own and felt proud of themselves as a result. Furthermore, many students mentioned experiencing improvements in several physical problems (e.g., constipation and facial acne), which made the participants hopeful that they would continue these better health behaviors after the assignment had finished. These experiences are expected to help make these nursing students more persuasive in helping patients successfully achieve behavioral changes in the future. This finding is similar to Lee et al. (2011), who found that the experiences helped students grow professionally as health promotion practitioners.

The transtheoretical model fits well the process used by nursing students to adopt health promotion behaviors. Classroom teaching and group discussions were conducted during the first 9 weeks of class, at which time the lecturer guides students to reflect and helps them identify their problematic behaviors. This period correlates to the precontemplation and contemplation stages in the transtheoretical model. In Week 10, the students write in their reflective journal the health behavior changes that they desire to make, their current lifestyle and problematic behaviors requiring analysis, and the health behavior changes that they will make in the subsequent 4-week period. This correlates to the preparation stage in the transtheoretical model. After the 4 weeks of practicing health-promoting behaviors, the nursing students begin to exhibit new behaviors and hope that they may continue adhering to these behaviors. This correlates to the action stage in the transtheoretical model. Therefore, this course design employed the transtheoretical model and enabled the students to further experience the process of behavioral change. This study may be used as a reference for designing nursing courses in the future to help students gain actual experience.

This study was a qualitative study. Therefore, the results reflected only the subjective experiences of nursing students during the 4-week behavior change assignment. Follow-up would be needed to determine their success in continuing their learned healthy behaviors after this 4-week period.

Conclusions

The results of this study indicate that experiential and reflective teaching designs help nursing students make actual health behavior changes and record their feelings, which assists them to better understand the process of behavioral change. Moreover, this process helps students learn methods to achieve behavioral change. Therefore, this experiential and reflective teaching course design may serve as a reference for designing related nursing courses. This course was designed to employ flipped teaching, which enhances the practical experience of nursing students, helping them be more persuasive in helping patients make behavioral changes in the future.

Acknowledgments

This study was supported by the Taiwan Nurses Association (TWNA-1071002). The authors express their gratitude to all of the participants who shared their valuable experiences in this study.

Author Contributions

Study conception and design: YYC
Data collection: YYC
Data analysis and interpretation: YYC, MCC
Drafting of the article: YYC, MCC
Critical revision of the article: YYC, MCC

References

Akın, A. (2012). The relationships between Internet addiction, subjective vitality, and subjective happiness. *Cyberpsychology, Behavior and Social Networking, 15*(8), 404–410. https://doi.org/10.1089/cyber.2011.0609

Bakouei, F., Seyedi-Andi, S. J., Bakhtiari, A., & Khafri, S. (2018). Health promotion behaviors and its predictors among the college students in Iran. *International Quarterly of Community Health Education, 38*(4), 251–258. https://doi.org/10.1177/0272684X18781780

Braun, V., & Clarke, V. (2006). Using thematic analysis in psychology. *Qualitative Research in Psychology, 3*(2), 77–101. https://doi.org/10.1191/1478088706qp063oa

Chang, C. C., Liao, J. Y., & Shia, H. (2014). The analysis on the assessment of freshman's health-promoting lifestyle and self-rated health in colleges and universities. *Journal of Healthy Life and Successful Aging, 6*(1), 43–62. (Original work published in Chinese)

Chang, H. C. (2016). Flipped teaching: The cultivation of self-learning ability and new education of library. *National Cheng Kung University Library Journal, 25*, 1–7. (Original work published in Chinese)

Chen, S. Y., Lai, C. C., Chang, H. M., Hsu, H. C., & Pai, H. C. (2016). Chinese version of psychometric evaluation of self-reflection and insight scale on Taiwanese nursing students. *The Journal of Nursing Research, 24*(4), 337–356. https://doi.org/10.1097/jnr.0000000000000132

Chen, W. L. (2010). Reflection skills: A guide for clinical teaching in nursing practice. *VGH Nursing Journal, 27*(3), 225–230. https://doi.org/10.6142/vghn.27.3.225 (Original work published in Chinese)

Chenh, C. Y., Yang, Y. H., Hone, Y. J., & Shieh, T. Y. (2002). The study of oral condition with oral hygiene knowledge, attitude and practice for university atudents in Kaohsiung City. *Taiwan Journal of Oral Medicine & Health Sciences, 18*(1), 27–38. https://doi.org/10.7059/tjomhs.200210.0027 (Original work published in Chinese)

Chou, W. P., Lee, K. H., Ko, C. H., Liu, T. L., Hsiao, R. C., Lin, H. F., & Yen, C. F. (2017). Relationship between psychological inflexibility and experiential avoidance and internet addiction: Mediating effects of mental health problems. *Psychiatry Research, 257*, 40–44. https://doi.org/10.1016/j.psychres.2017.07.021

Ganesan, S., Ravishankar, S. L., & Ramalingam, S. (2018). Are body image issues affecting our adolescents? A cross-sectional study among college going adolescent girls. *Indian Journal of Community Medicine, 43*(5), 42–46. https://doi.org/10.4103/ijcm.IJCM_62_18

Huang, Y. H., Hsieh, S. I., & Hsu, L. L. (2014). The effect of a scenario-based simulation communication course on improving the communication skills of nurses. *The Journal of Nursing, 61*(2), 33–43. https://doi.org/10.6224/JN.61.2.33 (Original work published in Chinese)

Hung, S. C., & Chiu, Y. C. (2011). A study on the lifestyle of college students at Lunghwa University of Science. *Sport Journal of Tainan University, 6*, 116–132. https://doi.org/10.29740/jpenut.201112.0010Technology (Original work published in Chinese)

Jiang, D., Zhu, S., Ye, M., & Lin, C. (2012). Cross-sectional survey of prevalence and personality characteristics of college students with internet addiction in Wenzhou, China. *Shanghai Archives of Psychiatry, 24*(2), 99–107. https://doi.org/10.3969/j.issn.1002-0829.2012.02.005

Kim, H. R., & Jang, Y. K. (2017). Flipped learning with simulation in undergraduate nursing education. *Journal of Nursing Education, 56*(6), 329–336. https://doi.org/10.3928/01484834-20170518-03

Kunst, E. L., Mitchell, M., & Johnston, A. N. B. (2017). Using simulation to improve the capability of undergraduate nursing students in mental health care. *Nurse Education Today, 50*, 29–35. https://doi.org/10.1016/j.nedt.2016.12.012

Lee, B. K., Yanicki, S. M., & Solowoniuk, J. (2011). Value of a health behavior change reflection assignment for health promotion learning. *Education for Health: Change in Learning & Practice, 24*(2), 1–13.

Lincoln, Y., & Guba, E. (1985). *Naturalistic inquiry.* Newbury Park, CA: Sage.

Lo, H. M., Chang, S. C., & Chen, W. X. (2014). The effectiveness of using reflective program for enhance core competency of nursing students. *The Journal of Health Sciences, 2*(2), 52–71. (Original work published in Chinese)

Mazhari, S. (2012). The prevalence of problematic internet use and the related factors in medical students, Kerman, Iran. *Addiction & Health, 4*(3–4), 87–94.

Ross, C., Mahal, K., Chinnapen, Y., Kolar, M., & Woodman, K. (2014). Evaluation of nursing students' work experience through the use of reflective journals. *Mental Health Practice, 17*(6), 21–27. https://doi.org/10.7748/mhp2014.03.17.6.21.e823

Šmídová, S., Švancara, J., Andrýsková, L., & Šimůnek, J. (2018). Adolescent body image: Results of Czech ELSPAC study. *Central European Journal of Public Health, 26*(1), 60–64. https://doi.org/10.21101/cejph.a4930

Tang, F. C., Su, W. L., & Huang, S. L. (2015). The level of health-promoting lifestyle and related factors among undergraduate students in central Taiwan. *Journal of Ergonomic Study, 17*(1), 27–38. https://doi.org/10.6273/jes.2015.17(01).03 (Original work published in Chinese)

Yang, C. F. (2014). The prevalence and psychological risk factors of internet addiction of college students in Taiwan. *Educational Journal of National Taichung University of Science and Technology, 34*(2), 95–130. (Original work published in Chinese)

Yao, M. Z., He, J., Ko, D. M., & Pang, K. (2014). The influence of personality, parental behaviors, and self-esteem on Internet addiction: A study of Chinese college students. *Cyberpsychology, Behavior and Social Networking, 17*(2), 104–110. https://doi.org/10.1089/cyber.2012.0710

Yeh, P. C. (2015). How to ensure the success of flipped classroom? The BTS scheme. *Secondary Education, 66*(2), 30–43. (Original work published in Chinese)

17

A Hierarchical Model of Occupational Burnout in Nurses Associated with Job-Induced Stress, Self-Concept and Work Environment

Ru-Wen LIAO[1] • Mei-Ling YEH[2]* • Kuan-Chia LIN[3] • Kwua-Yun WANG[4]

ABSTRACT

Background: Nurses may experience different levels of occupational burnout in different unit and hospital settings. However, pooling multilevel data in an analysis ignores independent, environmental, and sociocultural contexts of ecological validity.

Purpose: This study aimed to explore a hierarchical model of occupational burnout that is associated with job-induced stress, nurse self-concept, and practice environment in nurses working in different units and hospitals.

Methods: A cross-sectional study was conducted, and 2,605 nurses were recruited from seven hospitals. The outcomes were measured using the Maslach Occupational Burnout Inventory-Human Services Survey, Nurses' Self-Concept Instrument, Nurse Stress Checklist, and Nursing Work Index-Revised. Hierarchical Linear Modeling 6.0 software was used to conduct hierarchical analysis on the study data.

Results: On the nurse level, job-induced stress was a significant factor affecting emotional exhaustion ($\beta = 0.608$, $p < .001$) and depersonalization ($\beta = 2.439$, $p < .001$), whereas nurse self-concept was a significant factor affecting emotional exhaustion ($\beta = -0.250$, $p < .001$), depersonalization ($\beta = -1.587$, $p < .001$), and personal accomplishment ($\beta = 4.126$, $p < .001$). Furthermore, emotional exhaustion and depersonalization were significantly related to level of education ($\beta = 0.111$, $p < .01$; $\beta = 0.583$, $p < .05$). No significant unit-level associations were identified between occupational burnout and the factors of job-induced stress, nurse self-concept, and practice environment ($p > .05$). The intragroup correlation coefficient for emotional exhaustion was 2.86 ($p < .001$).

Conclusions/Implications for Practice: The findings of this study confirm that individual nurse characteristics are strong predictors of emotional exhaustion, depersonalization, and personal accomplishment as these relate to occupational burnout. In addition, nurse self-concept was identified as the most important predictor of all three aspects. In clinical practice, self-concepts about nursing may reduce occupational burnout. Nursing managers formulating new policies should consider nursing background and offer autonomous control over practice.

KEY WORDS:

occupational burnout, job-induced stress, self-concept, practice environment, nurse.

Introduction

Nursing has been ranked as the fourth most stressful profession (Jodas & Haddad, 2009). Nurses face many challenges, including managing complex medical care needs and keeping up to date on current best practices. Job satisfaction is influenced by the exercise of job autonomy and the receipt of sufficient support from the organization. Conflicts between nurses and physicians and between nurses and hospital administrators also sometimes occur. In the practice environment, nurses are often criticized, which leads to increased job-induced stress (Gasparino & Guirardello, 2015).

Job-induced stress, which may cause occupational burnout, has been recognized as a reality within the nursing profession for quite some time (Maslach & Leiter, 2016). Rates of professional burnout among nurses range between 29% and 36% in the United States (Aiken et al., 2010) and are 66% in Taiwan (Chou, Li, & Hu, 2014). Nursing care is a profession that requires striking an equitable balance between providing high-quality care to patients and managing personal emotions during periods of job-induced stress (Khamisa, Peltzer, Ilic, & Oldenburg, 2016).

Level of occupational burnout in nurses relates to job-induced stress, self-concept, and work environment and influences their practice efficacy and patient care (McHugh et al., 2013; Panunto & Guirardello Ede, 2013). The term "burnout" refers to an individual's feeling of being unable to cope with emotional stress, of being drained of energy and resources, and of exhaustion (Maslach & Leiter, 2016). According to Maslach, Schaufeli, and Leiter (2001), burnout consists of three dimensions: emotional exhaustion, depersonalization,

[1]PhD, RN, Vice Director, Department of Nursing, Taipei Tzu Chi Hospital, Buddhist Tzu Chi Medical Foundation • [2]PhD, DMS, RN, Professor, School of Nursing, National Taipei University of Nursing and Health Sciences • [3]PhD, Professor, Institute of Hospital and Health Care Administration, National Yang-Ming University • [4]PhD, RN, FAAN, Director, Rui Guang Healthcare Group, and Jointly Appointed Professor, School of Nursing, National Defense Medical Center.

and a reduced sense of personal accomplishment. Emotional exhaustion is a state of emotion and, sometimes, physical depletion. Depersonalization reflects feelings of detachment and having an impersonal response toward care recipients. These behaviors are associated with psychological strain and escape as a way of coping (Wilkinson, Whittington, Perry, & Eames, 2017). A reduced sense of personal accomplishment fosters a negative self-image, particularly in relation to one's work with service users (Maslach et al., 2001).

Burnout in nurses may be because of several factors, including critical decision making in the absence of complete information, facing life-threatening or traumatic situations, making rapid decisions regarding a complex disease, concerns over litigation, and pressures regarding patient safety and quality of care (Wu et al., 2014). One study found a moderate level of occupational burnout among South African nurses (van der Colff & Rothmann, 2014). Similarly, a study of nurses in Brazil found a moderate level of emotional exhaustion and depersonalization but a severe level of reduced personal accomplishment (Panunto & Guirardello Ede, 2013). In Taiwan, depersonalization levels are moderate, whereas emotional exhaustion and reduced personal accomplishment are severe (Shih et al., 2013).

The relationship between job-induced stress and burnout in nurses may be explained using Maslach's Burnout Model (Maslach et al., 2001), which relates exposure to environmental and situational stressors to job-induced stress. Job-induced stress contributes to negative burnout in nurses and is associated with low levels of job satisfaction. One study pointed out that nurses may be dissatisfied with their income, job promotions such as with a nursing clinical ladder level, and nurse–physician relationships (Khamisa et al., 2016). Moreover, being unable to share frustrations with others and not receiving positive feedback from colleagues or superiors have been shown to lead to feelings of exclusion and loneliness and then to burnout (Wu et al., 2014). Conversely, positive relationships with colleagues and superiors are protective factors against burnout (Wu et al., 2014).

Self-concept in nursing emphasizes the personal value that nurses derive from their work. One study showed that improving self-concept enhances job satisfaction and retention (Cowin, Johnson, Craven, & Marsh, 2008). Nurses with a poor self-concept are likely to exhibit behaviors that affect patient care negatively, whereas having a positive, professional self-concept facilitates a more positive attitude toward the self and even others (Arthur & Randle, 2007). Guided by a nurse-related self-concept, nurses working in hospital settings may create an environment that promotes active caring, mature work behaviors, and adherence to medical-team-proposed rules, which are all beneficial for the hospital.

With strong support from the work environment, nurses may become more passionate about delivering quality of care and about actively upgrading their care skills in a complex job environment. Control over the environment, supplemental nurse staffing, number of beds, and nonprofit ownership affect the risk of occupational burnout in nurses (McHugh

et al., 2013). In addition, autonomy, organizational support, and the nurse–physician relationship in the nursing practice environment are characteristics that drive the development of professional care ability and patient safety (Gasparino & Guirardello, 2015; Li et al., 2013). One study found organizational support from hospital managers to be important in achieving good nursing care through improving nurse autonomy, granting greater control over resources to nurses, and strengthening nurse–physician relations (Panunto & Guirardello Ede, 2013).

According to Maslach et al. (2001), situational factors in the workplace affect burnout in nurses. For instance, the level of occupational burnout varies among nurses who work in different units. Nursing units such as medical, surgical, pediatric, psychiatric, and burn wards are significantly meaningful in the interpersonal environment (Sahraian, Fazelzadeh, Mehdizadeh, & Toobaee, 2008). Nursing units with different patient severity levels, workloads, and nurse staffing numbers are affected by differing levels of nurse burnout (Bogaert, Clarke, Roelant, Meulemans, & Heyning, 2010). The work environment relates dynamically to the burnout experiences of nurses in the context of both their nursing unit and their hospital tier type. One study verified that nurses in medical and surgical units had the highest ratios of occupational burnout, followed by nurses in intensive care units (Gasparino & Guirardello, 2015).

Many studies have found that nurses who are younger, female, and not married have significantly higher incidences of occupational burnout (Lee, Yen, Fetzer, & Chien, 2015; Shih et al., 2013; Thomas, Kohli, & Choi, 2014). In addition, earning a lower salary, having a higher job position, having a higher education level, and bearing a heavier workload have been associated with higher levels of occupational burnout (Gallavan & Newman, 2013; Khamisa et al., 2016; Oyefeso, Clancy, & Farmer, 2008).

Occupational burnout among nurses is affected by a variety of factors that are associated with their unit and hospital. Thus, the pooling of multilevel data together in an analysis would ignore the independent, environmental, and sociocultural contexts of ecological validity. Therefore, this study aimed to explore a hierarchical model of occupational burnout associated with job-induced stress, the practice environment, and nurse self-concept among nurses in different units and hospitals.

Methods

Research Design and Participants

A cross-sectional study was conducted from January 10, 2015, to June 30, 2016. Figure 1 presents a three-level hierarchical model of occupational burnout. This study encompasses data from nurses (Level I, the nurse level) in six nursing units (Level II, the unit level). The participating organizations comprised seven hospitals (Level III, the hospital level) that were located in all four of Taiwan's principal geographic regions. A convenience sampling method was used for data collection. The inclusion criteria were nurses over 20 years

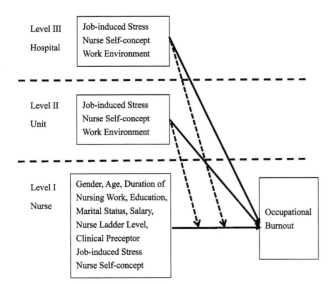

Figure 1. A hierarchical model of occupational burnout.

old who had been working full time in hospitals for at least 3 months. The exclusion criterion was currently working in an administrative capacity.

Ethical Consideration

This study was approved by the institutional review board of the Tri-Service General Hospital National Defense Medical Center (TSGHIRB 1-103-05-107) and by the administrators of the seven hospitals. Written informed consent was signed by and obtained from all of the participants, who were all volunteers, after they were given a detailed explanation of the purpose and procedures of this study. Confidentiality was maintained by assigning code numbers to each answer sheet. All of the participants were made aware that the data collected by the researcher would remain confidential and they would be free to withdraw at any time. The researcher distributed the questionnaires at 125 discrete nursing wards at six nursing units in the seven hospitals. The completed questionnaires were sealed in anonymous envelopes, dropped into reception boxes that were installed in each nursing ward, and then collected by the same researcher.

Measurements

Demographic characteristics

The demographic information collected included age, gender, years of nursing work, marital status (single or not single), educational level (university or above, or less than university), monthly salary (≤ US$1,335, US$1,336–US$1,670, or > US$1,670), nursing clinical ladder level (N vs. N1, N2, or N3–N4), and clinical nursing preceptor (no or yes).

Occupational burnout

Occupational burnout in the participants is widely measured using the Maslach Burnout Inventory-Human Services Survey

(MBI-HSS; Maslach et al., 2001). The Chinese version of the MBI-HSS (Huang, 2012) was used in this study. The MBI-HSS contains 22 items related to personal feelings and attitudes, which are categorized into three dimensions: emotional exhaustion (nine items), depersonalization (five items), and personal accomplishment (eight items). Emotional exhaustion defines the occupational burnout level of an individual according to their job and work overload, including exhaustion, weariness, and decrease in emotional energy. Depersonalization assesses the degree to which a respondent responds emotionally to those with whom they work. Personal accomplishment evaluates the degree to which the respondent feels a sense of accomplishment or success in their job. A 7-point Likert scale (0–6 points) is used to score these items, with a high score suggesting high levels of occupational burnout. The Cronbach's alphas of internal consistency reliability for the emotional exhaustion, depersonalization, and personal accomplishment dimensions were, respectively, .92, .93, and .93 in Huang (2012) and .87, .81, and .83 in this study.

Job-induced stress

Job-induced stress among hospital nurses was tested using the Nurse Stress Checklist, which is designed to measure stress in clinical working environments and includes nurses' physical and mental responses toward work and satisfaction after completion of work and individual professional ability (Benoliel, McCorkle, Georgiadou, Denton, & Spitger, 1990). The Chinese version of the Nurse Stress Checklist (Tsai & Chen, 1996) was used in this study. This checklist contains 47 items in four categories: personal response (18 items), work concern (13 items), competency (11 items), and incompletion of personal arrangement (five items). A 9-point Likert scale (0–8 points) was used to score these items, with a high score suggesting high levels of stress. The Cronbach's alphas of internal consistency reliability for the personal response, work concern, competency, and incompletion of personal arrangement categories were, respectively, .94, .91, .86, and .84 in Tsai and Chen (1996) and .95, .94, .92, and .87 in this study.

Nurse self-concept

Nurse self-concept was measured using the Nurses' Self-Concept Instrument, which is designed to test the subjective experiences of nurses, incorporating how they think and feel (beliefs reflected in questions encompassing both cognition and affect) about themselves in their nursing roles (Angel, Craven, & Denson, 2012). The Chinese version of the Nurses' Self-Concept Instrument (Chang & Yeh, 2016) was used in this study. The instrument contains 14 items that are divided into four categories: knowledge (four items), leadership (four items), care (three items), and staff relations (three items). The response alternative is an 8-point, forced-choice, Likert scale that ranges from 1 = *definitely false* to 8 = *definitely true*. Each item is scored using positive numbers, with a higher score indicating stronger endorsement of each item. The psychometric properties have been tested to show its favorable reliability and validity. The Cronbach's alphas of internal consistency reliability for care, knowledge, staff relations, and leadership were, respectively, .81, .91, .65, and .84 in Chang and Yeh (2016) and .83, .86, .88, and .90 in this study.

Nursing work environment

Nursing work environment was measured using the Nursing Work Index-Revised (NWI-R), which is widely used to identify the presence of certain characteristics in the work environment that contribute to the professional practice of nurses (Aiken & Patrician, 2000). The Chinese version of the NWI-R (Chao, Yuan, Wang, & Hsieh, 2008) was used in this study. The 57-item instrument includes four categories: autonomy in work (five items), nurse–physician relationships (three items), control over the practice setting (seven items), and organizational support (10 items). A 4-point Likert scale (1–4 points) was used. Higher scores on the NWI-R reflect a higher presence of positive attributes that are conducive to the practice of professionals. Scores higher than 2.5 indicate favorable professional practice environments, and scores below 2.5 indicate unfavorable practice environments. The Cronbach's alphas of internal consistency reliability for the autonomy, control over the practice setting, nurse–physician relationship aspect, and organizational support were, respectively, .76, .79, .85, and .71 in Chang and Yeh (2016) and .73, .79, .70, and .83 in this study.

Statistical Analysis

The predictors of demographic characteristics that were analyzed and controlled at the nurse level included age, gender, nursing work years, educational level, monthly salary, nursing clinical ladder level, and clinical nursing preceptor in six nursing units from seven hospitals. As these predictors may relate differently at the three different levels, the hierarchical model is an appropriate method of analysis. Multilevel regression analyses conducted using Hierarchical Linear Modeling (HLM) 6.0 software examined the predictors of occupational burnout at the nurse, unit, and hospital levels. Variations in analysis results were distinguished into between-group variation and within-group variation. Multilevel analysis was done when overall variation in the results was associated with intergroup variation, whereas overall variation in the results comes from within-group variation under conditions of large within-group heterogeneity. This study used the intragroup correlation coefficient (ICC) as a measure for the adoption of multilevel analysis. The formula for ICC is as follows: intergroup correlation coefficient = [intergroup variation / (intergroup variation + intragroup variation)]. If all of the observations are independent of one another, then the ICC approaches 0. At the other extreme, if all of the responses from the observations in all of the clusters are exactly correlated, then the ICC approaches 1 (Hox, 2002).

Results

Two thousand six hundred five nurses from 125 nursing wards at six nursing units in seven hospitals were enrolled as participants, with an overall response rate of 82.25%. Table 1 summarizes the demographic characteristics and work factors that potentially affect occupational burnout at Level I. The sample included 57 men and 2,548 women with an average age of 32.01 ± 7.89 years and an average of 9.55 ± 7.74 years of nursing work. Three fifths (59.9%) were single, 59.2% held a university level education or higher, and 38.4% and 26.2% worked in general wards and intensive care units, respectively. Mean scores were 26.51 ± 10.86 for emotional exhaustion, 10.63 ± 6.86 for depersonalization, 30.41 ± 9.07 for personal accomplishment, 5.37 ± 1.10 for

TABLE 1.
Level I Variables for Nurses

Variable	n	%
Age (years; M and SD)	32.01	7.89
Duration of nursing work (years; M and SD)	9.55	7.74
Gender		
Male	57	2.2
Female	2,548	97.8
Marital status		
Single	1,561	59.9
Not single	1,044	40.1
Educational level		
University or above	1,543	59.2
Under university	1,062	40.8
Nursing unit		
Outpatient department unit	259	9.9
General unit	1,000	38.4
Psychiatric unit	192	7.4
Intensive care unit	684	26.2
Special unit	325	12.5
Hemodialysis unit	145	5.6
Monthly salary (USD)		
≤ 1,335	856	32.9
1,336–1,670	964	37.0
> 1,670	785	30.1
Nursing ladder level		
N	655	25.2
N1	597	22.9
N2	1004	38.5
N3–N4	349	13.4
Clinical nursing preceptor		
No	1813	69.6
Yes	792	30.4
	M	SD
Occupational burnout		
Emotional exhaustion	26.51	10.86
Depersonalization	10.63	6.86
Personal accomplishment	30.41	9.07
Nurse self-concept	5.37	1.10
Job-induced stress	3.90	1.07
Work environment	2.85	0.35

nurse self-concept, 3.90 ± 1.07 for job-induced stress, and 2.85 ± 0.35 for work environment.

According to the results of the HLM analyses, no statistical significance was identified on the three-level model. The hospital level was ultimately removed from the HLM analyses because of the high collinearity among variables. Thus, a two-level model was then used in the analysis in the random intercept, random coefficient, and two-level models. However, the cross-level model did not converge because of multicollinearity between predictors.

Table 2 shows the results of emotional exhaustion for occupational burnout. Participants with a university or higher level of education, who earned a salary of more than US$1,670 per month, or who were N2 or N3–N4 had significance in the random intercept model and random coefficient model. Note that nurse self-concept and job-induced stress had significance based on the random intercept, random coefficient, and two-level models. However, nurse self-concept was negatively associated with emotional exhaustion.

Table 3 shows the results of the depersonalization aspect of occupational burnout. Nurses with a university or higher level of education or who earned a salary of more than US$1,670 per month had significance in the random

intercept model and random coefficient model. Note that the nursing clinical ladder levels N1 and N2, nurse self-concept, and job-induced stress all had significance in the three models. However, nurse self-concept was negatively associated with depersonalization.

Table 4 shows the results of personal accomplishment for occupational burnout. Nursing clinical ladder levels N1, N2, and N3–N4 had significance in the random intercept model and random coefficient model. However, a high ladder level was negatively associated with personal accomplishment. Note that nurse self-concept had significance in all three models and was positively associated with personal accomplishment.

As shown in Tables 2–4, the two-level model was identified as the optimal model for analysis. At the unit level, no significance was found in any aspect of occupational burnout. At the nurse level, the ICC for emotional exhaustion was 2.86 [0.042/(0.042 + 1.424) = 2.86%; $p < .001$], indicating 5.33% reliability in the unit mean difference. ICC for depersonalization was 3.48 [1.648/(1.648 + 45.692) = 3.48%; $p < .001$], indicating 4.42% reliability. ICC for personal accomplishment was 1.21 [1.006/(1.006 + 81.788) = 1.21%; $p < .001$], indicating 3.87% reliability. Because ICC was greater than 0, all of the observations were associated with each other.

TABLE 2.
Results of Hierarchical Models of Emotional Exhaustion

Fixed Effect	Random Intercept β	Random Intercept SE	Random Coefficient β	Random Coefficient SE	Two-Level β	Two-Level SE
Intercept	2.829***	0.088	1.610	0.247	−11.594	5.575
Level I						
Gender			0.090	0.131	0.087	0.137
Age			−0.006	0.007	−0.005	0.007
Years of nursing work			0.018*	0.007	0.018*	0.007
Marital status (single vs. not)			−0.084	0.045	−0.081	0.045
Educational level (university and above vs. under)			0.111**	0.041	0.109**	0.041
Monthly salary (US$; ≤ 1,335 vs. 1,336–1,670)			0.070	0.048	0.067	0.048
Monthly salary (US$; ≤ 1,335 vs. > 1,670)			0.129**	0.056	0.125**	0.056
Nurse ladder level (N vs. N1)			0.095	0.056	0.100	0.056
Nurse ladder level (N vs. N2)			0.185**	0.059	0.185**	0.059
Nurse ladder level (N vs. N3–N4)			0.084*	0.081	0.086	0.081
Nursing preceptor (no vs. yes)			−0.034	0.050	−0.035	0.050
Nurse self-concept			−0.250***	0.019	−0.250***	0.019
Job-induced stress			0.608***	0.018	0.607***	0.018
Level II						
Nurse self-concept					2.736	1.036
Job-induced stress					0.056	0.210
Work environment					0.975	0.634
Random effect						
Intergroup variation	0.042		0.015		0.006	
Intragroup variation	1.424		0.919		0.919	
Deviance			7240.160		7234.970	

*$p < .05$. **$p < .01$. ***$p < .001$.

TABLE 3.
Results of Hierarchical Models of Depersonalization

Fixed Effect	Random Intercept		Random Coefficient		Two-Level	
	β	SE	β	SE	β	SE
Intercept	10.006***	0.549	9.516	1.538	−24.985	78.245
Level I						
Gender			−0.306	0.804	−0.323	0.804
Age			−0.041	0.041	−0.040	0.041
Years of nursing work			−0.010	0.043	−0.012	0.044
Marital status (single vs. not)			−0.265	0.277	−0.265	0.278
Educational level (university or above vs. under)			0.583*	0.252	0.582*	0.252
Monthly salary (US$; ≤ 1,335 vs. 1,336–1,670)			0.582	0.297	0.589*	0.298
Monthly salary (US$; ≤ 1,335 vs. > 1,670)			0.772*	0.345	0.774*	0.346
Nurse ladder level (N vs. N1)			1.213**	0.345	1.218**	0.345
Nurse ladder level (N vs. N2)			1.721***	0.361	1.733***	0.361
Nurse ladder level (N vs. N3–N4)			0.698	0.500	0.721	0.501
Nursing preceptor (no vs. yes)			−0.423	0.307	−0.424	0.308
Nurse self-concept			−1.587***	0.115	−1.588***	0.115
Job-induced stress			2.439***	0.112	2.442***	0.112
Level II						
Nurse self-concept					1.008	8.781
Job-induced stress					−1.114	2.901
Work environment					11.781	15.520
Random effect						
Intergroup variation	1.648		0.942		1.872	
Intragroup variation	45.692		34.779		34.779	
Deviance			16655.442		16640.572	

*$p < .05.$ **$p < .01.$ ***$p < .001.$

Three aspects of occupational burnout showed greater variation among nursing units than among individual nurses.

Discussion

This study hypothesized a hierarchical model of occupational burnout that is associated with job-induced stress, nurse self-concept, and work environment among nurses working in six units of seven hospitals. Occupational burnout refers to emotional exhaustion, depersonalization, and a reduced sense of personal accomplishment. This study confirmed that these three categories were highly associated with the characteristics of individual nurses. These characteristics included years of nursing work, educational level, salary, and nursing clinical ladder level. Having an educational level of university or above and a ladder level of N2 were important predictors of occupational-burnout-related emotional exhaustion and depersonalization in this study, with number of years of nursing work also affecting this exhaustion. These findings are similar to other studies (Gallavan & Newman, 2013; Khamisa et al., 2016; Shih et al., 2013; Wu et al., 2014).

Nurse self-concept was the most important predictor of emotional exhaustion, depersonalization, and personal accomplishment in this study. Nurse self-concept related negatively to emotional exhaustion and depersonalization but positively to

personal accomplishment, indicating that nurses with a high self-concept of nursing are less susceptible to job burnout. Positive self-concept and job satisfaction among nurses may be helpful in reducing the degree of burnout in experienced nurses, as self-concept has been shown to mediate the relationship between job satisfaction and burnout (Nwafor, Immanel, & Obi-Nwosu, 2015). Nursing self-concept is relevant to how nurses think and feel about themselves. Moreover, self-concept is typically relatively stable between an individual's academic career and during his or her early professional career as a nurse (Arthur & Randle, 2007). Although self-concept is cultivated in nursing education, clinical continuing education should also pay attention to this issue. Very few studies have explored the professional self-concepts of nurses. This study provides evidence on nursing self-concepts from nurse populations across six nursing units at seven hospitals.

In addition to self-concept, job-induced stress was identified as an important predictor of the emotional exhaustion and depersonalization dimensions of occupational burnout, with those exhibiting higher job-induced stress having higher levels of occupational burnout. This finding is similar to other studies, supporting that job-induced stress contributes to burnout in nurses (Khamisa et al., 2016; Shih et al., 2013; Wu et al., 2014). The Institute of Labor, Occupational Safety and Health, Ministry of Labor (2013) has identified the occupational

TABLE 4.
Results of Hierarchical Models of Personal Accomplishment

Fixed Effect	Random Intercept		Random Coefficient		Two-Level	
	β	SE	β	SE	β	SE
Intercept	30.504***	0.461	9.553	1.974	−12.242	62.056
Level I						
Gender			−1.788	1.060	−1.850	1.060
Age			0.032	0.054	0.029	0.054
Years of nursing work			0.044	0.057	0.042	0.057
Marital status (single vs. not)			0.081	0.365	0.079	0.366
Educational level (university or above vs. under)			−0.586	0.333	−0.577	0.333
Monthly salary (US$; ≤ 1,335 vs. 1,336–1,670)			−0.103	0.389	−0.049	0.391
Monthly salary (US$; ≤ 1,335 vs. > 1,670)			0.261	0.450	0.334	0.454
Nurse ladder level (N vs. N1)			−1.168*	0.454	−1.166*	0.455
Nurse ladder level (N vs. N2)			−1.356**	0.475	−1.310**	0.476
Nurse ladder level (N vs. N3–N4)			−1.812**	0.657	−1.739**	0.661
Nursing preceptor (no vs. yes)			0.715	0.404	0.718	0.406
Nurse self-concept			4.126***	0.152	4.120***	0.152
Job-induced stress			0.015	0.147	0.030	0.148
Level II						
Nurse self-concept					5.999	12.001
Job-induced stress					−1.184	2.324
Work environment					1.753	7.003
Random effect						
Intergroup variation	1.006		0.453		1.021	
Intragroup variation	81.788		60.518		60.517	
Deviance			18085.621		18072.056	

*$p < .05$. **$p < .01$. ***$p < .001$.

stressors for nurses as compactness of job content, work interfering with personal time and life, stresses from the medical team, stresses from occupational hazards, stresses from nurse–patient–family relationships, stresses from assault, and stresses from powerlessness and patient deaths. Thus, the occupational burnout of nurses may be effectively minimized by reducing their perceived stress.

In addition, nursing clinical ladder level N2 was identified as an important predictor for depersonalization in this study. The clinical ladder system in Taiwan aims to improve the quality of patient care based on learning experience and on increasing the rewards and recognitions given to nurses in clinical practice. This study found that nurses at higher nursing clinical ladder levels and with more clinical situational experience had a less reduced sense of personal accomplishment than their novice-level peers. One study found that perceptions of a clinical ladder system correlated positively with job satisfaction and negatively with intention to leave (Chae, Ko, Kim, & Yoon, 2015), although other studies concluded the opposite (Chae et al., 2015; Hariyati, Igarashi, Fujinam, Susilaningsih, & Prayenti, 2017). The conflicting results may relate to the differing perceptions of nurses toward the clinical ladder system. Nurses in Taiwan with higher ladder levels are expected to take on more clinical responsibilities and to practice and guide new recruits, which may increase their

perceived pressures and lead to a lower sense of personal accomplishment.

This study found that longer nursing work years, a university or higher educational level, a monthly salary greater than 1,670 U.S. dollars, and a nursing clinical ladder level of N2–N4 were each associated with higher emotional exhaustion and occupational burnout. Moreover, a university or higher educational level, a monthly salary greater than 1,670 U.S. dollars, and a nursing clinical ladder level of N1–N2 were each associated with higher depersonalization burnout. Furthermore, nurses at higher ladder levels had a lower sense of personal accomplishment than their novice-level peers. Clinical nurses with more working experience, education, and income and a higher ladder level are often given more job responsibilities (Gallavan & Newman, 2013; Khamisa et al., 2016; Oyefeso et al., 2008; Shih et al., 2013; Wu et al., 2014). Thus, taking on heavier responsibilities and stress in more important roles may cause more frequent instances of more severe levels of burnout.

This study did not find evidence that the work environment is a predictor of nursing occupational burnout. This differs from Gasparino and Guirardello (2015), which indicated that unfavorable nursing care environments may cause development of burnout syndrome. In addition, this study did not support the idea that occupational burnout varies among different nursing units. Thus, the nursing unit may not be an important predictor of occupational burnout in nurses. This differs from Bogaert et al. (2010), which indicated that nurse perceptions about the environment of their nursing units potentially influence their job experiences and may be associated with occupation burnout. This may be because the three aspects of occupation burnout exhibited greater variation at the nursing unit level than at the individual nurse level. Better clarifying the relationship between units and occupational burnout will be important to further distinguishing the differences at the unit level.

Limitations

This study is affected by several limitations. First, the cross-sectional design of this study provided data at one time point only. Therefore, longitudinal follow-up of the relationships between occupational burnout and job-induced stress, self-concept, and the work environment was not conducted. Second, although this study included seven hospitals from all of Taiwan's main geographic regions, many regions were still not covered. Differences in medical culture may affect the responses of nurses toward their practice environment. Third, the hospital-level burnout model was found to have no statistical significance in this study, which may reflect the small number of hospitals that were included.

Conclusions/Implications for Practice

The findings of this study confirm that individual nurse characteristics predict the emotional exhaustion, depersonalization, and personal accomplishment dimensions of occupational burnout. Individual factors such as number of years working in nursing, educational level, income, nursing clinical ladder level, job-induced stress, and nurse self-concept were all identified as important predictors of occupational burnout. This study did not support that occupational burnout varied among nursing units, as occupational burnout variation between nursing units was greater than that between individual nurses. The findings suggest, in particular, that improving self-concept may effectively decrease perceived burnout in nurses, which may then improve overall patient care. In clinical practice, nurses holding a positive self-concept regarding nursing reduce their occupational burnout, which may help them provide a higher quality of care. A two-level hierarchical model appropriately fits the data, with no significance identified for any of the dimensions of occupational burnout at the unit level. A larger number of hospitals in the sample may be required to achieve the hypothesized hierarchical model.

Authors Contributions

Study conception and design: All authors
Data collection: RWL
Data analysis and interpretation: RWL, MLY, KCL
Drafting of the article: RWL, MLY
Critical revision of the article: RWL, MLY

References

Aiken, L. H., & Patrician, P. A. (2000). Measuring organizational traits of hospitals: The Revised Nursing Work Index. *Nursing Research, 49*(3), 146–153.

Aiken, L. H., Sloane, D. M., Cimiotti, J. P., Clarke, S. P., Flynn, L., Seago, J. A., ... Smith, H. L. (2010). Implications of the California nurse staffing mandate for other states. *Health Services Research, 45*(4), 904–921. https://doi.org/10.1111/j.1475-6773.2010.01114.x

Angel, E., Craven, R., & Denson, N. (2012). The nurses' self-concept instrument (NSCI): Assessment of psychometric properties for Australian domestic and international student nurses. *International Journal of Nursing Studies, 49*(7), 880–886. https://doi.org/10.1016/j.ijnurstu.2012.01.016

Arthur, D., & Randle, J. (2007). The professional self-concept of nurses: A review of the literature from 1992-2006. *Australian Journal of Advanced Nursing, 24*(3), 60–64.

Benoliel, J. Q., McCorkle, R., Georgiadou, F., Denton, T., & Spitger, A. (1990). Measurement of stress in clinical nursing. *Cancer Nursing, 13*(4), 221–228.

Bogaert, P. V., Clarke, S., Roelant, E., Meulemans, H., & Heyning, P. V. (2010). Impacts of unit-level nurse practice environment and burnout on nurse-reported outcomes: A multilevel modelling approach. *Journal of Clinical Nursing, 19*(11–12), 1664–1674. https://doi.org/10.1111/j.1365-2702.2009.03128.x

Chae, S. N., Ko, I. S., Kim, I. S., & Yoon, K. S. (2015). Effect of perception of career ladder system on job satisfaction, intention to leave among perioperative nurses. *Journal of Korean Academy of Nursing Administration, 21*(3), 233–242. https://doi.org/10.11111/jkana.2015.21.3.233

Chang, Y. C., & Yeh, M. L. (2016). Translation and validation of the Nurses' Self-Concept Instrument for college-level nursing students in Taiwan. *Nurse Education Today, 36*, 112–117. https://doi.org/10.1016/j.nedt.2015.08.009

Chao, W. C., Yuan, C. Y., Wang, M. H., & Hsieh, P. C. (2008). A study of perceived nursing work environment among nurses: An example of regional teaching hospitals in Taipei County. *Journal of Oriental Institute of Technology, 28_S*, 105–116. https://doi.org/10.30167/JOIT.200812.0012 (Original work published in Chinese)

Chou, L. P., Li, C. Y., & Hu, S. C. (2014). Job stress and burnout in hospital employees: Comparisons of different medical professions in a regional hospital in Taiwan. *BMJ Open, 4*, e004185. https://doi.org/10.1136/bmjopen-2013-004185

Cowin, L. S., Johnson, M., Craven, R. G., & Marsh, H. W. (2008). Causal modeling of self-concept, job satisfaction, and retention of nurses. *International Journal of Nursing Studies, 45*(10), 1449–1459. https://doi.org/10.1016/j.ijnurstu.2007.10.009

Gallavan, D. B., & Newman, J. L. (2013). Predictors of burnout among correctional mental health professionals. *Psychological Services, 10*(1), 115–122. https://doi.org/10.1037/a0031341

Gasparino, R. C., & Guirardello, E. B. (2015). Professional practice environment and occupational burnout among nurses. *Rev Rene, 16*(1), 90–96. https://doi.org/10.15253/2175-6783.2015000100012

Hariyati, R. T. S., Igarashi, K., Fujinam, Y., & Susilaningsih, F. S. Prayenti (2017). Correlation between career ladder, continuing professional development and nurse satisfaction: A case study in Indonesia. *International Journal of Caring Sciences, 10*(3), 1490–1497.

Hox, J. (2002). *Multilevel analysis: Techniques and applications.* Mahwah, NJ: Lawrence Erlbaum Associates.

Huang, C. C. (2012). *Research regarding influences on career occupational burnout of nurse aides in long-term care facilities through personality hardiness and work-family conflict* (Unpublished master's thesis). Taiwan, ROC: Meiho University. (Original work published in Chinese)

Institute of Labor, Occupational Safety and Health, Ministry of Labor. (2013). *A study on practice environment and physical and mental health of nurses in Taiwan.* Retrieved from https://laws.ilosh.gov.tw/ioshcustom/Web/YearlyReserachReports/Detail?id=2711 (Original work published in Chinese)

Jodas, D. A., & Haddad, M. C. L. (2009). Burnout syndrome among nursing staff from an emergency department of a university hospital. *Acta Paulista de Enfermagem, 22*(2), 192–197. https://doi.org/10.1590/S0103-21002009000200012 (Original work published in Portuguese)

Khamisa, N., Peltzer, K., Ilic, D., & Oldenburg, B. (2016). Work related stress, burnout, job satisfaction and general health of nurses: A follow-up study. *International Journal of Nursing Practice, 22*(6), 538–545. https://doi.org/10.1111/ijn.12455

Lee, H. F., Yen, M., Fetzer, S., & Chien, T. W. (2015). Predictors of burnout among nurses in Taiwan. *Community Mental Health Journal, 51*(6), 733–737. https://doi.org/10.1007/s10597-014-9818-4

Li, B., Bruyneel, L., Sermeus, W., Van den Heede, K., Matawie, K., Aiken, L., & Lesaffre, E. (2013). Group-level impact of work environment dimensions on burnout experiences among nurses: A multivariate multilevel probit model. *International Journal of Nursing Studies, 50*, 281–291. https://doi.org/10.1016/j.ijnurstu.2012.07.001

Oyefeso, A., Clancy, C., & Farmer, R. (2008). Prevalence and associated factors in burnout and psychological morbidity among substance misuse professionals. *BMC Health Services Research, 8*(1), 39–48. https://doi.org/10.1186/1472-6963-8-39

Panunto, M. R., & Guirardello Ede, B. (2013). Professional nursing practice: Environment and emotional exhaustion among intensive care nurses. *Revista Latino-Americana de Enfermagem, 21*(3), 765–772. https://doi.org/10.1590/S0104-11692013000300016

Maslach, C., & Leiter, M. P. (2016). Understanding the burnout experience: Recent research and its implications for psychiatry. *World Psychiatry, 15*(2), 103–111. https://doi.org/10.1002/wps.20311

Maslach, C., Schaufeli, W. B., & Leiter, M. P. (2001). Occupational burnout. *Annual Review of Psychology, 52*(1), 397–422. https://doi.org/10.1146/annurev.psych.52.1.397

McHugh, M. D., Kelly, L. A., Smith, H. L., Wu, E. S., Vanak, J. M., & Aiken, L. H. (2013). Lower mortality in magnet hospitals. *Medical Care, 51*(5), 382–388. https://doi.org/10.1097/MLR.0b013e3182726cc5

Nwafor, C. E., Immanel, E. U., & Obi-Nwosu, H. (2015). Does nurses' self-concept mediate the relationship between job satisfaction and burnout among Nigerian nurses. *International Journal of Africa Nursing Sciences, 3*, 71–75. https://doi.org/10.1016/j.ijans.2015.08.003

Sahraian, A., Fazelzadeh, A., Mehdizadeh, A. R., & Toobaee, S. H. (2008). Burnout in hospital nurses: A comparison of internal, surgery, psychiatry and burns wards. *International Nursing Review, 55*(1), 62–67. https://doi.org/10.1111/j.1466-7657.2007.00582.x

Shih, E. C., Chiu, H. H., Sun, C. A., Wei, C. Y., Chou, Y. C., & Yang, T. (2013). Impact of personal characteristics and work stress on job burnout among psychiatric nurses. *Innovative Journal of Medical and Health Science, 3*(4), 201–208.

Thomas, M., Kohli, V., & Choi, J. (2014). Correlates of job burnout among human services workers: Implications for workforce retention. *Journal of Sociology & Social Welfare, 41*(4), 69–90. Retrieved from http://scholarworks.wmich.edu/jssw/vol41/iss4/5

Tsai, S. L., & Chen, M. L. (1996). A test of the reliability and validity of nurse stress checklist. *Nursing Research, 4*(4), 355–362. (Original work published in Chinese)

van der Colff, J. J., & Rothmann, S. (2014). Burnout of registered nurses in South Africa. *Journal of Nursing Management, 22*, 630–642. https://doi.org/10.1111/j.1365-2834.2012.01467

Wilkinson, H., Whittington, R., Perry, L., & Eames, C. (2017). Examining the relationship between burnout and empathy in healthcare professionals: A systematic review. *Burnout Research, 6*, 18–29. https://doi.org/10.1016/j.burn.2017.06.003

Wu, H., Liu, L., Sun, W., Zhao, X., Wang, J., & Wang, L. (2014). Factors related to burnout among Chinese female hospital nurses: Cross-sectional survey in Liaoning Province of China. *Journal of Nursing Management, 22*, 621–629. https://doi.org/10.1111/jonm.12015

18

Effects of Team-Based Learning on the Core Competencies of Nursing Students

Kyung Eun Lee

ABSTRACT

Background: An important goal of nursing education is helping students achieve core competencies efficiently. One proposed way of improving nursing education is team-based learning (TBL).

Purpose: The aim of this study was to assess the comparative effectiveness of TBL and lecture-style classes in terms of teaching core competencies in nursing education, which include clinical competence skills, problem-solving ability, communication competencies, critical thinking ability, and self-leadership.

Methods: This quasi-experimental study enrolled 183 students as participants, with 95 and 88 in the experimental and control groups, respectively. These two groups attended 6 hours (2 hours weekly for 3 weeks) of TBL and lecture-style classes, respectively. Differences in core competencies between the two groups were compared before and after the intervention.

Results: The experimental group achieved significantly higher scores for clinical competence skills, communication competence, critical thinking ability, and self-leadership at posttest than at pretest, whereas the control group achieved significantly higher scores for clinical competence skills and critical thinking ability at posttest than at pretest. After the intervention, the experimental group had significantly better clinical competence skills, communication competence, and self-leadership than the control group.

Conclusion: TBL is an effective approach method to teaching core competencies in nursing education.

KEY WORDS:
team-based learning, competency, nursing education.

Introduction

Nursing education aims to develop competent nurses to provide professional nursing services in a rapidly changing nursing practice field (Mennenga & Smyer, 2010). Therefore, nursing students must have the knowledge, techniques, and attitudes necessary to effectively solve problems that are presented in various situations throughout their course of study. This discrete group of knowledge, techniques, and attitudes are the core competencies that nursing students must learn and achieve before graduation (Choi, 2016; Lee, Park, & Jeong, 2012). These core competencies include not only the perceptual capabilities that enable successful problem solving in clinical situations but also widely applicable and complex capabilities such as healthy attitudes toward the self, others, and the organization as well as effective social skills (Ko et al., 2013). More specifically, nursing students must become capable of integrated nursing skills delivery, possess knowledge of liberal arts and their major area, communicate and cooperate with various professional fields, exercise critical thinking, and exhibit self-leadership (Korean Accreditation Board of Nursing Education, 2012).

Therefore, in nursing education, helping students efficiently achieve these core competencies has become an important goal of education. However, traditional lecture-type classes (traditional instructor-centered teaching centered on the unilateral delivery of knowledge) are limited in achieving the goals of nursing education that are consistent with the demands of the times. This is because the instructor-centered nature of lecture-type classes is not suited to enhancing the abilities of students to manage issues in a flexible and creative manner. Therefore, introducing new education curricula that allow students to experience the process of integrating and applying knowledge autonomously in nursing education is necessary (Branson, Boss, & Fowler, 2016). Team-based learning (TBL) is one of many self-directed and active teaching–learning methods (Haidet et al., 2012).

The concept of TBL was introduced by Michaelsen as an instructional method wherein students acquire knowledge and then apply this knowledge to solve problems through discussions in small teams in a traditional lecture room (Michaelsen, Parmelee, McMahon, & Levine, 2008). This type of class structure allows students to receive continuous practice-related feedback as they solve applied problems through individual and cooperative study and iterative learning. In addition, mini-lectures are given by instructors to summarize the core contents (Haidet et al., 2012). TBL sets the scope and direction of learning by supplying prior reading material and allows students to check their level of understanding through quizzes that are administered during discussion, facilitating the active participation of students in

PhD, RN, Assistant Professor, Department of Nursing, Keimyung College University, Daegu, South Korea.

the class through feedback and motivating students to become active in organizing and acquiring knowledge (Haidet et al., 2012; Parmelee & Michaelsen, 2010). Overall, TBL is a set of teaching and learning methods that is deployed at education sites. TBL combines the strengths of individual and cooperative learning and relies on a system whereby groups lead conceptual learning to solve various problems (Michaelsen & Sweet, 2011; Parmelee & Michaelsen, 2010). Finally, TBL is an educational method wherein the learners become class leaders and the teacher becomes a facilitator and guides who designs and manages the learning process, acting not as a "knowledge deliverer" but as a "learning facilitator" (Vermette & Foote, 2001). These TBL characteristics make it effective for developing communication, problem solving, cooperation, and professional, clinical, and critical thinking skills (Parmelee & Michaelsen, 2010) through its active, cooperative, and problem-solving, team-learning-based process that enables learners to engage in classes through sufficient preparation. Therefore, we expect that TBL may play a positive role in strengthening the core capabilities of nursing students such as integrated nursing skills delivery, knowledge of liberal arts and their major area, communication and cooperation with various professional fields, critical thinking, and self-leadership. Furthermore, because of its teaching/learning-based approach, which allows a small number of instructors to lead classes comprising large numbers of students, TBL should be easy to apply in the current nursing education field, where most teaching still consists of lecture-based classes (Zgheib, Simaan, & Sabra, 2010).

Previous studies have shown TBL as effective in promoting academic achievement and satisfaction (Roh, Ryoo, Choi, Baek, & Kim, 2012), class satisfaction (Clark, Nguyen, Bray, & Levine, 2008; Oh, 2015), learning motivation (Han, 2013), learning attitude (Cheng, Liou, Tsai, & Chang, 2014; Han, 2013), critical thinking (Kim & Hong, 2015), problem-solving abilities (Kim & Hong, 2015; Oh, 2015), self-directed learning (Kim & Hong, 2015), and clinical competence skills (Mennenga, 2013) in nursing students. However, its application in nursing education has not been as widely adopted as in other health education fields, and few studies have assessed the effectiveness of TBL in nursing education.

In particular, the effectiveness of TBL in promoting the core competencies of nursing education remains unclear. Although fragmentary evidence exists for the effectiveness of TBL in promoting individual competencies such as communication competence, critical thinking, and problem-solving ability, no study has yet examined the effectiveness of TBL in enhancing the core competencies of nursing education as a whole. Accordingly, this study was designed to determine the effectiveness of TBL in enhancing nursing student mastery of these core competencies by developing and applying a TBL program for nursing students and comparing its effectiveness with that of traditional lecture-style classes.

Methods

Research Design
This quasi-experimental study applied a nonequivalent, control-group, pretest–posttest design. Our main aim was to compare clinical competence skills, problem-solving ability, communication competence, critical thinking ability, and self-leadership between the experimental group (receiving TBL) and the control group (receiving lectures).

Participants
The participants were senior nursing students of Yeungnam University in Daegu City, South Korea, who were taking an adult health nursing course and voluntarily agreed to participate after explaining of the study purpose, method, and expected effects. G*Power 3.1.9.2 was used to calculate the necessary sample size; for a two-tailed t test with a significance level of $\alpha = .05$, two groups, an effect size of $d = .05$, and a power of test = 0.90, 88 subjects per group, for a total of 176 subjects, were needed. One hundred eighty-nine students from two classes agreed to participate. Although 96 and 93 students were randomly assigned to the experimental group and the control group, respectively, only 183 students were selected as the final participants because of incomplete responses from one person in the experimental group and five in the control group. Despite these exclusions, the total number of participants in each group was sufficient.

Instruments
Core competencies
Core competencies represent the set of knowledge, skills, and attitudes that nursing students must have to effectively manage diverse and complex clinical situations and must master before graduation (Choi, 2016; Lee et al., 2012). In this study, core competencies specifically refer to clinical competence skills, problem-solving ability, communication competence, critical thinking ability, and self-leadership.

Clinical competence skills
We used an instrument that was developed by Yang and Park (2004) to measure the clinical competence skills of the participants. This instrument is composed of 19 items with six subscales: nursing process, nursing intervention, client education, observation, physical examination, and fundamental nursing. All items are rated on a 5-point scale, with higher scores representing higher clinical competency. The Cronbach's α measure of internal reliability for this instrument was .86 in its development study (Yang & Park, 2004) and .94 in this study.

Problem-solving ability
To measure the problem-solving ability of the participants, this study used a 25-item instrument that was developed by Lee (1978, as cited in Park & Woo, 1999) and modified

and supplemented by Park and Woo (1999). All of the items are rated on a 5-point scale, with higher scores indicating better problem-solving ability. The Cronbach's α was .89 at the time of instrument development and .89 in this study.

Communication competence

To measure the communication competence of the participants, this study used the Global Interpersonal Communication Competence Scale, which was modified by Hur (2003) by adding seven items to the eight items that were originally proposed by Rubin (1990) for assessing the communication competence construct. This scale is composed of 15 items, with higher scores indicating greater communication competence. The Cronbach's α was .72 in Hur's study and .88 in this study.

Critical thinking ability

To measure the critical thinking ability of the participants, this study used a critical thinking disposition instrument comprising 27 items (Yoon, 2004). This instrument is composed of the subscales of intellectual eagerness/curiosity, prudence, systematicity, intellectual fairness, healthy skepticism, and objectivity. All of the items are rated on a 5-point scale, with higher scores indicating better critical thinking ability. Cronbach's α was .84 at the time of instrument development and .92 in this study.

Self-leadership

To measure the self-leadership of the participants, this study used the Revised Self-Leadership Questionnaire that was developed by Houghton and Neck (2002) and modified and supplemented by Shin, Kim, and Han (2009) for Korean students. The instrument is composed of 35 items, and each is rated on a 5-point scale, with higher scores indicating greater self-leadership. The Cronbach's α was .73–.83 at the time of instrument development (Shin et al., 2009) and .89 in this study.

Research Procedure

We assigned students who voluntarily filled out the research participation agreement forms randomly into the test and control groups. The TBL intervention was administered to the experimental group, and the existing lecture-based course was administered to the control group. Each course was administered in one weekly 2-hour class for a period of 3 weeks. This study measured the clinical competence skills, problem-solving ability, communication competence, critical thinking ability, and self-leadership of all study participants using self-report surveys before and after the 3-week experiment. Each tool was used with the permission of its respective author(s).

The methods used to deliver TBL and lecture-based classes are described, respectively, below.

Team-based learning

TBL is a structured set of methods that are designed to maximize the outcomes of both individual students and

their teams through individual learning and interactions among team members (Haidet et al., 2012). During the preplanning phase, the lecture material, case studies in nursing, and questions for the individual readiness assurance test (IRAT) and group readiness assurance test (GRAT) were based on providing "nursing care for diabetic patients," a topic from the adult health nursing course. In the case study phase, we documented the cases based on clinical experience and adult nursing textbooks. To increase the validity of the TBL program, two professors of adult health nursing modified and supplemented the content.

The TBL instructional process was completed according to a standardized three-stage protocol: individual self-learning through reading assignments (first stage), assessment of readiness assurance through tests and feedback (second stage), and application of course contents (third stage). We applied four main principles throughout these stages: appropriate formation and operation of teams, giving responsibilities for assignments to both individuals and teams, promoting learning and team development through team assignments, and providing appropriate feedback on achievements (Haidet et al., 2012).

In the first stage (i.e., self-learning), the purpose and method of TBL were explained to the experimental group in an orientation that was held 1 week before the first session. Then, each learning objective and related content and materials were presented to group participants on a weekly basis during the 3-week TBL course. The experimental group participants attended the session after completing their self-learning of the provided learning material.

The second stage (readiness assurance) was completed by administering, consecutively, the IRAT, GRAT, between-group evaluations, and feedback consistent with the learning result. The seven IRAT and GRAT questions that were used to measure the level of understanding of the training contents were multiple-choice (with five possible responses for each question) and identical every week. Of the 100 minutes of the total session time, we assigned 10 minutes for the IRAT and 30 minutes for the GRAT. After this, each group of participants held learning evaluations and exchanged feedback with instructors based on the posted correct answers. The learning evaluation involved discussions among groups that were guided by the instructor. At that time, students checked the correct answers for each question, asked questions about wrong answers, and discussed the different opinions on these questions, whereas the professor provided feedback on the questions and on difficult parts of the prior reading material.

In the third stage (application of course contents), group discussions were completed in the last 30 minutes. Diabetic patient scenarios, which were developed based on actual hospital cases, were distributed to each team member, and then the class progressed with group discussions and presentations to the class utilizing concept maps, feedback among groups, and feedback by the instructor. During this time, the instructor took on the roles of both facilitator and information provider. Finally, peer evaluations were performed to assess the contribution of each member to the team.

Each team was composed of six to seven members, and each class had eight teams, thus totaling 16 teams for the two classes. The participants were randomly assigned to each group by drawing lots. The same groups were maintained through the end of the course.

Lecture-style classes
Lectures addressing the nursing care of diabetic patients, the same topic as the TBL, were administered by the researcher for 6 hours (2 hours per week for 3 weeks) in a traditional lecture format.

Data Analysis
The collected data were analyzed using SPSS 21.0 (IBM, Inc., Armonk, NY, USA). Descriptive statistics were calculated, including numbers and percentages for the general characteristics of both groups and means and standard deviations (SDs) for core competencies, including clinical competence skills, problem-solving ability, communication competence, critical thinking ability, and self-leadership. Homogeneity tests were conducted before the intervention using χ^2 test and independent t test for the general characteristics and core competencies of the two groups. The differences between the two groups after the intervention were tested using an independent t test. Changes in core competencies before and after the intervention in each group were determined using a paired t test.

Ethical Considerations
Before completing this study, permission from the institutional review board of our affiliated university was obtained (No. 40525-201404-HR-13-02). The study was completed only after explanations on the purpose, method, and expected effects of the study were given to potential participants and their written informed consent was obtained. In the explanation and agreement forms, we assured participants that the personal information that was obtained for this study would not be used for any other purpose, that there were no disadvantages to not participating, and that participants could withdraw at any point during the study.

Results

General Characteristics and Homogeneity Tests Between the Two Groups
The mean age of participants was 23.57 ($SD = 1.81$) years for the experimental group and 23.48 ($SD = 1.74$) years for the control group, with no significant difference between the groups. Most of the participants in both groups were female. Furthermore, both groups were relatively homogeneous in terms of personal relationship status, degree of

satisfaction with academic major, academic performance, and preferred learning method. In terms of the preferred learning method, it should be noted that 97.9% of the experimental group and 96.6% of the control group expressed a preference for lecture-style classes (Table 1).

Homogeneity Tests of Core Competencies Between the Two Groups Before the Intervention
There were no significant differences between the two groups before the intervention (pretest) in terms of clinical competence skills, problem-solving ability, communication competence, critical thinking ability, or self-leadership. Thus, the two groups were homogenous (Table 2).

Differences in Core Competencies Between the Two Groups After the Intervention
After the intervention, the mean scores for clinical competence skills, communication competence, and self-leadership in the experimental group were significantly higher than those in the control group, with all differences meeting statistical significance. Although problem-solving ability and critical thinking ability were also higher in the experimental group than in the control group, these differences did not meet statistical significance (Table 3).

Changes in Pretest–Posttest Core Competencies for the Two Groups
In the experimental group, the mean posttest scores for clinical competence skills, communication competence, critical thinking ability, and self-leadership were significantly higher than the respective pretest scores. By comparison, in the control group, only the posttest scores for clinical competence skills and critical thinking ability were higher than the respective pretest scores (Table 4).

Both groups achieved improvements in all of the core competencies after the intervention, with degree of score improvement higher in the experimental group than in the control group for each core competency category (Figure 1).

Discussion
This study was conducted to assess the effects of TBL on the core competencies that nursing students must master as a prerequisite to graduation. After applying TBL and lecture-style classes, the core competencies including clinical competence skills, problem-solving ability, communication competence, critical thinking ability, and self-leadership were evaluated.

There were no significant differences between the two groups at pretest in terms of general characteristics or core competencies. However, we noted improvements in both groups in all core

TABLE 1.

Homogeneity Test of General Characteristics Between the Two Groups (N = 183)

Item	Experimental Group (n = 95)		Control Group (n = 88)		t/χ^2	p
	n	%	n	%		
Age (M and SD)	23.57	1.81	23.48	1.74	0.347	.729
Gender					1.344	.511
Male	6	6.3	4	4.5		
Female	89	93.7	84	95.5		
Interpersonal relationship					0.977	.613
Good	53	55.8	51	58.0		
Neural	41	43.1	37	42.0		
Poor	1	1.1	0	0.0		
Satisfaction with major					0.101	.951
Satisfactory	47	49.5	45	51.1		
Neutral	41	43.1	36	40.9		
Unsatisfactory	7	7.4	7	8.0		
Academic achievement (average scores)					0.211	.976
90–100	4	4.2	3	3.4		
80–89	47	49.5	46	52.3		
70–79	41	43.1	36	40.9		
< 70	3	3.2	3	3.4		
Preferred learning method					0.292	.464
Lecture	93	97.9	85	96.6		
Other	2	2.1	3	3.4		

competencies after the intervention, with greater comparative improvements achieved by experimental group participants. The experimental group earned significantly higher scores for clinical competence skills, communication competence, critical thinking ability, and self-leadership at posttest than at pretest. By contrast, the control group earned significantly higher posttest scores for clinical competence skills and critical thinking ability only. In comparing the posttest results of the two groups, the experimental group earned significantly higher scores for clinical competence skills, communication competence, and self-leadership than the control group.

The clinical competence skills results in this study are consistent with those of Mennenga's (2013) study of nursing students. One possible explanation is that, although the

participants in neither group experienced clinical situations directly, experimental (TBL) group participants may have gained relatively stronger training in making clinical inferences because of their repeated learning and establishing clear answers through immediate feedback as they progressed through the three stages of preparation, readiness assurance, and application of course concepts.

It must be noted that directly comparing our findings on communication competence with other studies is difficult because of the lack of research on nursing students. Still, our results echo those of Hazel, Heberle, McEwen, and Adams (2013), who examined students of veterinary medicine and zootechny, and those of Baildinova et al. (2013), who examined medical students. Our findings regarding communication

TABLE 2.

Homogeneity Tests of Core Competencies Between the Two Groups: Pretest

Variable	Experimental Group (n = 95)		Control Group (n = 88)		t	p
	M	SD	M	SD		
Clinical competence skills	67.80	9.05	67.60	8.78	0.150	.881
Problem-solving ability	71.35	15.32	71.38	15.39	−0.012	.990
Communication competence	56.20	7.66	56.34	7.31	−0.127	.899
Critical thinking ability	96.18	12.63	95.83	12.91	0.185	.853
Self-leadership	125.83	16.72	125.24	15.73	0.247	.805

TABLE 3.

Differences in Core Competencies Between the Two Groups: Posttest

Variable	Experimental Group (*n* = 95)		Control Group (*n* = 88)		*t*	*p*
	M	*SD*	*M*	*SD*		
Clinical competence skills	75.28	9.26	72.18	7.51	2.478	.014
Problem-solving ability	74.76	20.84	72.53	16.89	0.789	.431
Communication competence	60.62	7.38	57.86	6.24	2.717	.007
Critical thinking ability	101.60	12.28	99.03	10.18	1.532	.127
Self-leadership	132.01	17.10	126.73	14.36	2.254	.025

competence may reflect how TBL centers on interactions via team activities, which facilitate active and open attitudes among students, promote desirable interactions among team members in asserting their opinions and listening to others, and facilitate communication among team members, teams, learners, and the instructor.

In terms of self-leadership, comparing our results with those of other studies is difficult due to the lack of existing studies on this topic. However, considering that self-leadership refers to the exertion of one's influence over the self to improve self-direction and self-motivation and that self-leadership is formed through experience of autonomy and may be improved through learning and education (Stewart, Courtright, & Manz, 2011), it may be that the self-leadership scores were improved through the active learning process that is inherent to TBL. Specifically, self-leadership may have improved through the active seeking

by participants of knowledge and learning via preclass individual study and active participation in team activities.

Conversely, although problem-solving ability and critical thinking ability improved after the intervention in both groups, the posttest differences between the two groups were not significant. Notably, in a study by Oh (2015), when nursing students were given 6 hours (3 hours per session for 2 weeks) of TBL, their problem-solving ability was significantly greater than that of their peers who had received lecture-style classes. However, the score for critical thinking ability was not significantly higher in the experimental group in this study. This is similar to the findings of Oh but different from that of Kim and Hong (2015), who taught a TBL curriculum to nursing students for 2 hours per week for 6 weeks (total = 12 hours) and found improvements in both problem-solving and critical thinking abilities. Although substantial comparison of this study's results with

TABLE 4.

Pretest–Posttest Changes in Core Competencies for Each of the Two Groups

Variable	Intervention				*t*	*p*
	Before		After			
	M	*SD*	*M*	*SD*		
Clinical competence skills						
Experimental group	67.80	9.05	75.28	9.26	7.963	<.001
Control group	67.60	8.78	72.18	7.51	5.259	<.001
Problem-solving ability						
Experimental group	71.35	15.32	74.76	20.84	1.817	.072
Control group	71.38	15.39	72.53	16.89	0.668	.506
Communication competence						
Experimental group	56.20	7.66	60.62	7.38	5.728	<.001
Control group	56.34	7.31	57.86	6.24	2.098	.039
Critical thinking ability						
Experimental group	96.18	12.63	101.60	12.28	4.241	<.001
Control group	95.83	12.91	99.03	10.18	2.582	.011
Self-leadership						
Experimental group	125.83	16.72	132.01	17.10	3.562	.001
Control group	125.24	15.73	126.73	14.36	0.928	.356

Note. Experimental group (*n* = 95); Control group (*n* = 88).

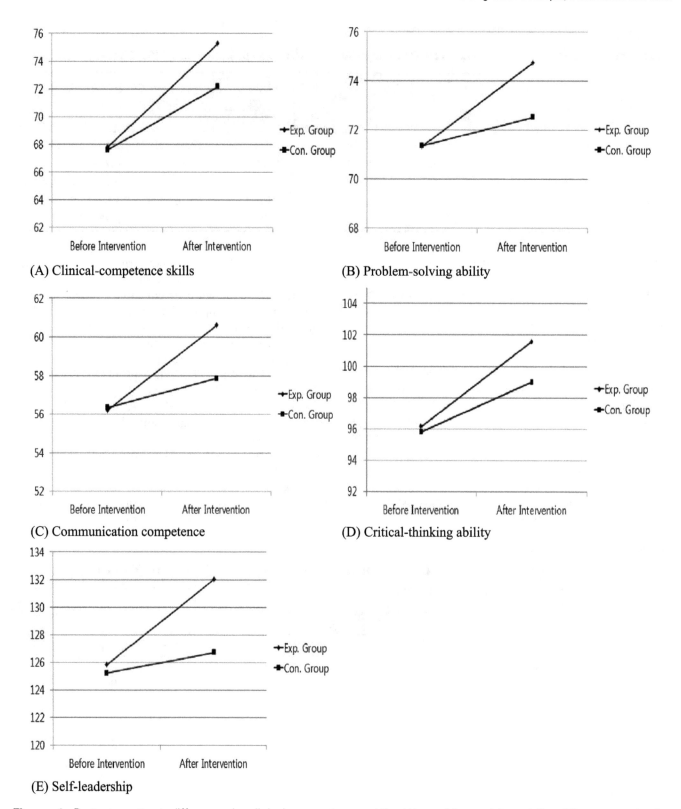

Figure 1. Pretest–posttest difference in clinical competence skills (A), problem-solving ability (B), communication competence (C), critical thinking ability (D), and self-leadership (E) for the two groups. Exp. Group = experimental group; Con. Group = control group.

other studies is not possible (due to the lack of equivalent prior studies on this issue), intervention duration of this study was too short to improve problem-solving or critical thinking ability when considering the studies of Kim and Hong (2015), and Oh (2015). Accordingly, because of inadequate research on optimal TBL duration, this issue should be studied in the future.

In summary, this study found TBL to be more effective than lecture-style classes in terms of strengthening the core competencies of nursing students. Compared with the typical lecture-based classes, where knowledge is delivered to students by instructors unilaterally, TBL curricula effectively develop the core competencies that are required of nursing students before graduation (Choi, 2016; Lee et al., 2012) such as self-leadership and clinical competence skills, problem-solving ability, and critical thinking ability by integrating and applying their knowledge that is based on course materials that they have studied in advance. In addition, TBL enhances communication competence via interactions among team members (Haidet et al., 2012; Parmelee & Michaelsen, 2010). Furthermore, previous studies targeting nursing students have shown TBL to be an effective teaching–learning method in nursing education, as it enhances the academic achievement and satisfaction of nursing students (Roh et al., 2012), improves class satisfaction (Clark et al., 2008; Oh, 2015), and elicits positive learning attitudes from students (Cheng et al., 2014; Han, 2013) while also reinforcing self-directed learning (Kim & Hong, 2015).

However, the foremost significance of TBL is that a single instructor is able to lead a number of students in a single, team-based class within the lecture-based classroom environments that still prevail in the field of nursing education. Thus, TBL is a method that enables nursing students to master the required core competencies effectively before graduating while maintaining the current quality of education and consistency in evaluation without requiring additional facilities or human resources (Lee et al., 2012).

Nevertheless, TBL has not yet been widely adopted in current nursing education. One possible reason is that TBL is affected by certain negative perceptions, as it requires instructors to develop IRAT/GRAT questions and teaching scenarios and imposes additional academic burdens on students due to self-directed learning and active participation requirements. Therefore, for TBL to be more actively adopted in nursing education, instructors will require a suitable curriculum and sufficient time to prepare the management of TBL sessions and students should be provided with sufficient information on the TBL processes in addition to learning content. Furthermore, students will need sufficient time to conduct self-directed learning in advance using preclass assignments or regular class sessions. To success fully adopt TBL, it will be necessary to take the abovementioned preparatory steps to reduce the related burdens to instructors and students.

The limitations of this study include the short duration of the intervention period and the inclusion of nursing students from only one university. Nevertheless, the significance of this study lies in its finding that TBL is an effective strategy for teaching core competencies in nursing education.

Conclusion and Suggestions

This study investigated the effect of TBL on the core competencies that nursing students must master as a prerequisite for graduation by comparing the results of a TBL course and a traditional lecture-style course in terms of the clinical competence skills, problem-solving ability, communication competence, critical thinking ability, and self-leadership of participants.

Pretest differences in these core competencies were not significant between TBL and lecture-style courses. After the intervention, the participants in the TBL group earned significantly higher scores for clinical competence skills, communication competence, and self-leadership than their lecture-group peers. Degree of improvement in each core competencies was greater in the TBL group than the lecture group. Furthermore, the TBL group had significantly larger increases in posttest scores for each of the core competencies than the lecture group.

Therefore, TBL is recommended as an effective method of teaching core competencies to nursing students. More research is needed to identify the optimal length of related TBL programs.

References

Baildinova, K., Zhunusova, A., Kuanysheva, A., Maukayeva, S., Kozhanova, S., Zhanaspayev, M., ... Orazalina, A. (2013). Analysis of efficiency of team based learning (TBL) technology. *European Scientific Journal, 9*(10), 296–298.

Branson, S., Boss, L., & Fowler, D. L. (2016). Team-based learning: Application in undergraduate baccalaureate nursing education. *Journal of Nursing Education and Practice, 6*(4), 59–64. doi:10.5430/jnep.v6n4p59

Cheng, C. Y., Liou, S. R., Tsai, H. M., & Chang, C. H. (2014). The effects of team-based learning on learning behaviors in the maternal–child nursing course. *Nurse Education Today, 34*(1), 25–30. doi:10.1016/j.nedt.2013.03.013

Choi, E. H. (2016). Nursing competency and debriefing evaluation according to satisfaction in simulation practice. *International Journal of Bio-Science and Bio-Technology, 8*(2), 333–340. doi:10.14257/ijbsbt.2016.8.2.31

Clark, M. C., Nguyen, H. T., Bray, C., & Levine, R. E. (2008). Team-based learning in an undergraduate nursing course. *Journal of Nursing Education, 47*(3), 111–117. doi:10.3928/01484834-20080301-02

Haidet, P., Levine, R. E., Parmeless, D. X., Crow, S., Kennedy, F., Kelly, P. A., ... Richards, B. F. (2012). Perspective: Guidelines for reporting team-based learning activities in the medical and health sciences education literature. *Academic Medicine, 87*(3), 292–299. doi:10.1097/ACM.0b013e318244759e

Han, S. J. (2013). The impact of TBL (team-based learning) on nursing students. *Journal of Convergence, 11*(11), 595–602. doi:10.14400/JDPM.2013.11.11.595 (Original work published in Korean)

Hazel, S. J., Heberle, N., McEwen, M.-M., & Adams, K. (2013). Team-based learning increases active engagement and enhances development of teamwork and communication skills in a first-year course for veterinary and animal science undergraduates. *Journal of Veterinary Medical Education, 40*(4), 333–341. doi:10.3138/jvme.0213-034R1

Houghton, J. D., & Neck, C. P. (2002). The revised self-leadership questionnaire: Testing a hierarchical factor structure for self-leadership. *Journal of Managerial Psychology, 17*(8), 672–691. doi:10.1108/02683940210450484

Hur, K. H. (2003). Construction and validation of a global interpersonal communication competence scale. *Korean Journal of Journalism & Communication Studies, 47*(6), 380–408. (Original work published in Korean)

Kim, E. H., & Hong, S. J. (2015). The effects of team-based learning on core competencies in undergraduate nursing students. *Advanced Science and Technology Letters, 115*, 73–78. doi:10.14257/astl.2015.115.15

Ko, J. K., Chung, M. S., Choe, M. A., Park, Y. I., Bang, K. S., Kim, J. A., … Jang, H. Y. (2013). Modeling of nursing competencies for competency-based curriculum development. *The Journal of Korean Academic Society of Nursing Education, 19*(1), 87–96. doi:10.5977/jkasne.2013.19.1.87 (Original work published in Korean)

Korean Accreditation Board of Nursing Education. (2012). *Nursing core competencies.* Retrieved from http://kabone.or.kr/HyAdmin/view.php?&ss[sc]=1&ss[kw]=????&bbs_id=kab01&page=&doc_num=307 (Original work published in Korean)

Lee, S. K., Park, S. N., & Jeong, S. H. (2012). Nursing core competencies needed in the fields of nursing practice for graduates in nursing. *Journal of Korean Academy of Nursing Administration, 18*(4), 460–473. doi:10.11111/jkana.2012.18.4.460 (Original work published in Korean)

Mennenga, H. A. (2013). Student engagement and examination performance in a team-based learning course. *The Journal of Nursing Education, 52*(8), 475–479. doi:10.3928/01484834-20130718-04

Mennenga, H. A., & Smyer, T. (2010). A model for easily incorporating team-based learning into nursing education. *International Journal of Nursing Education Scholarship, 7*, Article 4. doi:10.2202/1548-923X.1924

Michaelsen, L., Parmelee, D., McMahon, K. K., & Levine, R. E. (Eds.). (2008). *Team-based learning for health professions education: A guide to using small groups for improving learning.* Sterling, VA: Stylus.

Michaelsen, L. K., & Sweet, M. (2011). Team-based learning. *New Directions for Teaching and Learning, 128*, 41–51. doi:10.1002/tl.467

Oh, H. S. (2015). The effects of team-based learning on outcome based nursing education. *Journal of Digital Convergence, 13*(9), 409–418. doi:10.14400/jdc.2015.13.9.409 (Original work published in Korean)

Park, J. H., & Woo, O. K. (1999). The effects of problem-based learning on problem solving process by learner's metacognitive level. *Journal of Educational Technology, 15*(3), 55–81. (Original work published in Korean)

Parmelee, D. X., & Michaelsen, L. K. (2010). Twelve tips for doing effective team-based learning (TBL). *Medical Teacher, 32*(2), 118–122. doi:10.3109/01421590903548562

Roh, Y. S., Ryoo, E. N., Choi, D. W., Baek, S. S., & Kim, S. S. (2012). A survey of student perceptions, academic achievement, and satisfaction of team-based learning in a nursing course. *The Journal of Korean Academic Society of Nursing Education, 18*(2), 239–247. doi:10.5977/jkasne.2012.18.2.239

Rubin, R. B. (1990). Communication competence. In G. Phillips & J. Wood (Eds.), *Speech communication: Essays to commemorate the 75th anniversary of the speech communication association* (pp. 94–129). Carbondale, IL: Southern Illinois University Press.

Shin, Y. K., Kim, M. S., & Han, Y. S. (2009). A study on the validation of the Korean version of the revised self-leadership questionnaire (RSLQ) for Korean college students. *The Korean Journal of School Psychology, 6*(3), 377–393. doi:10.16983/kjsp.2009.6.3.377 (Original work published in Korean)

Stewart, G. L., Courtright, S. H., & Manz, C. C. (2011). Self-leadership: A multilevel review. *Journal of Management, 37*(1), 185–222. doi:10.1177/0149206310383911

Vermette, P., & Foote, C. (2001). Constructivist philosophy and cooperative learning practice: Toward integration and reconciliation in secondary classrooms. *American Secondary Education, 30*(1), 26–37.

Yang, J. J., & Park, M. Y. (2004). The relationship of clinical competency and self-directed learning in nursing students. *The Journal of Korean Academic Society of Nursing Education, 10*(2), 271–277. (Original work published in Korean)

Yoon, J. (2004). *Development of an instrument for the measurement of critical thinking disposition: In nursing* (Unpublished doctoral dissertation). The Catholic University, Korea. (Original work published in Korean)

Zgheib, N. K., Simaan, J. A., & Sabra, R. (2010). Using team based learning to teach pharmacology to second year medical students improves student performance. *Medical Teacher, 32*(2), 130–135. doi:10.3109/01421590903548521

19

Determinants of Workplace Bullying Types and their Relationship with Depression Among Female Nurses

Ying-Ying KO[1] • Yi LIU[2] • Chi-Jane WANG[3] • Hsiu-Yun LIAO[4] • Yu-Mei LIAO[5] • Hsing-Mei CHEN[3]*

ABSTRACT

Background: Workplace bullying is commonly experienced by nurses worldwide.

Purpose: This study was conducted to examine the determinants of different types of workplace bullying and their relationship to depression in female nurses.

Methods: A cross-sectional correlational study was employed, and 484 female nurses from a large medical center in southern Taiwan completed the questionnaire. Data were analyzed using logistic regression analysis.

Results: Being unmarried and working in medical/surgical units were found to be the major determinants of work-related bullying, whereas being unmarried was found to be the single determinant of person-related and physical-intimidation bullying. Moreover, work-related and person-related bullying were both found to be significant determinants of depression.

Conclusions/Implications for Practice: Nursing administrators should establish workplace-bullying prevention and management strategies by setting reasonable and equal workloads for nurses, assigning tasks equitably, and building depression-related support and consultation groups.

KEY WORDS:
workplace bullying, depression, marital status, nurse.

Introduction

Workplace bullying (WB) refers to repeated and continuous verbal insults or hurtful behaviors by one or more coworkers at least once per week for at least 6 months (Einarsen, Hotel, Zapf, & Cooper, 2011). WB encompasses a wide range of negative acts, including work-related, person-related, and physical intimidation behaviors (Einarsen, Hotel, & Notelaers, 2009). Work-related bullying includes assigning too many, too few, or too simple tasks as well as criticizing an individual's work persistently. Person-related bullying includes slander, social isolation, and gossiping about an individual. Physical-intimidation bullying includes physical violence or the threat of physical violence. WB is common in nursing, with a prevalence ranging from 27.3% to 86.5% across various countries (Etienne, 2014; Rayan, Sisan, & Baker, 2019; Tsai, Han, Chen, & Chou, 2014; Wilson, 2016).

Nurse administrators are aware of WB, and researchers have conducted studies to examine related issues. However, WB remains chronically prevalent in nursing practice (Rutherford, Gillespie, & Smith, 2018). One reason for this may be the multifactorial nature of the causes of WB. Several factors have been shown to be associated with WB, including economic conditions, workload, lack of interpersonal skills, lack of management skills, the hierarchical nature of the nursing field, and nurses not feeling empowered (Wilson, 2016). However, the causes and consequences of WB vary among the several different types of WB behaviors (Wright & Khatri, 2015). Wright and Khatri have argued that work-related bullying may be a product of staffing shortages, workplace design, policies, and/or organizational structures. Moreover, they suggested that person-related bullying is negatively associated with age and that physical-intimidation bullying is positively associated with age. In terms of the consequences of WB, person-related bullying has been significantly correlated with psychological/behavioral responses and medical errors, whereas work-related bullying has been associated only with psychological/behavioral responses. However, physical-intimidation bullying has not been shown to have a significant relationship with either of these outcomes (Wright & Khatri, 2015).

Previous studies have found that women face a higher risk of experiencing WB than men (Ling, Young, Shepherd, Mak, & Saw, 2016; Workplace Bullying Institute, 2017) and that WB occurs at similar frequencies in male-dominated and female-dominated workplaces (Chatziioannidis, Bascialla, Chatzivalsama, Vouzas, & Mitsiakos, 2018). Nurses are viewed as an oppressed group in the healthcare field. As the large

[1]MSN, RN, NP, Department of Nursing, Kaohsiung Medical University Hospital, Kaohsiung Medical University, Taiwan, ROC • [2]PhD, RN, Associate Professor, School of Nursing, Kaohsiung Medical University, Taiwan, ROC • [3]PhD, RN, Associate Professor, Department of Nursing, College of Medicine, National Cheng Kung University, Taiwan, ROC • [4]MSN, RN, Teaching Assistant, School of Nursing, Kaohsiung Medical University, Taiwan, ROC • [5]MSN, RN, Supervisor, Department of Nursing, Kaohsiung Medical University Hospital, Kaohsiung Medical University, Taiwan, ROC.

majority of nurses are female, WB has generally been reported more often by nurses than by other healthcare professionals (Evans, 2017). However, female nurses may view bullying behaviors as normal and allow these behaviors to continue (Szutenbach, 2013). Although many studies have examined WB among nurses, few have focused on female nurses only.

Depression is characterized by symptoms of low mood such as sadness, loss of interest or pleasure, and feelings of worthlessness (Bianchi, Schonfeld, & Laurent, 2015). Research studies have found that up to 50% of nurses experience depressed moods (Chuang & Yang, 2011; Letvak, Ruhm, & McCoy, 2012). Depression is commonly viewed as a consequence of WB (Fang et al., 2018; Kivimäki et al., 2003; Yildirim, 2009). However, a large-scale study did not find that exposure to bullying behavior at baseline predicted depression 1 year later (Reknes et al., 2014). It is possible that different types of bullying behavior tend to result in different levels of depression severity. Additional research studies are needed to determine the relationship between depression and types of WB.

In Taiwan, most nurses are female as well as tend to be young and unmarried (Lee, Yen, Fetzer, & Chien, 2015), which may be important predictors of WB. However, previous studies have not focused on bullying in relation to depression in female nurses. This study aimed to examine the determinants of WB types and their relationship with depression among female nurses. The hypothesis of this study is that demographics and work-related factors are correlated with WB variables in female nurses. However, different WB-related variables may result in different levels of depression severity.

Methods

Design

A cross-sectional, correlational research design was employed. Data were collected from November 2012 to May 2013.

Setting and Sample

A convenience sample of nurses was recruited from a large medical center and two of its affiliated hospitals in southern Taiwan. The inclusion criteria were female nurses who were 20 years old or older and who had worked as a nurse for at least 6 months. Two questions about having had a diagnosis of major depression/mental illness and the time of the most recent diagnosis were used to exclude nurses who were diagnosed with major depression or other mental illness before entering the nursing profession.

G-Power software (Faul, Erdfelder, Buchner, & Lang, 2009) was used to calculate the sample size needed for a multiple linear regression analysis with an α of .05, a power of .80, a small effect size of .05, and 12 variables. A sample size of 358 participants was recommended. Considering the sensitive nature of the WB issue, we expected to encounter a low response rate and to have an invalid questionnaire rate of up to 60%. Thus, 513 questionnaires were distributed, with 509 questionnaires returned and 23 questionnaires excluded

because of missing data, resulting in a return rate of 99.2%. Two participants were excluded because of a diagnosis of major depression before entering the nursing profession. A post hoc power analysis of a logistic regression analysis with an α of .05 yielded an odds ratio of 1.89 of marital status for WB (H0 = .277 and X parm μ of .66) and an odds ratio of 1.91 of WB for depression (H0 = .298 and X parm μ of 1.81, with a σ of 0.76). A sample size of 484 yielded a power of .87–.99.

Instruments

Demographic and work-related data

The demographic data included age, gender, marital status (yes/no), and education ("junior college" or "bachelor's degree or above"). Work-related data included years worked as a nurse, job title (registered nurse or not), working unit (medical/surgical, critical/emergent care unit, other), and shift assignment (fixed/rotating).

Negative Acts Questionnaire–Revised

WB was measured using the Negative Acts Questionnaire–Revised (NAQ-R) developed by Einarsen and Raknes (1997). The NAQ-R includes 22 items covering three types of bullying: work-related (seven items), person-related (12 items), and physical intimidation (three items). Each question is scored from 1 to 5 (never, sometimes, every month, every week, and every day for the past 6 months; Einarsen et al., 2009). The total possible score for the NAQ-R ranges from 22 to 110, with a higher score indicating that the individual has been the target of more severe WB during the most recent 6-month period. To conduct comparisons between WB types, the total score for each type was converted to a 1- to 5-point score by summing the scores of the items for that type and then dividing by the number of type items. In a previous study of 511 nurses, the Cronbach's α for the English version was .88 (Simons, 2008).

The NAQ-R was translated into Mandarin Chinese for this study. The translation was guided by knowledge about cultural equivalences between the original and translated versions (Flaherty et al., 1988). The English version was first forward-translated into Mandarin Chinese by the principal investigator. A nurse who was familiar with both English and Taiwanese cultures was invited to review the translated version. The research team then held a consensus meeting to confirm the translated version. Then, a Taiwanese-American doctoral student who was not familiar with the NAQ-R was asked to back-translate the questionnaire into English. To finalize the Chinese version, the original developer, Dr. Einarsen, was invited to examine the difference between the original and translated versions. Regarding the internal consistency reliability, Cronbach's α was .95 for the overall scale and .77, .68, and .88 for the three WB types (work-related, person-related, and physical intimidation), respectively.

Taiwanese Depression Questionnaire

Depression was measured using the Taiwanese Depression Questionnaire (TDQ; Lee, Yang, Lai, Chiu, & Chau, 2000).

The 18-item self-report questionnaire includes three domains: cognitive, emotional, and physical. Participants were asked to answer questions about their depressive symptoms over the past 6 months using a 4-point Likert scale (0 = *never or rarely* to 3 = *usually*). The total possible score ranges from 0 to 54, with a total score of 19 or more indicating the presence of clinically significant depressive symptoms (John Tung Foundation, 2004). The TDQ has been validated using the Chinese version of the Center for Epidemiologic Studies Depression Scale and has shown a high correlation coefficient of .92 (Lee et al., 2000). The Cronbach's α for this study was .94.

Data Collection and Ethical Considerations

Approval to conduct this study was obtained from the institutional review board of the affiliated facilities (KMUH-IRB-20120179). The primary researcher, an intensive care unit nurse, contacted each head nurse of the ward of the three hospitals and made appointments to discuss the study during the staff meetings. Next, nurses were approached and invited to participate. The primary researcher explained the study protocol and gave the informed consent form to the nurses. Those who consented to participate then received a package that included the questionnaire, the consent form, a return stamped envelope, and a small token of appreciation. The participants were asked to return the questionnaire within 1 week.

Data Analysis

Data were analyzed using SPSS 18.0 for Windows (SPSS, Inc., Chicago, IL, USA). Descriptive statistics were calculated for each variable. A Kolmogorov–Smirnov test showed that the scores on the NAQ-R (Z = 3.81, p = .000) and TDQ (Z = 1.97, p = .001) were not normally distributed, even after data transformation. Therefore, a nonparametric analytical method applied via a logistic regression analysis was used to examine the major factors associated with the three types of bullying and the relationship between these factors and depression. The goodness of fit for the model was assessed using the Hosmer–Lemeshow test.

Results

Demographic and Work-Related Data

The mean age of the sample of nurses was 31.1 (SD = 6.5) years, ranging from 21 to 53 years. The mean number of years having worked as a nurse was 8.9 (SD = 6.9). As shown in Table 1, most of the participants were unmarried at the time of the study (66.1%), had a bachelor's degree or above (90.5%), were registered nurses (89.9%), worked in the medical/surgical ward (59.9%), and worked rotating shifts (72.1%).

Workplace Bullying

The mean total score on the NAQ-R was 34.5 (SD = 13.3), with 27.7% (n = 134) of the participants meeting the

TABLE 1.
Demographic Variables

Variable	M	SD
Age (years)	31.1	6.5
Years employed as a nurse	8.9	6.9
	n	%
Marital status		
Married	164	33.9
Single	320	66.1
Education		
Junior college	46	9.5
Bachelor's degree or above	438	90.5
Job title		
Registered nurse	435	89.9
Other (nurse practitioner, head nurse)	49	10.1
Working unit		
Medical/surgical ward	290	59.9
Critical and emergent care unit	150	31.0
Other (pediatrics, hemodialysis, etc.)	44	9.1
Shift assignment		
Fixed	135	27.9
Rotating	349	72.1

definition of experiencing WB at least once per week for a period of 6 months (Table 2). Regarding the 22 NAQ-R items, 79 participants (16.3%) reported that they encountered one or more of these items on a daily basis, whereas 98 (20.2%) experienced one or more of these items on a weekly basis. Twenty-two nurses reported never having experienced bullying behaviors. Across the three types, work-related bullying scored the highest, and physical-intimidation bullying scored the lowest. The three bullying behaviors with the highest scores were "Having your opinions and views ignored" (2.0 ± 1.0), "Being exposed to an unmanageable workload" (1.9 ± 1.0), and "Being given tasks with unreasonable or impossible targets or deadlines" (1.9 ± 1.0).

TABLE 2.
WB (NAQ-R) and Depression (TDS) Scores (N = 484)

Variable	M	SD
NAQ-R (total score)	34.52	13.30
Work-related WB	1.81	0.76
Person-related WB	1.48	0.62
Physical-intimidation WB	1.39	0.66
TDS	14.09	10.48
Yes (TDS ≥ 19; n and %)	144	29.8
No (TDS < 19; n and %)	340	70.2

Note. WB = workplace bullying; NAQ-R = Negative Acts Questionnaire–Revised; TDS = Taiwanese Depression Scale.

Depression

The mean overall depression score was 14.1 (*SD* = 10.5). One hundred forty-four (29.8%) nurses revealed clinically significant symptoms of depression (John Tung Foundation, 2004). The three most commonly reported symptoms were "I feel very annoyed" (1.3 ± 0.9), "I feel that my memory is not good" (1.2 ± 0.9), and "My body feels tired, weak, and lacking in energy" (1.2 ± 1.0).

Determinants of Workplace Bullying

The logistic regression analysis (Table 3) showed that the major determinants of work-related bullying were being single (OR = 1.89, 95% CI [1.08, 3.33]) and working in a medical/surgical unit (Wald statistic = 6.08, *p* = .48). Being single was the only determinant of person-related bullying (OR = 3.51, 95% CI [1.57, 7.89]) and of physical-intimidation bullying (OR = 15.52, 95% CI [2.00, 120.69]).

Workplace Bullying and Depression

As expected, depression was significantly associated with work-related bullying (OR = 1.91, 95% CI [1.14, 3.20]) and person-related bullying (OR = 3.89, 95% CI [1.99, 7.61]). However, physical-intimidation bullying (OR = 1.23, 95% CI [0.50, 3.03]) was not associated with depression among the participants in this study (Table 4).

Discussion

This study found that being single and working in a medical/surgical nursing unit were the major determinants of nurses experiencing work-related bullying. Furthermore, being single was the only determinant of nurses experiencing person-related

TABLE 4.

Association Between Workplace Bullying Domains and Depression

Domain	B	SE	Wald	p	Odds Ratio	95% CI
Work related	0.65	0.26	5.97	.015	1.91	[1.14, 3.20]
Person related	1.36	0.34	15.71	.000	3.89	[1.99, 7.61]
Physical intimidation	0.21	0.46	0.21	.648	1.23	[0.50, 3.03]

Note. Hosmer–Lemeshow test for model fit: χ^2 = 0.63, *p* = .429.

and physical-intimidation bullying. Work-related and person-related bullying were identified as significant determinants of depression in nurses, whereas physical-intimidation bullying was not.

Approximately 27.7% of the participants had experienced one or more of the NAQ-R items (bullying behaviors) over the previous 6-month period. Of the three domains, work-related bullying had the highest score, followed by person-related bullying. These results are different from the findings of Wright and Khatri (2015); Obeidat, Qan'ir, and Turaani (2018); and Lin, Hsiao, Lin, Yang, and Chung (2018), which all found person-related bullying to be the most common type of bullying in Columbia, Jordan, and Taiwan, respectively. However, the findings of this study are similar to those of another study conducted in Taiwan with 708 nurses (Tsai et al., 2014). This may indicate that the context of WB may differ among different cultures and settings. In the nursing profession, it remains common for nurses to work extended hours, complain of heavy workloads

TABLE 3.

Logistic Regression Analysis for the Three Domains of Workplace Bullying

Predictive Variable	Work Related		Personal Related		Physical Intimidation	
	Odds Ratio	95% CI	Odds Ratio	95% CI	Odds Ratio	95% CI
Age	1.00	[0.91, 1.09]	0.95	[0.84, 1.06]	1.12	[0.97, 1.30]
Years worked as a nurse	1.00	[0.92, 1.10]	1.05	[0.94, 1.18]	0.91	[0.78, 1.06]
Marital status (yes[a]/no)	1.89*	[1.08, 3.33]	3.51**	[1.57, 7.89]	15.52*	[2.00, 120.69]
Education						
Junior college[a]/bachelor's or above	0.62	[0.30, 1.31]	1.35	[0.45, 4.07]	2.20	[0.28, 17.41]
Job title						
Registered nurse (no[a]/yes)	0.52	[0.22, 1.20]	0.66	[0.19, 2.33]	0.42	[0.43, 4.17]
Working unit	Wald = 6.08*					
Medical/surgical ward[a]						
Critical/emergent unit	0.60	[0.36, 1.02]	0.77	[0.41, 1.45]	0.91	[0.39, 2.13]
Others	0.40	[0.15, 1.06]	0.73	[0.24, 2.20]	0.39	[0.05, 3.10]
Shift (fixed[a]/rotating)	0.83	[0.46, 1.49]	0.84	[0.41, 1.70]	0.92	[0.34, 2.48]

Note. Hosmer–Lemeshow test for model fit: work-related (χ^2 = 13.31, *p* = .102), personal-related (χ^2 = 5.51, *p* = .702), and physical intimidation (χ^2 = 9.96, *p* = .268).
[a]Referent group.
*p < .05. **p < .01.

with unequal pay, experience conflicts with medical team members, and feel disrespected or unappreciated (Ke, Wang, & Hsu, 2016). These feelings may lead to experiences or perceptions of work-related bullying (Kao, 2011).

The participants in this study who were unmarried were more likely to experience all types of WB. No other studies have been found that support this finding. However, Tai et al. (2014) found that unmarried nurses reported less family support than married nurses. Another study on flight attendants found that greater social support was associated with less WB (Tian, 2009). Therefore, social support may be a factor that helps nurses mitigate WB. Notably, it seems that the occurrence of WB is relatively low in countries with strong gender equality protections and values prevailing (Mikkelsen & Einarsen, 2001). In Taiwan, many nurses leave their jobs after marriage because of the full-time work requirements and the nature of shift work. Thus, it is common to allow married nurses to take fewer night shifts and to be assigned less paperwork in consideration of their childcare responsibilities. As a result, unmarried nurses may work more night shifts, serve as support personnel for urgent or emergent events, and perform more non-patient-care activities (Wang, Huang, Lu, & Ho, 2007) and thus feel less supported and subsequently more bullied. These findings suggest that nurses should be fairly and properly rewarded based on job performance rather than on non-work-related standards such as marital status.

Working in medical/surgical units was shown in this study to be a primary determinant of work-related WB, echoing Vessey, Demarco, Gaffney, and Budin's (2009) study on 303 nurses. One study found that nurses who worked in medical/surgical units reported greater job stress, fatigue, and intention to leave than those in other units (Tsai et al., 2014). Medical/surgical units are typically very busy for nurses because of the high patient-to-nurse ratio and the greater severity of illnesses and injuries treated. As a result, WB may be higher in these units, which may in turn endanger patient care quality and patient safety (Lin et al., 2018). Therefore, it is imperative to regularly review and adjust related human resource allocation mechanisms as well as the manpower for the units with higher levels of patient illness severity and acuity.

Depression was prevalent (29.8%) among the participants in this study and was found to be significantly associated with work-related and person-related bullying. This finding is consistent with previous studies showing an association between WB and psychological problems (Bardakçı & Günüşen, 2016; Wright & Khatri, 2015). Moreover, Wright and Khatri's study found only work-related and person-related bullying (not physical-intimidation bullying) to be correlated with psychological responses such as depression, indicating that different mechanisms may exist for different types of WB and depression.

Person-related bullying was associated in this study with the highest risk of depression, although work-related bullying had the highest score of the three types of WB. This

indicates that person-related bullying behaviors such as spreading gossip and rumors, being the target of practical jokes, and being ignored or excluded, all of which are instigated primarily by peers, have the strongest impact on depression (Wright & Khatri, 2015). Bullying experiences often lead to perseverative and intrusive thoughts and cause psychological distress in victims (Verkuil, Atasayi, & Molendijk, 2015). This finding supports that nurse administrators should work to create a professional, trusting, and supportive work environment by encouraging nurses to respect each other, practice good communication behaviors, and bring interpersonal conflicts into the open and address them promptly (Wilson, 2016). Counseling sessions are needed to help victims learn to be assertive in bullying events (Becher & Visovsky, 2012). Colleague support and personal skills to build resilience and hope may help deter person-related bullying and the development of depression (Wilson, 2016).

It is possible that, because nurses are usually taught to be responsible and to follow orders, their superiors, with the support of the administration, may practice work-related bullying in terms of assigning unmanageable workloads or requiring compliance with unreasonable deadlines. Therefore, it is important for empowered administrators to review manpower, workplace design, policies, and organizational structures to determine whether these factors promote bullying. Nurses should be educated to recognize an optimal workload as well as work-related bullying. In addition, bullying behaviors that are perceived by the nurse should be openly discussed at staff meetings (Wright & Khatri, 2015).

Study Limitations

The study was affected by several limitations. First, it included only nurses from one large medical center and two affiliated hospitals in southern Taiwan who had at least 6 months of work experience in nursing. Thus, the sample may not be representative of the entire population of nurses. The use of a self-report questionnaire may have led responses to be affected by recall bias. The study used a cross-sectional design, and as a result, conclusions cannot be drawn regarding the causal relationships between the associated variables. Finally, the incidence and severity of WB may have been underestimated in this study because of the sensitive nature of this issue, which may encourage underreporting or avoidance of discussion.

Conclusions

In this study, work-related and person-related bullying were associated with depression, whereas physical-intimidation bullying was not associated with depression, suggesting that exposure to certain WB behaviors may not significantly increase depression risk. Other outcome measures should be considered in the future to better understand the effect of physical-intimidation bullying.

Overall, the findings suggest that nursing educators and administrators should aggressively develop WB prevention and management strategies such as a WB reporting system and regular seminars that address bullying-related topics such as communication skills, conflict resolution, obtaining peer support, and consultation channels. WB should be handled in a timely manner to ensure protection and confidentiality. The development of written policies for zero tolerance of WB at the organizational level should be accelerated to provide a safe working environment for nurses. Finally, establishment of a legal system at the national level is needed to protect against bullying.

To prevent and reduce depression, psychological advisory departments should be established that randomly assess the emotional state of nurses to ensure the early detection of depression. WB should be managed based on the level of severity perceived by nurses rather than on the prevalence and frequency of bullying behaviors (Ma, Wang, & Chien, 2017). It is necessary to help nurses learn how to manage difficult people and situations by practicing constructive coping strategies, learning assertiveness techniques, and developing personal resources and support.

Acknowledgments

This study was funded by the Kaohsiung Medical University Hospital, Kaohsiung Medical University (Grant number KUMH101-M180).

Author Contributions

Study conception and design: YYK, HMC
Data collection: YYK, HYL, YML, HMC
Data analysis and interpretation: YYK, YL, CJW, HMC
Drafting of the article: YYK, YL, CJW, HMC
Critical revision of the article: YYK, HMC

References

Bardakçı, E., & Günüşen, N. P. (2016). Influence of workplace bullying on Turkish nurses' psychological distress and nurses' reactions to bullying. *Journal of Transcultural Nursing, 27*(2), 166–171. https://doi.org/10.1177/1043659614549073

Becher, J., & Visovsky, C. (2012). Horizontal violence in nursing. *Medsurg Nursing, 21*(4), 210–213.

Bianchi, R., Schonfeld, I. S., & Laurent, E. (2015). Burnout-depression overlap: A review. *Clinical Psychology Review, 36,* 28–41. https://doi.org/10.1016/j.cpr.2015.01.004

Chatziioannidis, I., Bascialla, F. G., Chatzivalsama, P., Vouzas, F., & Mitsiakos, G. (2018). Prevalence, causes and mental health impact of workplace bullying in the neonatal intensive care unit environment. *BMJ Open, 8*(2), e018766–e018766. https://doi.org/10.1136/bmjopen-2017-018766

Chuang, H. H., & Yang, S. F. (2011). An analysis of the relationship between job burnout and organizational commitment among staff nurses: A case study in a regional teaching hospital in Central Taiwan. *Cheng Ching Medical Journal, 7*(2), 51–60. https://doi.org/10.30156/CCMJ.201104.0006 (Original work published in Chinese)

Einarsen, S., Hotel, H., & Notelaers, G. (2009). Measuring exposure to bullying and harassment at work: Validity, factor structure and psychometric properties of the Negative Acts Questionnaire–Revised. *Work & Stress, 23*(1), 24–44. https://doi.org/10.1080/02678370902815673

Einarsen, S., Hotel, H., Zapf, D., & Cooper, C. L. (2011). The concept of bullying at work: The European tradition. In S. Einarsen, H. Hotel, D. Zapf, & C. L. Cooper (Eds.), *Bullying and harassment in the workplace: Development in theory, research, and practice* (2nd ed., pp. 3–39). New York, NY: Taylor & Francis.

Einarsen, S., & Raknes, B. (1997). Harassment in the workplace and the victimization of men. *Violence and Victims, 12*(3), 247–263. https://doi.org/10.1891/0886-6708.12.3.247

Etienne, E. (2014). Exploring workplace bullying in nursing. *Workplace Health and Safety, 62*(1), 6–11. https://doi.org/10.3928/21650799-20131220-02

Evans, D. (2017). Categorizing the magnitude and frequency of exposure to uncivil behaviors: A new approach for more meaningful interventions. *Journal of Nursing Scholarship, 49*(2), 214–222. https://doi.org/10.1111/jnu.12275

Fang, H., Zhao, X., Yang, H., Sun, P., Li, Y., Jiang, K., ... Wu, Q. (2018). Depressive symptoms and workplace-violence-related risk factors among otorhinolaryngology nurses and physicians in northern China: A cross-sectional study. *British Medical Association Journals, 8*(1), e019514. https://doi.org/10.1136/bmjopen-2017-019514

Faul, F., Erdfelder, E., Buchner, A., & Lang, A.-G. (2009). Statistical power analyses using G*Power 3.1: Tests for correlation and regression analyses. *Behavior Research Methods, 41*(4), 1149–1160. https://doi.org/10.3758/BRM.41.4.1149

Flaherty, J. A., Gaviria, F. M., Pathak, D., Mitchell, T., Wintrob, R., Richman, J. A., & Birz, S. (1988). Developing instruments for cross-cultural psychiatric research. *The Journal of Nervous and Mental Disease, 176*(5), 257–263.

John Tung Foundation. (2004). *Taiwanese depression scale.* Retrieved from http://www.jtf.org.tw/overblue/taiwan1/

Kao, C. C. (2011). Multi-aspects of nursing manpower in Taiwan. *Cheng Ching Medical Journal, 7*(3), 41–46. https://doi.org/10.30156/CCMJ.201107.0005 (Original work published in Chinese)

Ke, Y. T., Wang, H. H., & Hsu, S. C. (2016). Improving the issue of nurses' delay of off-duty from work through organizational transformation. *Leadership Nursing, 17*(4), 58–70. (Original work published in Chinese)

Kivimäki, M., Virtanen, M., Vartia, M., Elovainio, M., Vahtera, J., & Keltikangas-Järvinen, L. (2003). Workplace bullying and the risk of cardiovascular disease and depression. *Occupational and Environmental Medicine, 60*(10), 779–783. https://doi.org/10.1136/oem.60.10.779

Lee, H. F., Yen, M., Fetzer, S., & Chien, T. W. (2015). Predictors of burnout among nurses in Taiwan. *Community Mental Health Journal, 51*(6), 733–777. https://doi.org/10.1007/s10597-014-9818-4

Lee, Y., Yang, M. J., Lai, T. J., Chiu, N. M., & Chau, T. T. (2000). Development of the Taiwanese Depression Questionnaire. *Chang Gung Medical Journal, 23*(11), 688–694.

Letvak, S., Ruhm, C. J., & McCoy, T. (2012). Depression in hospital-employed nurses. *Clinical Nurse Specialist, 26*(3), 177–182. https://doi.org/10.1097/NUR.0b013e3182503ef0

Lin, Y. H., Hsiao, S. S., Lin, C. F., Yang, C. Y., & Chung, M. H. (2018). Exploration of the association between workplace bullying and attitudes toward patient safety in female nurses. *The Journal of Nursing, 65*(1), 51–60. https://doi.org/10.6224/JN.201802_65(1).08

Ling, M., Young, C. J., Shepherd, H. L., Mak, C., & Saw, R. P. M. (2016). Workplace bullying in surgery. *World Journal of Surgery, 40*(11), 2560–2566. https://doi.org/10.1007/s00268-016-3642-7

Ma, S. C., Wang, H. H., & Chien, T. W. (2017). Hospital nurses' attitudes, negative perceptions, and negative acts regarding workplace bullying. *Annals of General Psychiatry, 16*, 33. https://doi.org/10.1186/s12991-017-0156-0

Mikkelsen, E. G., & Einarsen, S. (2001). Bulling in Danish work-life: Prevalence and health correlates. *European Journal of Work and Organizational Psychology, 10*(4), 393–413. https://doi.org/10.1080/13594320143000816

Obeidat, R. F., Qan'ir, Y., & Turaani, H. (2018). The relationship between perceived competence and perceived workplace bullying among registered nurses: A cross sectional survey. *International Journal of Nursing Studies, 88*, 71–78. https://doi.org/10.1016/j.ijnurstu.2018.08.012

Rayan, A., Sisan, M., & Baker, O. (2019). Stress, workplace violence, and burnout in nurses working in King Abdullah Medical City during Al-Hajj season. *The Journal of Nursing Research, 27*(3), e26. https://doi.org/10.1097/jnr.0000000000000291

Reknes, I., Pallesen, S., Magerøy, N., Moen, B. E., Bjorvatn, B., & Einarsen, S. (2014). Exposure to bullying behaviors as a predictor of mental health problems among Norwegian nurses: Results from the prospective SUSSH-survey. *International Journal of Nursing Studies, 51*(3), 479–487. https://doi.org/10.1016/j.ijnurstu.2013.06.017

Rutherford, D. E., Gillespie, G. L., & Smith, C. R. (2018). Interventions against bullying of prelicensure students and nursing professionals: An integrative review. *Nursing Forum, 54*(1), 84–90. https://doi.org/10.1111/nuf.12301

Simons, S. (2008). Workplace bullying experienced by Massachusetts registered nurses and the relationship to intention to leave the organization. *Advances in Nursing Science Journal, 31*(2), E48–E59. https://doi.org/10.1097/01.ANS.0000319571.37373.d7

Szutenbach, M. P. (2013). Bullying in nursing: Roots, rationales, and remedies. *Journal of Christian Nursing, 30*(1), 16–23. https://doi.org/10.1097/CNJ.0b013e318276be28

Tai, S. Y., Lin, P. C., Chen, Y. M., Hung, H. C., Pan, C. H., Pan, S. M., ... Wu, M. T. (2014). Effects of marital status and shift work on family function among registered nurses. *Industrial Health, 52*(4), 296–303. https://doi.org/10.2486/indhealth.2014-0009

Tian, C. C. (2009). *A correlational study among workplace bullying and job vigor of cabin crew by using social support as moderating variable* (Unpublished master's thesis). Southern Taiwan University of Technology, Tainan, Taiwan, ROC. (Original work published in Chinese)

Tsai, S. T., Han, C. H., Chen, L. F., & Chou, F. H. (2014). Nursing workplace bullying and turnover intention: An exploration of associated factors at a medical center in southern Taiwan. *The Journal of Nursing, 61*(3), 58–68. https://doi.org/10.6224/JN.61.3.58 (Original work published in Chinese)

Verkuil, B., Atasayi, S., & Molendijk, M. L. (2015). Workplace bullying and mental health: A meta-analysis on cross-sectional and longitudinal data. *PLoS ONE, 10*(8), e0135225. https://doi.org/10.1371/journal.pone.0135225

Vessey, J. A., Demarco, R. F., Gaffney, D. A., & Budin, W. C. (2009). Bullying of staff registered nurses in the workplace: A preliminary study for developing personal and organizational strategies for the transformation of hostile to healthy workplace environments. *Journal of Professional Nursing, 25*(5), 299–306. https://doi.org/10.1016/j.profnurs.2009.01.022

Wang, C. L., Huang, C. Y., Lu, K. Y., & Ho, M. Y. (2007). A study of the social support and job stress among nursing staff. *VGH Nursing Journal, 24*(1), 59–68. https://doi.org/10.6142/VGHN.24.1.59 (Original work published in Chinese)

Wilson, J. L. (2016). An exploration of bullying behaviors in nursing: A review of the literature. *British Journal of Nursing, 25*(6), 303–306. https://doi.org/10.12968/bjon.2016.25.6.303

Workplace Bullying Institute. (2017). *2017 WBI U.S. workplace bullying survey.* Retrieved from https://www.workplacebullying.org/wbiresearch/wbi-2017-survey/

Wright, W., & Khatri, N. (2015). Bullying among nursing staff: Relationship with psychological/behavioral responses of nurses and medical errors. *Health Care Management Review, 40*(2), 139–147. https://doi.org/10.1097/HMR.0000000000000015

Yildirim, D. (2009). Bullying among nurses and its effects. *International Nursing Review, 56*(4), 504–511. https://doi.org/10.1111/j.1466-7657.2009.00745.x

20

Evidence-Based Practice Curriculum Development for Undergraduate Nursing Students: The Preliminary Results of an Action Research Study in Taiwan

Hsiao-Ying HUNG[1] • Yu-Wen WANG[1] • Jui-Ying FENG[2] • Chi-Jane WANG[3] • Esther Ching-Lan LIN[3] • Ying-Ju CHANG[4]*

ABSTRACT

Background: Equipping undergraduate nursing students with sufficient competence in evidence-based practice (EBP) is essential to meeting future practice needs. Integrating necessary EBP knowledge and skills systematically into the formal curriculum allows students to obtain better learning experience and outcomes. However, in Taiwan, a systematic nursing curriculum that integrates EBP concepts across the 4-year nursing baccalaureate program has not yet been developed. Moreover, engaging students in the clinical application of evidence remains a key challenge facing nursing education.

Purpose: This study aimed to construct an EBP undergraduate nursing curriculum and develop clinical scenarios that support EBP teaching.

Methods: Three cycles of action research, incorporating both focus group interviews and questionnaire surveys, were applied to construct and evaluate the appropriateness and feasibility of the EBP nursing curriculum and relevant teaching strategies.

Results: An EBP nursing curriculum was constructed that integrates the three levels of learning objectives and corresponding learning outcomes, teaching content, and learning activities. Scenario activities were developed to familiarize students with the EBP process and to maximize their learning with regard to the clinical application of evidence. Next, a preliminary evaluation showed the appropriateness and feasibility of the developed curriculum, which was shown to foster the EBP competency of students and increase their confidence and positive attitudes toward EBP.

Conclusions/Implications for Practice: A systematic EBP bachelor nursing curriculum with effective pedagogical strategies was developed. The associated process and the elicited information may offer a valuable reference for other nursing schools.

KEY WORDS:
baccalaureate nursing education, curriculum design, evidence-based practice, teaching strategies, undergraduate nursing students.

Introduction

Evidence-based practice (EBP) is valued widely in clinical environments. Implementation of EBP facilitates effective clinical decision making and superior patient outcomes through the integration of the best available evidence, expert opinions, and patient preferences (Melnyk, Fineout-Overholt, Gallagher-Ford, & Kaplan, 2012). Therefore, EBP competency is an essential requirement for healthcare professionals (Tilson et al., 2011).

Developing EBP competency in nurses requires their acquiring competencies in areas such as informatics literacy, research methodology, and statistics to provide a requisite foundation for further learning. Therefore, cultivating EBP competency rarely achieves remarkable results after only a few courses or a short-term continuing education program (Melnyk & Fineout-Overholt, 2014). Nursing scholars have proposed that EBP teaching should be introduced early in undergraduate nursing education and EBP concepts should be integrated throughout the undergraduate nursing curriculum to connect multiple levels of prerequisite knowledge to equip undergraduate nursing students with the EBP competencies necessary to satisfy future practice needs (Melnyk, 2013; Nickerson & Thurkettle, 2013).

In response, a number of EBP curricula have been proposed in Western countries. However, shortcomings in these curricula include the integration of EBP concepts into limited aspects of the nursing curriculum (Bloom, Olinzock, Radjenovic, & Trice, 2013; Finotto, Carpanoni, Turroni, Camellini, & Mecugni, 2013), unresolved uncertainties regarding the

[1]MSN, RN, Doctoral Student, Department of Nursing, College of Medicine, National Cheng Kung University • [2]PhD, RN, Professor, Department of Nursing, College of Medicine, National Cheng Kung University • [3]PhD, RN, Associate Professor, Department of Nursing, College of Medicine, National Cheng Kung University • [4]PhD, RN, Professor, Institution of Allied Health Sciences and Department of Nursing, College of Medicine, National Cheng Kung University, and Director, Department of Nursing, National Cheng Kung University Hospital, College of Medicine, National Cheng Kung University.

applicability/adequacy of these curricula in actual teaching contexts (Rolloff, 2010), and ambiguities regarding how to integrate EBP content into professional nursing courses (Finotto et al., 2013). In addition, these curricula expect that undergraduate students will attain desired competencies in critical appraisal and the synthesis of research evidence by their third year (Bloom et al., 2013; Rolloff, 2010). On the basis of the abovementioned uncertainties and the different cultural contexts, it is uncertain whether these curricula would be appropriate for teaching nursing students in Taiwan.

In Taiwan, EBP is not only strongly emphasized in clinical practice but also valued in nursing academia (Mu, Tsay, & Chang, 2013). However, a national survey revealed that EBP teaching has been primarily conducted either independently or as one or two stand-alone lectures during nursing courses, with the teaching of clinical applications of evidence identified as the major challenge in EBP teaching (Hung, Huang, Tsai, & Chang, 2015). Therefore, developing a curriculum that integrates EBP concepts and teaches students how to apply evidence in clinical practice is an urgent issue in Taiwan.

In addition to selecting the essential EBP knowledge and skills for inclusion in undergraduate nursing curricula, educators must consider effective strategies to enhance the affective domain learning of EBP to foster a positive attitude toward EBP in students (Ryan, 2016). Generally, the steps for EBP, including search for evidence, formulation of answerable questions, and the critical appraisal and integration of available evidence, are considered to be essential EBP knowledge and skills that students must learn and master (Levin & Feldman, 2012). Several studies have shown that, although classroom teaching improves their EBP knowledge and skills, students should also enrich their EBP experience in clinical settings to enhance their attitudes toward EBP and their confidence in implementing EBP (Brown, Kim, Stichler, & Fields, 2010; Zhang, Zeng, Chen, & Li, 2012). However, the creation of a positive EBP learning experience in a clinical setting for students may be challenging. This is because transforming evidence into practice involves multiple complex factors such as the readiness of students and nurses as well as organizational readiness (Coomarasamy & Khan, 2004; Saunders & Vehviläinen-Julkunen, 2016; Solomons & Spross, 2011), which may increase the difficulties in enabling students to experience the implementation of EBP in clinical settings. Simulation-based teaching may offer a solution for surmounting these obstacles to EBP teaching. Simulation-based teaching has been reported as an effective teaching method in nursing education (Cant & Cooper, 2010) in terms of improving critical thinking ability and self-confidence in nurses (Alamrani, Alammar, Alqahtani, & Salem, 2018). In EBP teaching, Meeker, Jones, and Flanagan (2008) found that simulating clinical patient care scenarios enables students with limited clinical experience to practice formulating clinical problems and developing feasible solutions. Therefore, simulated patient care scenarios may be a useful teaching strategy for students to learn EBP skills and practice implementing EBP.

Therefore, the purpose of this study was to construct an EBP curriculum by systematically integrating EBP essential knowledge and skills into a 4-year undergraduate nursing curriculum and developing clinical scenarios to support EBP teaching.

Methods

Design

Action research (AR) has been shown as an effective approach to improve teaching quality and solve curriculum problems, with teachers applying self-reflection to identify problems and develop solutions that improve their education practice (Kemmis, McTaggart, & Nixon, 2014). Accordingly, AR was applied to develop and evaluate the undergraduate EBP nursing curriculum in this study.

AR usually involves an iterative cycle that starts from the identification of initial problems and then works to formulate possible solutions (planning), take appropriate actions (action), and reflect on the process to further plan and guide the iteration process in the next cycle (observation and reflection; Kemmis et al., 2014) to help participants improve their practice. In following this approach, the first cycles of this AR study started by identifying the need to construct a nursing curriculum that integrates EBP concepts. Subsequent iterative cycles proceeded forward based on the reflections of the participants in the prior cycle. Three iterative AR cycles were conducted in a department of nursing at a research-based university in southern Taiwan from July 2011 to August 2014, with approval from the institutional review board (A-ER-101-127).

Setting

This study was carried out in a department of nursing that offers a 4-year baccalaureate nursing program and enrolls approximately 40 students each year. One hundred twenty-eight credits, including professional nursing and general education credits as well as 1,016 hours of clinical practicum, are required to earn a bachelor of nursing degree. Nineteen educators worked in this department. All of these educators had EBP teaching experience in clinical settings, and 12 had received EBP training from the Taiwan Joanna Briggs Institute Collaborating Center.

Participants

Eleven nursing teachers with EBP teaching experience, 68 third- and fourth-year undergraduate students with EBP learning experience, and three external EBP education experts with Joanna Briggs Institute "Train the Trainer" certification participated in this study.

Data Collection

AR may require that qualitative and quantitative data complement each other to provide comprehensive information about what to do and how to proceed through the AR cycles (Bryman, 2012). Accordingly, this study collected information using focus group interviews, external course-review documents, and questionnaire surveys.

The focus group interview was the main method used to inform and guide the three AR cycles in this study. During the three AR cycles, focus group interviews were held repeatedly to collect the observations and reflections of participants. These focus groups were moderated by the chief researcher (Y. J. Chang), who was also a teacher in the department of nursing. All of the group meetings were audio-recorded and then transcribed verbatim for use in the analysis.

Self-developed, external course-review documents were applied in the first cycle that comprised items reflecting the design of the preliminary EBP curriculum. These documents, including learning objectives, learning outcomes, teaching content, and learning activities, were mailed to the external experts with a request that they judge the completeness and appropriateness of the curriculum. Completeness was defined as an EBP curriculum that contained the overall concepts of EBP, whereas appropriateness indicated whether the design of the teaching content and learning activities matched expected learning outcomes and learning objectives. The experts were asked to rate each item in the documents on a 4-point scale, with 1 = *very inappropriate* and 4 = *very appropriate*.

The "EBP Attitude Questionnaire," applied in Cycle 3, was adopted from parts of the EBP Knowledge, Attitude, and Behavior Questionnaire that was developed previously to assess the EBP knowledge, attitudes, and behaviors of nurses after participating in an EBP training program. The content validity index of this questionnaire is .86, whereas the internal consistency earned a Cronbach α of .74 (Lee, Wang, & Chang, 2011). This questionnaire consists of 10 items that are scored using a 4-point Likert scale, with 1 = *strong disagreement* and 4 = *strong agreement*. The total possible score range is 10–40, with higher scores indicating more positive attitudes toward EBP.

Action Research Process

In response to the American Association of Colleges of Nursing (2008) appeal that baccalaureate nursing students should acquire sufficient EBP competency before they graduate, the participating department of nursing determined that applying empirical scientific strategies to explore, answer, and resolve clinical practice problems should be a core competency of undergraduate students. However, before this study, relevant EBP elements were only taught in certain courses. Therefore, the first cycle of AR in this study (planning stage) began after identifying the need to develop an EBP nursing curriculum. In this cycle (July 2011–August 2012), six EBP-experienced teachers in charge of core nursing courses were grouped by the chief researcher. In the group, the chief researcher used a series of questions regarding EBP curriculum design to encourage the participating teachers to discuss and share their recommendations. Then, focus groups were

held repeatedly to confirm these recommendations and to continue discussing other elements of the EBP curriculum not yet covered or agreed upon (action stage). Three focus group interviews were held in the first cycle. After framing the preliminary EBP curriculum, three external EBP education experts validated this curriculum using the external course-review documents (observation and reflection stage).

The second cycle (August 2012–July 2013) began after obtaining the reflections of the participants on the first cycle, with the goal of evaluating the feasibility of the preliminary EBP curriculum in an actual teaching context (planning stage). Four teachers who were responsible for teaching core nursing courses, four teachers in charge of students' clinical practicum, and 32 third- and fourth-year students participated in this cycle. Because the EBP course was not a compulsory course at the time, before implementation of the preliminary EBP curriculum, a coordination meeting was held with the participating teachers to discuss how to implement the related teaching content and learning activities. Afterward, the preliminary EBP curriculum was implemented for two consecutive semesters (action stage). At the end of each semester, focus groups were held to characterize the experiences of the teachers and students for the purpose of further modifying the EBP curriculum. Overall, two teacher focus groups and two student focus groups were conducted during this cycle (observation and reflection stage).

The third cycle commenced (August 2013–July 2014) after the preliminary EBP curriculum was modified based on the reflections of participants in the second cycle. This cycle included three tasks: (a) implement the entire modified EBP curriculum, (b) continually assess the feasibility of the modified EBP curriculum, and (c) evaluate the impact of the EBP curriculum on the EBP competency and attitudes of students toward EBP. Before implementation, the modified EBP curriculum was submitted to the nursing department's curriculum committee and presented at the departmental meeting for approval. After obtaining support from the dean and the committee, the researchers communicated with the teachers in charge of each designated course to characterize their needs for EBP teaching and share their experiences from the previous cycles of EBP teaching (planning stage). Subsequently, the modified EBP curriculum was implemented for two consecutive semesters (action stage). At the end of each semester, focus groups were held to evaluate the feasibility of the curriculum, and the EBP attitude questionnaire was used to assess the impact of the EBP curriculum on student attitudes. Eleven teachers and 61 third- and fourth-year students participated in this cycle. Two teacher focus groups and two student focus groups were held during this cycle (observation and reflection stage). The goal of each cycle, the data collection methods used, and information on the participants are outlined in Figure 1.

Data Analysis

The verbatim transcripts were analyzed using deductive qualitative content analysis based on the categories that previous studies had formulated or on theories designed to code the

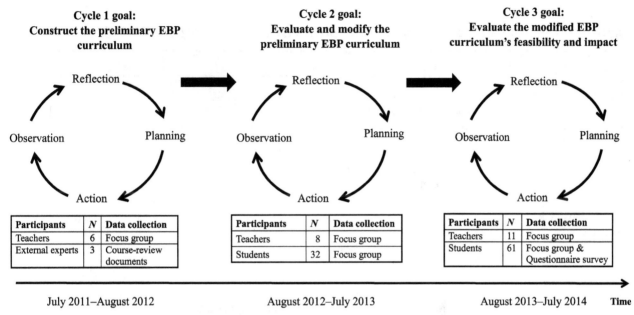

Figure 1. The process used to develop the undergraduate evidence-based practice (EBP) curriculum.

transcript (Hsieh & Shannon, 2005; Vaismoradi, Turunen, & Bondas, 2013). Thus, relevant elements of curriculum design were used as schemes to code the transcripts.

The external course-review documents were analyzed using the concept of content validity index (Polit, Beck, & Owen, 2007). The content of items that received either a score of 3 or 4 from the experts on a 4-point scale in the external course-review documents was deemed to be appropriate. All of the items were rated as appropriate by the three external experts in this study.

The questionnaire survey regarding student EBP attitudes in the third cycle was analyzed using a paired t test, with significant differences between the pretest and posttest scores set at $p < .05$.

Results

Cycle 1: Preliminary Evidence-Based Practice Curriculum Construction and Simulated Scenario Development

The participating teachers considered that EBP education should be conducted along with instruction in relevant background knowledge. Accordingly, three levels of learning objectives with corresponding learning outcomes, teaching content, and learning activities were developed and embedded into the core nursing courses for students of different academic years. The overall preliminary curriculum framework is shown in Tables 1 and 2.

Learning objectives and learning outcomes of each level

As shown in Table 1, as the first- and second-year students were beginners in the nursing field and only starting to

acquire basic knowledge related to nursing, biomedical, and behavioral sciences, Level 1 teaching focused on developing the ability of students to ask questions and acquire information literacy and literature comprehension to support subsequent EBP learning. After students had acquired nursing knowledge and begun to synthesize learned knowledge and skills related to solving clinical care problems during their third year, Level 2 teaching advanced the abilities of students to search in synthesized databases and integrate evidence to address clinical care problems. When the students entered their last year and began acquiring knowledge related to research methodology, they were guided to analyze and identify the obstructions to nursing professionalism. Therefore, Level 3 teaching focused on critical evidence appraisal and on encouraging students to reflect on the outcomes of research evidence. The expected learning outcomes were set according to the learning objectives of each level (Table 1).

Teaching content and core courses at each level

To help students achieve the learning objectives and outcomes listed in Table 1, corresponding teaching content was developed and core nursing courses were integrated based on their original teaching elements to deliver the EBP teaching content appropriately for each level (Table 2).

Introduction to Nursing and Fundamentals of Nursing were designated as the two core courses for Level l. Because Introduction to Nursing is the first course to help students gain insight into the nursing profession and to teach elements of credible source searches, this course was designed to introduce the basic concepts of EBP and to teach students how to perform a general database search. In addition, the nursing processes taught in Fundamentals of Nursing, which emphasize the integration of knowledge of basic medicine, physical assessment, and human development as a strategy for

TABLE 1.

Learning Objectives and Learning Outcomes of the Developed EBP Curriculum

Level of Objective	Learning Outcome	Corresponding Course		Academic Year
		Core Course	Practicum	
Level 1 Apply search strategy to explore nursing issues	• Ask background questions • Search for evidence in medical databases • Comprehend descriptive research articles → Comprehend English medical literature[a]	1. Introduction to Nursing 2. Fundamentals of Nursing	None 3. Fundamentals of Nursing Practicum[a]	First & second
Level 2 Apply EBP steps to solve clinical care issues	• Ask foreground questions • Search for evidence in synthesized databases • Comprehend quantitative research articles	1. Adult Health Nursing	2. Adult Health Nursing I & II Practicum 3. Maternal Nursing Practicum 4. Pediatric Nursing Practicum	Third
Level 3 Critically appraise and evaluate clinical application of research	• Appraise research articles • Evaluate the outcome of the clinical application of research evidence	1. Introduction to Nursing Research 2. Seminar of Nursing Profession	3. Psychiatric Nursing Practicum 4. Community Health Nursing Practicum 5. Nursing Elective Practicum	Fourth

Note. EBP = evidence-based practice.
[a]Revised contents during Cycle 2.

identifying specific patient care problems, echoed elements of the background-question-raising procedure introduced in the EBP steps. Therefore, the teaching content of the nursing processes in this course was modified to emphasize the background questions associated with patient care issues.

Adult Health Nursing was designated as the core course for Level 2 because the objectives of this course help enable students to apply the nursing process to identify patient problems and further develop evidence-based interventions that satisfy patient needs, which are relevant to the expected learning objectives of Level 2. In addition, because the understanding of the experiences and values of patients is also emphasized in our curriculum, the lecture content of this course was further enhanced to include quantitative and qualitative types of foreground question formulation, a synthesized database search for identifying quantitative and qualitative evidence, and the integration of evidence.

Introduction to Nursing Research and Seminar of the Nursing Profession were designated as the two core courses for Level 3. Introduction to Nursing Research aims to increase student competence in evaluating research articles and their clinical application, whereas Seminar of the Nursing Profession aims to guide students to discuss nursing professionalism and critically analyze the factors affecting the development of the nursing profession and the practice of nursing. These teaching

objectives are relevant to the expected learning objectives of Level 3. Thus, Introduction to Nursing Research was designed to integrate the previously learned EBP knowledge and to teach the appraisal of research evidence and application. Finally, the issues related to the vision of EBP, clinical dilemmas of EBP, and the role of nurses in disseminating EBP were added to the lectures of the Seminar of the Nursing Profession.

Learning activities at each level

Various individual and group learning activities were developed for classroom and practicum courses to provide students with opportunities to practice EBP content (Table 2). In particular, assignments consisting of clinical care scenarios and EBP processes were developed to familiarize students with the EBP steps. The scenario assignments were developed according to the concept of critically appraised topics (Sadigh, Parker, Kelly, & Cronin, 2012) and commenced with a simulated nursing scenario followed by instructions that were designed to guide students to think about the scenarios and complete each EBP step. The simulated nursing scenarios were developed preliminarily by the research team and then reviewed and modified by the participating teachers.

In addition, the original care-report assignments of the practicum were modified to emphasize the identification of

TABLE 2.
Preliminary Lecture Topics and Learning Activities of the Developed EBP Curriculum

Level of Objective/Course	Lecture Topic	Learning Activity
Level 1		
1. Introduction to Nursing	• Introduction to EBP • General medical databases search	◊ Searching for literature
2. Fundamentals of Nursing	• Background questions of patients' health	◊ Individual EBP reference reading assignments ◊ Group report of raising background questions based on scenarios
Level 2		
1. Adult Health Nursing	• Formulating foreground questions (PICO/Pico) • Synthesis database search • Literature synthesis • Discussion on the clinical application of evidence	◊ Certification of literature search ◊ Group report of foreground questions, searching strategy, reading, and synthesis of literature based on scenarios
2. Adult Health Nursing I & II Practicum	None	◊ Individual EBP case report
3. Maternal Nursing Practicum	None	◊ Individual literature report
4. Pediatric Nursing Practicum	None	◊ Individual EBP case report
Level 3		
1. Introduction to Nursing Research	• Critical appraisal of research articles • Clinical application of evidence	◊ Group report focusing on synthesis of research evidence and discussion on evidence clinical application
2. Seminar of the Nursing Profession	• Current state and vision of EBP • Barriers to implementing EBP • Clinical dilemma of EBP • Nursing role of disseminating EBP	◊ Group report of designated nursing professional issues
3. Psychiatric Nursing Practicum	None	◊ Individual EBP case report
4. Community Health Nursing Practicum	None	◊ Individual EBP family report
5. Nursing Elective Practicum	None	◊ Evidence-based case analysis

Note. EBP = evidence-based practice; PICO = Patient/Problem, Intervention, Comparison, and Outcome; Pico = Population, Phenomena of Interest, and Context.

nursing problems, the development of evidence-based interventions, and the application of interventions consistent with evidence and patient preferences.

Initial evaluation and other reflections

After establishing the preliminary EBP curriculum, three external EBP experts were invited to verify its completeness and appropriateness. Although the external experts approved the preliminary EBP curriculum, they recommended that the feasibility of the three-level learning scheme be assessed through actual implementation in lectures and practicums.

Moreover, in addition to providing perspectives for constructing the concrete and visible curriculum framework, the participating teachers, on the basis of their experience, reported that guiding students to form answerable questions was the biggest challenge in EBP teaching. The reason behind this difficulty may be that Taiwanese students are accustomed to learning passively and receiving what is taught. Therefore, creating a learning climate in which students are encouraged to ask questions and learn

actively was important to the successful implementation of the EBP curriculum.

Cycle 2: Evaluation and Modification of the Preliminary Evidence-Based Practice Curriculum

After the preliminary EBP curriculum was implemented for two consecutive semesters, the teachers and students agreed with the learning objectives of the curriculum. However, some learning outcomes, teaching content, and learning activities required further modification, and certain teaching elements needed to be added. These modifications are summarized in Tables 1 and 3.

The modification of learning outcomes for Level 1

The teachers reported that they preferred guiding students to read appropriate literature according to clinical issues pertinent to their own interests rather than confining them to reading a preassigned type of research article. Therefore, the learning outcomes for Level 1 were revised (Table 1).

TABLE 3.
Modified Lecture Topics and Learning Activities of the Developed EBP Curriculum

Level of Objective/Course	Lecture Topic	Learning Activity
Level 1		
1. Introduction to Nursing	• Introduction to EBP • General medical database search	◊ Searching for literature
2. Fundamentals of Nursing	• Background questions of patients' health	◊ Group report of raising background questions based on scenarios
3. Fundamentals of Nursing Practicum[a]	None	◊ Individual EBP reference reading assignment[a]
Level 2		
1. Adult Health Nursing (I)[a]	• Characteristics of background and foreground problems (basic concepts of PICO)[a] • Synthesis database search	◊ Certification of synthesis database search
2. Adult Health Nursing (II)[a]	• Formulating foreground questions (PICO/Pico) • Literature synthesis • Discussion on the clinical application of evidence	None
3. Adult Health Nursing I & II Practicum	None	◊ Group EBP report based on scenarios[a]
4. Maternal Nursing Practicum	None	◊ Group EBP report based on scenarios[a]
5. Pediatric Nursing Practicum	None	◊ Group EBP report based on scenarios[a]
Level 3		
1. Introduction to Nursing Research	• Critical appraisal of research articles • Current state of evidence utilization[a]	◊ Group report focusing on synthesis of research evidence and discussion on evidence clinical application
2. Seminar of Nursing Profession	• Current state and vision of EBP • Barriers to implementing EBP • Clinical dilemma of EBP • Nursing role of disseminating EBP	◊ Group report of designated nursing professional issues
3. Psychiatric Nursing Practicum	None	◊ Individual EBP case report
4. Community Health Nursing Practicum	None	◊ Individual EBP family report
5. Nursing Elective Practicum	None	◊ Evidence-based case analysis

Note. EBP = evidence-based practice; PICO = Patient/Problem, Intervention, Comparison, and Outcome; Pico = Population, Phenomena of Interest, and Context.
[a]Revised lecture topic or learning activity during Cycle 2.

The modification of teaching content for Levels 2 and 3

By evaluating the performance of students on the scenario assignments, the teachers found that, despite the classroom lectures, students still had difficulty formulating foreground questions. A possible reason for this difficulty was that students were not equipped with sufficient background knowledge, which caused them to ask background questions related to patient problems rather than foreground questions. Therefore, the teachers concluded that Level 2 teaching should be conducted in two phases to simultaneously build the background knowledge of students as a foundation for formulating foreground questions while strengthening the understanding of students of different types of clinical problems. Furthermore, because the application of evidence to practice could not be directly experienced in Introduction to Nursing Research, the course content was also revised to

include discussions of the current state of evidence utilization in clinical settings (Table 3).

The modification of learning activities

Because the third-year students had limited EBP knowledge, the teachers decided that the learning activities of Level 2 should all be handled as group work to facilitate better learning outcomes. In addition, the teachers concluded that the scenario assignments should also be handled as learning activities for the clinical practicum. One reason for this change was that time was limited for students to practice the EBP scenario assignments in the classroom. Another reason was that the design of the scenario assignments was based on common clinical patient care problems, and the teachers thought that practicing the scenario assignments in a clinical setting would give students better opportunities to correlate these scenarios with actual patient care and to observe the application of EBP. Other modifications of the learning activities are shown in Table 3.

Other reflections

The teachers perceived that EBP teaching in this stage of nursing education was challenging and time consuming, especially when guiding students through each EBP step in the scenario assignments. To support future EBP teaching, teachers suggested that graduate-level teaching assistants could help students search, understand, and integrate research evidence. In addition, self-learning supplementary materials consisting of examples on the differences between background and foreground questions, formulating PICO/PIco (Patient/Problem, Intervention, Comparison, and Outcome, or Population, Phenomena of Interest, and Context) frameworks, learning search strategies, understanding levels of evidence and resources, applying various research methodologies, and providing guidance for reading various types of research articles should be developed and shared on a digital teaching platform to help students complete additional self-learning exercises whenever necessary. Another important suggestion proposed by the participating teachers was to better engage the EBP learning motivation of students. To this point, integrating EBP concepts into events that students are likely to encounter in their lives may be an effective approach.

Cycle 3: Evaluation of the Feasibility and Impact of the Modified Evidence-Based Practice Curriculum

After the modified EBP curriculum was implemented comprehensively for two consecutive semesters, the teachers

and students generally approved of the modified EBP curriculum. By evaluating the progress of students through the learning activities and designated assignments, the teachers concluded that the students were able to achieve most of the expected learning outcomes. Moreover, the students were satisfied with their own performance, especially with regard to reviewing and integrating literature, and also expressed that the EBP learning experiences raised their level of inquiry and truth-seeking motivation and improved their confidence in clinical settings. Furthermore, the pretest and posttest questionnaires (Table 4) that were completed by 57 students revealed that the students earned significantly higher posttest scores after receiving the EBP education, which indicates that they had a more positive attitude toward EBP than before they completed the courses ($p < .004$).

Other reflections

Although the teachers were satisfied with the performance of the students, they believed that some effort should be made toward improving the students' insufficient understandings of foreground and background questions as well as their weaknesses in interpreting statistical results in research articles, using synthesized databases, and appraising and applying evidence. Therefore, clarifying the definition of foreground and background questions, providing reliable resources for answering foreground and background questions, and enhancing students' comprehension of the application of critical appraisal tools and holistic thinking about the risks, ethics, and safety issues involved in using evidence were proposed for use as teaching elements of EBP education. Furthermore, including strategies for interpreting the

TABLE 4.

Impact of the Developed EBP Curriculum on the EBP Attitudes of Students (N = 57)

Item	Pretest		Posttest	
	Mean	SD	Mean	SD
1. I think that EBP can solve clinical problems and difficulties.	3.3	0.5	3.3	0.6
2. I think that healthcare professionals should be equipped with EBP knowledge and skills.	3.4	0.5	3.6	0.5
3. I think that EBP can reduce the occurrence of medical errors.	3.1	0.6	3.2	0.6
4. I think that, if nurses can implement EBP in their daily clinical care, they can prevent mistakes.	3.3	0.5	3.3	0.6
5. I believe that the integration of research results can be used as clinical practice guidelines.	3.4	0.5	3.6	0.5
6. I think EBP is just a theory and that it cannot be applied in clinical care.	3.1	0.7	2.8	0.9
7. I think that evidence searching can facilitate my professional development.	3.4	0.5	3.4	0.5
8. I think that findings of a single study do not represent the true facts.	3.2	0.5	3.3	0.6
9. I think that EBP has been valued by medical institutions.	2.9	0.7	3.0	0.7
10. I think that learning EBP skills will help me a lot during my clinical practicum.	3.2	0.5	3.4	0.6
Total score[a]	30.7	4.8	32.8	3.5

Note. EBP = evidence-based practice.
[a]Total mean score of pretest and posttest was compared with a paired *t* test, and the result was *t* = 3.03, *p* = .004.

statistical results of research articles in biostatistics courses and for repetitive practice in searching the databases in other nursing courses was also suggested.

The participating teachers further suggested that clinically answerable questions (PICO/PIco format) that had been formulated and processed could be used as effective teaching resources to save time when guiding students to form answerable questions and to identify appropriate literature for helping students learn subsequent EBP steps. In addition, other support resources such as faculty development and additional teaching manpower should be engaged to more fully promote implementation of the EBP curriculum.

Discussion

A systematic EBP undergraduate nursing curriculum with three levels of learning objectives and corresponding learning outcomes, teaching content, and learning activities was developed. Our EBP curriculum was organized in a vertical structure from basic to advanced, simple to complex, and group cooperative learning to individual independent learning to build the EBP knowledge and competency of students progressively. Furthermore, interprofessional nursing courses were integrated in a horizontal structure to collaboratively assist students to achieve the learning objective of each level. This curriculum was designed not only to deliver relevant EBP knowledge but also to coordinate with various learning activities (the clinical scenario assignments, in particular) to deepen student comprehension of the EBP process and consolidate their EBP knowledge. A preliminary evaluation found that this curriculum successfully fostered the EBP competency of students, increased their confidence in clinical practice, and promoted their adoption of a positive attitude toward EBP.

Possible reasons for the effectiveness of the developed curriculum are that its design emphasized that EBP teaching be conducted in parallel with the accumulation of background knowledge (Nickerson & Thurkettle, 2013) and that it incorporated multiple pedagogical strategies, including lectures, group collaboration, and linking academic learning with clinical practice, in an effort to maximize EBP learning (Christie, Hamill, & Power, 2012). Furthermore, the findings of this study suggest that allowing students to practice EBP scenario assignments during the clinical practicum may greatly and positively impact their attitudes toward EBP. The reason for this effect is that working on these assignments during the clinical practicum not only provides students with opportunities to learn and experience how to judge the feasibility of available evidence in clinical practice through faculty guidance and role modeling but also enables students to visualize the impact of EBP on clinical care. These learning experiences have been shown to improve student attitudes toward EBP (Brown et al., 2010). Moreover, as undergraduate nursing students should be expected to be users of evidence in future clinical practice settings, the teaching elements addressing the clinical application of

evidence such as critical appraisal instruments that guide students in analyzing the clinical applicability of research evidence (Nadelson & Nadelson, 2014) and synthesized databases that allow students to instantly obtain the pre-appraised and integrated evidence (Ahmadi, Baradaran, & Ahmadi, 2015) were also emphasized in this curriculum. These efforts may enable students to better experience the feasibility and importance of EBP and lead to a more positive attitude toward EBP and greater confidence in practicing EBP in the clinical practicum.

Nevertheless, our teachers stated that EBP teaching was still replete with challenges that require multiple strategies and sufficient investments of resources. Although most teachers in this study had received EBP training, teachers still strongly perceived a need for advanced teaching skills and knowledge. A possible explanation for this finding is that, despite the growing emphasis in the literature on the importance of developing the EBP competency of nursing students, relatively little attention has been paid to developing the knowledge and skills of faculty that will be necessary to integrate EBP concepts into nursing courses and clinical practicums and to teach EBP more effectively (Levin, 2014). Workshops, small group activities, short courses, peer mentoring, and online resources are proposed as feasible strategies for faculty to acquire and exchange effective EBP teaching strategies (Snell, 2014). These methods could be considered in future work to enhance the EBP teaching competency of faculty.

Furthermore, adequate resources are indispensable to curriculum implementation (Iwasiw & Goldenberg, 2014). Despite the initial idea of the researchers of this study to integrate existing teaching elements of the original professional courses into the teaching of EBP to lessen the burden on teachers, the participating teachers still expressed the need for more resources to support their teaching. Establishing interprofessional teaching partnerships (such as collaboration with librarians to better teach on the use electronic databases and with clinical professionals to better teach on the application of evidence) may be considered as potentially supportive EBP teaching resources (Levin & Feldman, 2012).

Finally, this study identified showing effective leadership as important for constructing and implementing a new curriculum (Long et al., 2014) because related preparatory work had already begun on the construction of this EBP curriculum. In the present case, a faculty member (Y. J. Chang), who had received in-depth EBP training and had administrative experience, led the curriculum team. The contributions of this leader included seeking funding from the institution to support EBP training for faculty members, participating in the program committees to promote a consensus among teachers to set EBP as a core competency for nursing students, and convening the teacher groups that were responsible to design the EBP curriculum. During curriculum implementation, this project leader worked continuously with the faculty as a mentor and shared knowledge about EBP teaching. This leadership was, in this study, and will continue to be a key factor in constructing and implementing an effective EBP curriculum.

Limitations

As a preliminary study, this study created the framework for a systematic EBP curriculum and tested its feasibility and effectiveness on the EBP competency of students, mainly using subjective methods. This evaluation approach may not be sufficient to reflect the viability or effectiveness of a specific curriculum in practice (Iwasiw & Goldenberg, 2014). Therefore, we suggest that a future study be conducted to combine objective and subjective methods to continuously assess the appropriateness of the EBP curriculum and evaluate its impact on multiple domains of the EBP competency of students.

Conclusions

By integrating EBP concepts into a 4-year baccalaureate nursing program, this study developed a systematic and effective EBP nursing curriculum with valuable pedagogical content and strategies. The developed curriculum successfully increased the competency and confidence of the students, which positively impacted their attitudes toward EBP. The process of developing and implementing the EBP curriculum and the resulting information generated may provide a valuable reference for other nursing schools.

Acknowledgments

This study was funded by the Ministry of Science and Technology in Taiwan (grants of NSC 101-2511-S-006-002-MY2). The authors would like to thank all of the participating teachers in this study who donated their efforts and time to support the development and implementation of this curriculum.

References

Ahmadi, S.-F., Baradaran, H. R., & Ahmadi, E. (2015). Effectiveness of teaching evidence-based medicine to undergraduate medical students: A BEME systematic review. *Medical Teacher, 37*(1), 21–30. https://doi.org/10.3109/0142159X.2014.971724

Alamrani, M. H., Alammar, K. A., Alqahtani, S. S., & Salem, O. A. (2018). Comparing the effects of simulation-based and traditional teaching methods on the critical thinking abilities and self-confidence of nursing students. *The Journal of Nursing Research, 26*(3), 152–157. https://doi.org/10.1097/jnr.0000000000000231

American Association of Colleges of Nursing. (2008). *The essentials of baccalaureate education for professional nursing practice.* Washington, DC: Author.

Bloom, K. C., Olinzock, B. J., Radjenovic, D., & Trice, L. B. (2013). Leveling EBP content for undergraduate nursing students. *Journal of Professional Nursing, 29*(4), 217–224. https://doi.org/10.1016/j.profnurs.2012.05.015

Brown, C. E., Kim, S. C., Stichler, J. F., & Fields, W. (2010). Predictors of knowledge, attitudes, use and future use of evidence-based practice among baccalaureate nursing students at two universities. *Nurse Education Today, 30*(6), 521–527. https://doi.org/10.1016/j.nedt.2009.10.021

Bryman, A. (2012). *Social research methods* (4th ed.). Oxford, England: Oxford University Press.

Cant, R. P., & Cooper, S. J. (2010). Simulation-based learning in nurse education: Systematic review. *Journal of Advanced Nursing, 66*(1), 3–15. https://doi.org/10.1111/j.1365-2648.2009.05240.x

Christie, J., Hamill, C., & Power, J. (2012). How can we maximize nursing students' learning about research evidence and utilization in undergraduate, preregistration programmes? A discussion paper. *Journal of Advanced Nursing, 68*(12), 2789–2801. https://doi.org/10.1111/j.1365-2648.2012.05994.x

Coomarasamy, A., & Khan, K. S. (2004). What is the evidence that postgraduate teaching in evidence based medicine changes anything? A systematic review. *BMJ, 329*(7473), 1017. https://doi.org/10.1136/bmj.329.7473.1017

Finotto, S., Carpanoni, M., Turroni, E. C., Camellini, R., & Mecugni, D. (2013). Teaching evidence-based practice: Developing a curriculum model to foster evidence-based practice in undergraduate student nurses. *Nurse Education in Practice, 13*(5), 459–465. https://doi.org/10.1016/j.nepr.2013.03.021

Hsieh, H. F., & Shannon, S. E. (2005). Three approaches to qualitative content analysis. *Qualitative Health Research, 15*(9), 1277–1288. https://doi.org/10.1177/1049732305276687

Hung, H. Y., Huang, Y. F., Tsai, J. J., & Chang, Y. J. (2015). Current state of evidence-based practice education for undergraduate nursing students in Taiwan: A questionnaire study. *Nurse Education Today, 35*(12), 1262–1267. https://doi.org/10.1016/j.nedt.2015.05.001

Iwasiw, C. L., & Goldenberg, D. (2014). *Curriculum development in nursing education* (3rd ed.). Sudbury, MA: Jones & Bartlett Learning.

Kemmis, S., McTaggart, R., & Nixon, R. (2014). *The action research planner: Doing critical participatory action research* (1st ed.). Singapore: Springer. https://doi.org/10.1007/978-981-4560-67-2

Lee, C. Y., Wang, W. F., & Chang, Y. J. (2011). The effects of evidence-based nursing training program on nurses' knowledge, attitude, and behavior. *New Taipei Journal of Nursing, 13*(1), 19–31. https://doi.org/10.6540/NTJN.2011.1.003 (Original work published in Chinese).

Levin, R. F. (2014). Mentoring faculty for success. *Research and Theory for Nursing Practice, 28*(4), 274–277. https://doi.org/10.1891/1541-6577.28.4.274

Levin, R. F., & Feldman, H. R. (2012). *Teaching evidence-based practice in nursing* (2nd ed.). New York, NY: Springer.

Long, C. R., Ackerman, D. L., Hammerschlag, R., Delagran, L., Peterson, D. H., Berlin, M., & Evans, R. L. (2014). Faculty development initiatives to advance research literacy and evidence-based practice at CAM academic institutions. *The Journal of Alternative and Complementary Medicine, 20*(7), 563–570. https://doi.org/10.1089/acm.2013.0385

Meeker, M. A., Jones, J. M., & Flanagan, N. A. (2008). Teaching undergraduate nursing research from an evidence-based practice perspective. *Journal of Nursing Education, 47*(8), 376–379. https://doi.org/10.3928/01484834-20080801-06

Melnyk, B. M. (2013). Educational programming in undergraduate and graduate academic curricula: Friend or foe to accelerating evidence-based practice? *Worldviews on Evidence-Based Nursing, 10*(4), 185–186. https://doi.org/10.1111/wvn.12020

Melnyk, B. M., & Fineout-Overholt, E. (2014). *Evidence-based practice in nursing & healthcare: A guide to best practice* (3rd ed.). Philadelphia, PA: Lippincott Williams & Wilkins.

Melnyk, B. M., Fineout-Overholt, E., Gallagher-Ford, L., & Kaplan, L. (2012). The state of evidence-based practice in US nurses: Critical implications for nurse leaders and educators. *The Journal of Nursing Administration, 42*(9), 410–417. https://doi.org/10.1097/NNA.0b013e3182664e0a

Mu, P. F., Tsay, S. F., & Chang, L. Y. (2013). Factors associated with evidence-based nursing promotion in Taiwan. *VGH Nursing, 30*(2), 130–143. https://doi.org/10.6142/VGHN.30.2.130 (Original work published in Chinese).

Nadelson, S., & Nadelson, L. S. (2014). Evidence-based practice article reviews using CASP tools: A method for teaching EBP. *Worldviews on Evidence-Based Nursing, 11*(5), 344–346. https://doi.org/10.1111/wvn.12059

Nickerson, C. J., & Thurkettle, M. A. (2013). Cognitive maturity and readiness for evidence-based nursing practice. *Journal of Nursing Education, 52*(1), 17–23. https://doi.org/10.3928/01484834-20121121-04

Polit, D. F., Beck, C. T., & Owen, S. V. (2007). Is the CVI an acceptable indicator of content validity? Appraisal and recommendations. *Research in Nursing & Health, 30*(4), 459–467. https://doi.org/10.1002/nur.20199

Rolloff, M. (2010). A constructivist model for teaching evidence-based practice. *Nursing Education Perspectives, 31*(5), 290–293.

Ryan, E. J. (2016). Undergraduate nursing students' attitudes and use of research and evidence-based practice—An integrative literature review. *Journal of Clinical Nursing, 25*(11–12), 1548–1556. https://doi.org/10.1111/jocn.13229

Sadigh, G., Parker, R., Kelly, A. M., & Cronin, P. (2012). How to write a critically appraised topic (CAT). *Academic Radiology, 19*(7), 872–888. https://doi.org/10.1016/j.acra.2012.02.005

Saunders, H., & Vehviläinen-Julkunen, K. (2016). The state of readiness for evidence-based practice among nurses: An integrative review. *International Journal of Nursing Studies, 56*, 128–140. https://doi.org/10.1016/j.ijnurstu.2015.10.018

Snell, L. (2014). Faculty development for curriculum change: Towards competency-based teaching and assessment. In Y. Steninert (Ed.), *Faculty development in the health professions* (pp. 265–285). Dordrecht, the Netherlands: Springer.

Solomons, N. M., & Spross, J. A. (2011). Evidence-based practice barriers and facilitators from a continuous quality improvement perspective: An integrative review. *Journal of Nursing Management, 19*(1), 109–120. https://doi.org/10.1111/j.1365-2834.2010.01144.x

Tilson, J. K., Kaplan, S. L., Harris, J. L., Hutchinson, A., Ilic, D., Niederman, R., … Zwolsman, S. E. (2011). Sicily statement on classification and development of evidence-based practice learning assessment tools. *BMC Medical Education, 11*, 78. https://doi.org/10.1186/1472-6920-11-78

Vaismoradi, M., Turunen, H., & Bondas, T. (2013). Content analysis and thematic analysis: Implications for conducting a qualitative descriptive study. *Nursing & Health Sciences, 15*(3), 398–405. https://doi.org/10.1111/nhs.12048

Zhang, Q., Zeng, T., Chen, Y., & Li, X. (2012). Assisting undergraduate nursing students to learn evidence-based practice through self-directed learning and workshop strategies during clinical practicum. *Nurse Education Today, 32*(5), 570–575. https://doi.org/10.1016/j.nedt.2011.05.018

21

Predictors of Palliative Care Knowledge Among Nursing Students in Saudi Arabia

Ahmad E. ABOSHAIQAH

ABSTRACT

Background: Societal aging, a concern in many countries worldwide, is increasing the demand for quality palliative care in Saudi Arabia. Nursing education is responsible for providing nursing students with high levels of knowledge and competency related to palliative care.

Purpose: The aim of this study was to investigate the predictors of palliative care knowledge among nursing students in Saudi Arabia.

Methods: A convenience sample of 409 nursing students from one public academic institution and one private academic institution in Saudi Arabia was surveyed from November to December 2017 in this descriptive, cross-sectional study. The 20-item Palliative Care Quiz for Nursing was used to collect the data. Descriptive statistics were used to fully describe the demographic characteristics and palliative care knowledge of the participants. One-way analysis of variance and t test were used to examine the associations between palliative care knowledge and the demographic characteristics. Multiple regression analysis was conducted to identify the significant demographic predictors of this knowledge.

Results: The mean score of the participants was 5.23 ($SD = 3.24$, range = 0–12), indicating poor palliative care knowledge. The participants lacked palliative care knowledge in terms of palliative care principles and philosophy, management of pain and other symptoms, and psychosocial and spiritual care. Being enrolled in a private university, being in the second year of a nursing program, having attended palliative care education sessions outside a university setting, and attending a palliative care course in the nursing program were identified as significant predictors of higher palliative care knowledge.

Conclusions/Implications for Practice: This study may be used as a basis for formulating education policies and interventions to enhance palliative care education and clinical training among nursing students and ensure the quality of palliative care not only in Saudi Arabia but also in other countries.

KEY WORDS:
nursing, nursing education, nursing students, palliative care, palliative care knowledge.

Introduction

Societal aging is a concern in countries around the world, including Saudi Arabia. As aging progresses, the incidence of illnesses with no direct cure and terminal-stage diseases peaks. Thus, patients must receive competent care to meet their needs, which increases the demand for quality palliative care. Nurses are a frontline provider in clinical settings of healthcare, including palliative nursing. Nurses ensure that palliative care is delivered safely, effectively, and compassionately (Borneman, 2011). Unfortunately, palliative care knowledge among nurses remains poor, and high-quality palliative care remains a major challenge (Prem et al., 2012).

Despite the demand for palliative care among patients in Saudi Arabia, the development and expansion of this field have been slow. Advancements in palliative care in this country are hindered by several challenges, including an insufficient nursing workforce with palliative care specialization (Alshammary, Abdullah, Duraisamy, & Anbar, 2014). With a shortage of qualified local nurses, Saudi Arabia continues to rely on foreign nurses to meet the demands of its increasing population (Aldossary, While, & Barriball, 2008; Cruz, 2017). Hence, the greatest challenge to training future Saudi nurses to address the nursing shortage and to enhance palliative care is nursing education. Furthermore, palliative care not only is limited to physical pain but also encompasses the emotional, psychological, social, and spiritual dimensions (Aljawi & Harford, 2012). Cultural and religious backgrounds impact the attitudes toward and methods of palliative care rendered by healthcare workers as well as how patients accept a specific palliative care intervention (Steinberg, 2011). Being the global center of the Islamic faith, with most of the population embracing Muslim culture and beliefs, Saudi Arabia may have different issues and considerations with regard to palliative care than those countries that are predominantly Christian. However, limited studies have been conducted to examine the palliative care knowledge of Muslim nursing students from predominantly Muslim countries. Therefore,

PhD, RN, Associate Professor, College of Nursing, King Saud University, Saudi Arabia.

this study aimed to establish baseline data on the palliative care knowledge of Saudi nursing students, who are educated and trained to care for clients who mostly embrace Islamic beliefs and Muslim culture. This study may serve as a basis for the enhancement of the policies and context of nursing curricula in Saudi Arabia and other Muslim countries.

Background

Palliative care focuses on the comfort of patients, especially those in their end-of-life phase (Henoch et al., 2017). Palliative care and hospice aim to improve the quality of life of adults and children with life-limiting diseases and medical conditions and to reduce their suffering and the suffering of their families. With the increasing rates of mortality and aging worldwide, improved standards of palliative care are necessary. According to the World Health Organization, the mortality rate of the global population is increasing significantly because of life-limiting disease categories (Glover, Garvan, Nealis, Citty, & Derrico, 2017). In Saudi Arabia, the population is aging rapidly, and approximately 27.3% of the population, including children over 15 years old, adults, and the older adults with life-limiting conditions, is in need of palliative care (Usta, Aygin, & Sağlam, 2016).

Palliative care is linked with a culture and religion of both patients and healthcare workers (Steinberg, 2011). How clients perceive and respond to their illness, how they accept palliative care interventions, and how they handle their end-of-life decision making are all influenced greatly by their belief system, which is anchored in their cultural and religious backgrounds (Williams, Donovan, Stajduhar, & Spitzer, 2015). Furthermore, the attitudes of patients and healthcare workers and the approaches to delivering palliative care differ significantly among religions and cultures. For instance, Saudi Arabia, where most families live together or nearby as extended family groups, families typically prefer to care for dying relatives at home (Sarhill, LeGrand, Islambouli, Davis, & Walsh, 2001). One study found that most Muslims prefer dying at home or in a holy place such as in a mosque or in Makkah or Medina (Tayeb, Al-Zamel, Fareed, & Abouellail, 2010). From the Saudi perspective, "faith and belief, self-esteem and image to friends and family, and satisfaction about family security after the death of the patient" are the elements that determine a "good death" (Tayeb et al., 2010). The high value placed on modesty is another unique consideration for palliative care in Saudi Arabia, reflecting the preference placed by families and individuals on receiving care from healthcare workers of the same gender. Touching the hand of a patient of the opposite gender requires permission from that patient. Furthermore, Muslim patients believe that death is predetermined by Allah. Thus, discussions about prognosis and life expectancy should take this into consideration. Other considerations that need to be attended to when caring for Muslim patients include the extended hospital visits by large numbers of family members and friends who advocate on the patient's behalf regarding his or her performance of the Salah (the five daily

prayers) and adherence to dietary considerations (e.g., the avoidance of pork products and fasting during Ramadan; Aljawi & Harford, 2012). Hence, understanding the unique cultural backgrounds and belief systems of patients and their families may aid in providing the best quality palliative care to patients and their families (Steinberg, 2011).

Nurses play a pivotal role in caring for patients with life-limiting illnesses. To effectively manage these patients, nursing students should have proper education, knowledge, perception, and attitudes related to palliative care (Henoch et al., 2017). Moreover, nursing students must be adequately educated and trained to be competent in the different components of palliative care, including pain and physical symptoms management, holistic nursing care, and psychosocial support to patients and their families (Seow & Bainbridge, 2018). However, palliative care education among nursing students is currently inadequate. According to Kirkpatrick, Cantrell, and Smeltzer (2017), only 57.9% of nursing undergraduates receive sessions on palliative care during their education, whereas 42.1% have low or no understanding of palliative care and pain management. These populations constitute a large number of nursing graduates who become healthcare providers without proper palliative care training, thereby posing a serious threat to the standards and quality that should be delivered to patients with terminal illnesses.

Nursing undergraduates must be knowledgeable of the goal of palliative care to improve the quality of life of patients with life-threatening progressive or terminal illnesses (Hold, Blake, & Ward, 2015). Nursing education is a key element to prepare nurses to deliver good quality, lifelong palliative care (Ferrell, Malloy, Mazanec, & Virani, 2016). Nursing students must undergo comprehensive training and courses that include lessons designed to ensure that nurses have the knowledge and skills necessary to provide appropriate, high-quality care to seriously ill and dying patients (Zeinah, Al-Kindi, & Hassan, 2013). Educating nursing students on palliative care starting from the early stages of nursing education may help improve their capability to perform major palliative care tasks, including consulting patients and relatives on all outpatient and inpatient care options (e.g., inpatient hospice and palliative care unit); coordination and information of all those involved in the care and integration of voluntary services; creation of individualized treatment plans; development of crisis management abilities; provision of symptom relief through medication, devices, and other measures; and provision of psychosocial support to patients and relatives (Alshammary et al., 2014).

The significance of palliative care for patients with fatal illnesses indicates the necessity of educating and training Saudi Arabian nursing students to improve patient care quality and nursing practices. However, the lack of understanding and adequate knowledge of palliative care remains one of the foremost problems in palliative care improvement. In Saudi Arabia, determining whether nursing students receive adequate training and education on palliative care during their academic and prepractice years is difficult (Hold et al., 2015).

The aim of this study was to investigate the predictors of palliative care knowledge among nursing students in Saudi Arabia.

Methods

Design, Samples, and Settings

This descriptive, cross-sectional study used a convenience sample of 409 nursing students from one public and one private academic institutions in Riyadh, Saudi Arabia. The two educational institutions were selected because of their large number of registered nursing students. The total population was 582 nursing students (public university = 363, private university = 219). Using the total population of the nursing students in the two universities, the researcher calculated the sample size using a Survey Monkey sample size calculator (https://www.surveymonkey.com/mp/sample-size-calculator/). A sample size of 232 nursing students was determined to be necessary to achieve a 95% confidence interval and 5% margin of error. To ensure the maximum sample size was obtained, 500 questionnaires were distributed. Of these questionnaires, 409 surveys were completed and retrieved, giving a response rate of 81.8%.

The inclusion criteria were as follows: (a) registered in the regular Bachelor of Science in Nursing program at one of the two institutions; (b) in the second, third, fourth, or internship year; and (c) full-time student. Students in the first year were excluded because they are still taking preparatory classes, taking general courses, and not sufficiently exposed to nursing courses. In addition, those students who were under the direct supervision of the researcher were excluded from the study.

Measurement

A survey approach was used to gather data. A two-part survey questionnaire was utilized to gather data about the demographic profile of the participants and to assess their knowledge of palliative care. The first part consisted of questions that were constructed by the researcher to obtain data on demographic characteristics, which included year of study (second, third, fourth, and internship year), gender, whether they had received educational sessions on palliative care in the last 5 years outside the university (yes/no), and whether a palliative care course had been given in their nursing program (yes/no).

The second part of the questionnaire was the Palliative Care Quiz for Nursing (PCQN; Ross, McDonald, & McGuinness, 1996), which is based on the Canadian Palliative Care Curriculum. The tool is composed of 20 questions, and the three possible responses included "true," "false," or "don't know." Scores were obtained by summing the number of correct answers, with a range of total possible scores from 0 to 20, with higher scores corresponding to higher levels of palliative care knowledge. The PCQN measures the three theoretical dimensions of "philosophy and principles of palliative care" using four items (possible scores = 0–4),

"pain and symptoms management" using 13 items (possible scores = 0–13), and "psychosocial and spiritual care" using three items (possible scores = 0–3). The authors of the original scale reported the validity of the tool, with an acceptable alpha of .78 and a correlation coefficient (r) of .56 on a test–retest confirming its reliability (Ross et al., 1996). Although this tool was originally developed to assess the palliative care knowledge of practicing nurses, previous studies have used it to quantify palliative care knowledge among populations of nursing students (Al Qadire, 2014; Khraisat, Hamdan, & Ghazzawwi, 2017; Pope, 2013). The English version of the tool was utilized in this study, because English is the medium of instruction and the mode of communication used at both of the target universities. The reliability of the PCQN in the current sample was tested using the Kuder and Richardson Formula 20. The computed alpha was .70, which indicated an adequate internal consistency of the tool in the present sample.

Data Collection Procedure

Data collection was performed from November to December 2017 by the researcher. Before data were collected, the researcher visited both of the universities to coordinate and formulate plans for recruitment and data collection. Recruitment was carried out 2 weeks before the scheduled data collection, and the students were approached during their free time. Posters regarding the study were placed in strategic places in the universities. The researcher coordinated with the instructors of each class to take 25 minutes of their time at the end of their lectures. The instructors were then asked to leave the room during the entire data collection period. The students were provided adequate information about the study. After signing the informed consent form, the students were handed the questionnaire and given 15–20 minutes to complete. After the allotted time, the researcher collected the questionnaires. The answered questionnaires were kept in a locked cabinet until the data collection period had ended.

Ethical Considerations

The research protocol was reviewed and approved by the institutional review board of King Saud University College of Medicine (Project No. E-17-2633). Permission to conduct the study was given by the deans of the colleges of nursing of the two universities. The researcher provided the students with necessary information about the study, their rights (e.g., voluntary participation, right to withdraw before completing the questionnaire, and right of confidentiality), and their expected responsibilities as participants. Adequate time was provided to the students to ask questions about the study. Written informed consent was provided by the students to confirm their voluntary participation. Students were asked to not write anything that would identify them in the questionnaire. To protect the students from possible coercion or undue influence, students of the researcher were excluded from participation, data were collected while the instructors were not present, confidentiality was assured, and students were informed that their class performance would not be affected by their decision to participate or not.

Data Analysis

Statistical tests were conducted using SPSS Version 22.0 (IBM, Armonk, NY, USA). The demographic characteristics of the participants were fully described using descriptive statistics. The palliative care knowledge of the participants was shown in terms of means, standard deviations, frequency counts, and percentages. One-way analysis of variance with Tukey's honestly significant difference tests and t tests were performed to examine the associations between the participants' demographic variables and their knowledge, with the predictors of palliative care knowledge identified using standard multiple linear regression.

Results

As shown in Table 1, most participants were enrolled in the public university (55.3%), were female (69.4%), had participated in nonuniversity sessions on palliative care during the last 5 years (58.2%), and were not able to attend a palliative care course at their nursing school (65.5%). A high proportion of the participants were registered in the fourth year of their nursing program (33.7%), with 26.7% registered in their second year and 19.8% registered, respectively, in their third year and internship year.

Palliative Care Knowledge

The mean score for palliative care knowledge was 5.23 (SD = 3.24), with scores ranging from 0 to 12, indicating a

TABLE 1.
Demographic Characteristics of the Participants (N = 409)

Demographic	n	%
Type of university		
Private	183	44.7
Public	226	55.3
Year of study		
Second	109	26.7
Third	81	19.8
Fourth	138	33.7
Internship	81	19.8
Gender		
Female	284	69.4
Male	125	30.6
Received a nonuniversity educational session on palliative care during the last 5 years		
No	171	41.8
Yes	238	58.2
Attended a palliative care course at your nursing school		
No	268	65.5
Yes	141	34.5

generally poor knowledge of palliative care. Only 40 participants (9.8%) answered at least 50% of the questions correctly, whereas 90.2% obtained scores lower than 10. Table 2 shows the percentage of correct and incorrect answers achieved by the participants for each item. The range of correct responses for each item was 8.6%–54.0%. Item 4, "Adjuvant therapies are important in managing pain," yielded the highest number of correct responses (54.0%) and was the only item that was answered correctly by more than 50% of the participants. Item 13, "The use of placebos is appropriate in the treatment of some types of pain," received the lowest percentage of correct answers (8.6%), followed by Item 5, "It is crucial for family members to remain at the bedside until death" (12.7%). In terms of the three theoretical dimensions, most of the items in the "pain and symptoms management" dimension received a higher frequency of correct responses than the items in the dimensions of "philosophy and principles of palliative care" and "psychological and spiritual care.". The "philosophy and principles of palliative care" dimension earned a mean score of 0.79 (SD = 0.72, range = 0–3), whereas the dimensions "pain and symptoms management" and "psychosocial and spiritual care" received mean scores of 3.89 (SD = 2.62, range = 0–10) and 0.54 (SD = 0.77, range = 0–3), respectively. Thus, the participants lacked palliative care knowledge in the realms of palliative care principles and philosophy, management of pain and other symptoms, and psychosocial and spiritual care.

Table 3 summarizes the association between participant demographic characteristics and palliative care knowledge. The participants enrolled in the private university had significantly higher scores than their peers enrolled in the public university (t = 5.62, p < .001). Moreover, those in their fourth year had significantly lower scores than those in their second year (F = 3.48, p = .016). Those who had received nonuniversity educational sessions on palliative care during the last 5 years (t = -5.06, p < .001) and those who had attended a palliative care course at their nursing school (t = -5.23, p < .001) showed significantly higher palliative care knowledge than their peers who had not. Thus, these findings suggest that all of the examined demographic characteristics, with the exception of gender, were significantly associated with level of palliative care knowledge.

Predictors of Palliative Care Knowledge Among the Participants

The PCQN scores were entered into a regression model, with demographic characteristics designated as the predictor variables. The regression model was statistically significant, F(7, 401) = 12.64, p < .001, accounting for approximately 16.6% of the variance in palliative care knowledge (R^2 = .181, adjusted R^2 = .166). In Table 4, type of university, year of study, attending a nonuniversity educational session on palliative care during the last 5 years, and attending a university palliative care course are all identified as significant predictors of palliative care knowledge. The scores of the public university

TABLE 2.

Palliative Care Knowledge Among the Participants (N = 409)

Item	Correct Answer		Incorrect Answer	
	n	%	n	%
Philosophy and principles of palliative care				
1. Palliative care is only appropriate in situations where there is evidence of a downward trajectory or deterioration. (F)	73	17.8	336	82.2
9. The provision of palliative care requires emotional detachment. (F)	79	19.3	330	80.7
12. The philosophy of palliative care is compatible with that of aggressive treatment. (T)	123	30.1	286	69.9
17. The accumulation of losses makes burnout inevitable for those who work in palliative care. (F)	50	12.2	359	87.8
Pain and symptoms management				
2. Morphine is the standard used to compare the analgesic effect of other opioids. (T)	151	36.9	258	63.1
3. The extent of the disease determines the method of pain treatment. (F)	74	18.1	335	81.9
4. Adjuvant therapies are important in managing pain. (T)	221	54.0	188	46.0
6. During the last days of life, drowsiness associated with electrolyte imbalance may decrease the need for sedation. (T)	137	33.5	272	66.5
7. Drug addiction is a major problem when morphine is used on a long-term basis for the management of pain. (F)	77	18.8	332	81.2
8. Individuals who are taking opioids should also follow a bowel regime (laxative treatment). (T)	139	34.0	270	66.0
10. During the terminal stages of an illness, drugs that can cause respiratory depression are appropriate for the treatment of severe dyspnea. (T)	147	35.9	262	64.1
13. The use of placebos is appropriate in the treatment of some types of pain. (F)	35	8.6	374	91.4
14. High-dose codeine causes more nausea and vomiting than morphine. (T)	147	35.9	262	64.1
15. Suffering and physical pain are identical. (F)	83	20.3	326	79.7
16. Demerol (pethidine) is not an effective analgesic for the control of chronic pain. (T)	87	21.3	322	78.7
18. Manifestations of chronic pain are different from those of acute pain. (T)	165	40.3	244	59.7
20. Pain threshold is lowered by fatigue or anxiety. (T)	130	31.8	279	68.2
Psychosocial and spiritual care				
5. It is crucial for family members to remain at the bedside until death occurs. (F)	52	12.7	357	87.3
11. Men generally reconcile their grief more quickly than women. (F)	88	21.5	321	78.5
19. The loss of a distant relationship is easier to resolve than the loss of one that is close or intimate. (F)	80	19.6	329	80.4

Note. The T (True) or F (False) at the end of each item is the correct answer in that item.

participants were 1.31 points (*t* = –4.16, *p* < .001, 95% CI [–1.92, –0.69]) lower than those studying at the private university. The mean knowledge score for fourth-year nursing students was 1.77 points lower than the mean score for second-year nursing students (*t* = –4.30, *p* < .001, 95% CI [–2.58, –0.96]). Furthermore, the mean knowledge scores for those who had attended a nonuniversity palliative care educational session during the last 5 years (*t* = 3.20, *p* < .001, 95% CI [0.50, 2.09]) and those who had attended a university palliative care course (*t* = 3.34, *p* < .001, 95% CI [0.53, 2.06]) earned an average of 1.29 points more than their peers who had not.

Discussion

This study assessed palliative care knowledge among nursing students enrolled in private and public universities in Saudi Arabia. The mean PCQN score of participants was 5.23, and only 9.8% of the participants answered more than 50% of the questions correctly. This result suggests that the palliative care knowledge of Saudi Arabian nursing students is

inadequate. Previous studies conducted in other countries report similarly low knowledge among nursing students, although the mean score in this study was even lower than in those previous studies (Al Qadire, 2014; Karkada, Nayak, & Malathi, 2011). The mean score reported for nursing students in the southeastern United States was 12.19 (*SD* = 2.58; Pope, 2013). Furthermore, the present results indicate considerable misconceptions regarding palliative care. For example, 91.4% thought that placebos were appropriate for the treatment of some types of pain, and 87.3% believed that family members should remain at the bedside until a patient's death. The findings of the study also revealed that the participants had very low knowledge of the three theoretical dimensions of palliative care that are measured by the PCQN. Knowledge of palliative care philosophy and principles as well as of psychological and spiritual care were observed to be poorer compared with the dimension of pain and symptom management.

The low scores reported in this study may be associated with the inadequate curricular content related to palliative care at the two targeted universities. Although the curricular

TABLE 3.

Association Between the Demographic Profile and Palliative Care Knowledge of Participants (N = 409)

Demographic	M (SD)	t/F	p
Type of university			
Private	6.17 (2.77)	5.62	< .001***
Public	4.46 (3.39)		
Year of study[a]			
Second	5.88 (3.14)	F = 3.48	.016*
Third	5.01 (3.07)		
Fourth	4.64 (3.62)		
Internship	5.57 (2.66)		
Gender			
Female	5.30 (3.20)	0.64	.521
Male	5.07 (3.35)		
Received a nonuniversity educational session on palliative care during the last 5 years			
No	4.30 (3.10)	−5.06	< .001***
Yes	5.90 (3.18)		
Attended a palliative care course at your nursing school			
No	4.64 (3.02)	−5.23	< .001***
Yes	6.35 (3.37)		

[a]Second year versus fourth year (p = .014).
*p < .05. ***p < .001.

content of the two universities was not examined in this study, 65.5% of the participants reported not having received formal palliative care training from their nursing school. The literature supports the essentiality of palliative care nursing education in improving the knowledge, practice, and attitudes of nurses regarding palliative care (Al Qadire, 2014; Gillan, van der Riet, & Jeong, 2014). However, nursing students continue to feel unprepared to deal with issues related to death and dying

because they receive inadequate related education. This phenomenon is supported by a literature review conducted by Gillan et al. (2014), who found insufficient end-of-life content in nursing books and deficient palliative care content in undergraduate nursing curricula. Furthermore, the poor knowledge of the participants regarding palliative care philosophy and principles support the need to improve the curricular content of palliative care courses in nursing education. Basic principles of palliative care such as defining the concept, the objectives and essence of palliative care, and the philosophical underpinnings of palliative care should be reinforced in curricula. Notably, the study also revealed poor knowledge in the psychosocial and spiritual care dimension of palliative care. This finding may relate to cultural considerations. For instance, more than three fourths of the participants believed that family members should remain at the bedside until patient death. This misconception may be rooted in the close family ties that are typical in Saudi culture and society as well as the Saudi belief that caring for a dying family member is the responsibility of the family (Aljawi & Harford, 2012). Moreover, despite being a religious and spiritual country, several studies have reported poor spiritual care competencies for Saudi nursing students. Similar studies have reported that the incompetence of nursing students in this area is related to the inadequacy of curricular contents focusing on spirituality in relation to health and spiritual nursing care (Cruz, Alshammari, Alotaibi, & Colet, 2017; Cruz, Alshammari, & Colet, 2017). Hence, spiritual care should be included in the nursing curriculum in the country, either integrated into existing courses such as the Fundamentals of Nursing or added as a separate course dealing specifically with this topic.

In addition, the poor level of palliative care knowledge may relate to the underdevelopment and unpopularity of palliative care in Saudi Arabia, where palliative care is given less emphasis than other nursing specializations. Despite the advancements in palliative care introduced in the country, further efforts are still required to achieve the optimal level of palliative care. Increased awareness among public and health professionals and support from the authorities are

TABLE 4.

Predictors of Palliative Care Knowledge Among the Participants (N = 409)

Predictor Variable	B	SE b	β	t	p	95% CI
Type of university	−1.31	0.32	−0.20	−4.16	<.001***	[−1.92, −0.69]
Year of study (reference group = second)						
Third	−0.12	0.45	−0.01	−0.26	.796	[−1.00, 0.76]
Fourth	−1.77	0.41	−0.26	−4.30	<.001***	[−2.58, −0.96]
Internship	−0.08	0.45	−0.01	−0.18	.856	[−0.97, 0.81]
Gender	0.26	0.32	0.04	0.80	.424	[−0.38, 0.90]
Received a nonuniversity educational session on palliative care during the last 5 years	1.29	0.40	0.20	3.20	.001**	[0.50, 2.09]
Attended a palliative care course at your nursing school	1.29	0.39	0.19	3.34	.001**	[0.53, 2.06]

**p < .01. ***p < .001.

necessary to fully maximize the palliative care specialty in the country (Zeinah et al., 2013). Moreover, investment and improvement of education among healthcare professionals regarding palliative care remains a great challenge that requires immediate action (Alshammary et al., 2014).

The knowledge of palliative care among the nursing students in this study was associated with and predicted by several demographic characteristics. The levels of palliative knowledge among the private university nursing students, second-year nursing students, those who had received nonuniversity educational sessions on palliative care during the past 5 years, and those who had attended a palliative care course in their nursing school were all significantly higher than those of their peers. These demographic characteristics significantly predicted the level of palliative care knowledge among the participants. The higher level of knowledge among the participants who were enrolled in the private university may relate to differences in the content of the nursing curriculum between the two universities. The percentages of the participants who had received nonuniversity palliative care training during the last 5 years (66.1% vs. 51.8%) and who had taken a palliative care course at their nursing school (39.3% vs. 30.5%) were higher among the private university students than the public university students. Although this variation may also explain the difference, this finding could not be compared with results of other studies because of the lack of studies comparing the palliative care knowledge between private and public university students. However, this result has important implications for nursing education in Saudi Arabia and worldwide. Nursing education in Saudi Arabia should have unified curricular contents to address the needs of the nursing students in the country, regardless of university type.

The levels of knowledge of the participants who were in their second year were higher than those of the participants in their fourth year. This finding differs from previous findings showing that the palliative care knowledge of nursing students steadily increases as they progress through their nursing program (Al Qadire, 2014). This difference may be attributed to the integration of palliative care concepts into the course on Fundamentals of Nursing, which is currently taken by second-year students. The information regarding this concept, as partially discussed in the Fundamentals of Nursing, is still fresh among these students. Spiritual care, a part of palliative care, is also integrated and taught in Arabic and Islamic courses, which are part of the preparatory years and the second year of the nursing program (Cruz, Alshammari, Alotaibi, et al., 2017; Cruz, Alshammari, & Colet, 2017).

The levels of knowledge among the nursing students who had received a nonuniversity palliative care educational session during the past 5 years and those who had attended a palliative care course at the university were higher than those of the students without similar experiences. The impacts of palliative care training programs on the knowledge, attitudes, beliefs, and practices of nurses and other healthcare professionals have been studied previously. For instance, a multicenter study on bedside nurses in intensive care units initially implemented and evaluated a palliative care professional development program, reporting that the palliative care skills of nurses who undergo this training were improved and that their ability to identify palliative care needs and to create plans to address such needs was enhanced (Anderson et al., 2017). Another study that examined the effects of a palliative care training program on physiotherapists reported significant improvements in palliative care knowledge, attitudes, beliefs, and practices (Kumar, Jim, & Sisodia, 2011). Considering the importance of palliative care courses in the nursing program, Dobbins (2011) and Kirkpatrick et al. (2017) showed the positive impact of these courses on students' palliative care knowledge. Palliative care education is a critical factor in preparing nursing students for end-of-life care, which may be the most important aspect of nursing students' attitudes toward caring for the dying (Gillan et al., 2014). Nursing undergraduate training should incorporate considerable amounts of both didactic and clinical contents on palliative care to ensure that nursing students are properly prepared (Barrere, Durkin, & LaCoursiere, 2008). Thus, nursing faculty members have a unique opportunity and valuable contribution to enhance the provision of care among patients with serious illnesses and their families by giving effective education that ensures the development of students' palliative care competencies (Ferrell et al., 2016).

Limitations

This study has several limitations, which should be considered when interpreting the results. The study was conducted only in two universities that were located in the central region of Saudi Arabia. Moreover, the use of convenience sampling may affect the generalizability of findings. The curriculum content and the type of educational and training program that the students attended were not thoroughly elucidated in the study. Future studies should consider examining these variables in detail to explain their influence on student knowledge.

Conclusions and Implications

The study provides significant information on the palliative care knowledge of nursing students in Saudi Arabia. The students manifested levels of palliative care knowledge that were significantly lower than the levels reported in previous studies of this issue around the world. Being enrolled in a private university, being in the second year of a nursing program, attending nonuniversity palliative care educational sessions, and attending a university palliative care course in the nursing program were all identified as significant predictors of increased levels of palliative care knowledge.

The findings may be used as a basis for establishing educational policies and interventions to enhance palliative care education among nursing students and to ensure the quality of palliative care in Saudi Arabia and elsewhere. Several recommendations to improve nursing education in Saudi Arabia and in other countries follow. First, nursing education must provide a nursing curriculum with adequate palliative care content to properly prepare nursing students for their future roles. Second, palliative care nursing must be integrated into the nursing curriculum and must emphasize the different dimensions of palliative care such as palliative care philosophy and principles, pain and symptom management, and psychosocial and spiritual care. Moreover, cultural and religious considerations affecting the provision of palliative care should be emphasized in palliative care courses to avoid misconceptions. Third, nursing institutions in Saudi Arabia should adopt uniform curricular content on palliative care to address the knowledge gap between nursing students studying at private and public universities. Fourth, spiritual care nursing should be integrated into the nursing curriculum in Saudi Arabia. Fifth, additional learning opportunities such as palliative care training and seminars should be provided to students to strengthen their palliative care knowledge and competencies. Sixth, palliative care concepts should be reinforced in the clinical area to fill in the gap between classroom and clinical learning and to ensure the continuous learning of the students as they progress in their nursing program.

Acknowledgment

This study was funded by the Deanship of Scientific Research at King Saud University, Saudi Arabia, through Research Group No. RG-1436017.

References

Al Qadire, M. (2014). Knowledge of palliative care: An online survey. *Nurse Education Today, 34*(5), 714–718. https://doi.org/10.1016/j.nedt.2013.08.019

Aldossary, A., While, A., & Barriball, L. (2008). Health care and nursing in Saudi Arabia. *International Nursing Review, 55*(1), 125–128. https://doi.org/10.1111/j.1466-7657.2007.00596.x

Aljawi, D. M., & Harford, J. B. (2012). Palliative care in the Muslim-majority countries: The need for more and better care. In E. Chang (Ed.), *Contemporary and innovative practice in palliative care* (Chap. 9, pp. 137–151). Rijeka, Croatia: InTech. https://doi.org/10.5772/32452

Alshammary, S. A., Abdullah, A., Duraisamy, B. P., & Anbar, M. (2014). Palliative care in Saudi Arabia: Two decades of progress and going strong. *Journal of Health Specialties, 2*(2), 59–60. https://doi.org/10.4103/1658-600X.131749

Anderson, W. G., Puntillo, K., Cimino, J., Noort, J., Pearson, D., Boyle, D., & Pantilat, S. Z. (2017). Palliative care professional development for critical care nurses: A multicenter program.

American Journal of Critical Care, 26*(5), 361–371. https://doi.org/10.4037/ajcc2017336

Barrere, C. C., Durkin, A., & LaCoursiere, S. (2008). The influence of end-of-life education on attitudes of nursing students. *International Journal of Nursing Education Scholarship, 5*(1), 1–18. https://doi.org/10.2202/1548-923X.1494

Borneman, T. (2011). Palliative care nursing. *Current Problems in Cancer, 35*(6), 351–356. https://doi.org/10.1016/j.currproblcancer.2011.10.009

Cruz, J. P. (2017). Quality of life and its influence on clinical competence among nurses: A self-reported study. *Journal of Clinical Nursing, 26*(3–4), 388–399. https://doi.org/10.1111/jocn.13402

Cruz, J. P., Alshammari, F., Alotaibi, K. A., & Colet, P. C. (2017). Spirituality and spiritual care perspectives among baccalaureate nursing students in Saudi Arabia: A cross-sectional study. *Nurse Education Today, 49*, 156–162. https://doi.org/10.1016/j.nedt.2016.11.027

Cruz, J. P., Alshammari, F., & Colet, P. C. (2017). Psychometric properties of the Spiritual Care-Giving Scale–Arabic version in Saudi nursing students. *Journal of Holistic Nursing, 35*(2), 175–184. https://doi.org/10.1177/0898010116647804

Dobbins, E. H. (2011). The impact of end-of-life curriculum content on the attitudes of associate degree nursing students toward death and care of the dying. *Teaching and Learning in Nursing, 6*(4), 159–166. https://doi.org/10.1016/j.teln.2011.04.002

Ferrell, B., Malloy, P., Mazanec, P., & Virani, R. (2016). CARES: AACN's new competencies and recommendations for educating undergraduate nursing students to improve palliative care. *Journal of Professional Nursing, 32*(5), 327–333. https://doi.org/10.1016/j.profnurs.2016.07.002

Gillan, P. C., van der Riet, P. J., & Jeong, S. (2014). End of life care education, past and present: A review of the literature. *Nurse Education Today, 34*(3), 331–342. https://doi.org/10.1016/j.nedt.2013.06.009

Glover, T. L., Garvan, C., Nealis, R. M., Citty, S. W., & Derrico, D. J. (2017). Improving end-of-life care knowledge among senior baccalaureate nursing students. *American Journal of Hospice and Palliative Medicine, 34*(10), 938–945. https://doi.org/10.1177/1049909117693214

Henoch, I., Melin-Johansson, C., Bergh, I., Strang, S., Ek, K., Hammarlund, K., & Browall, M. (2017). Undergraduate nursing students' attitudes and preparedness toward caring for dying persons—A longitudinal study. *Nurse Education in Practice, 26*, 12–20. https://doi.org/10.1016/j.nepr.2017.06.007

Hold, J. L., Blake, B. J., & Ward, E. N. (2015). Perceptions and experiences of nursing students enrolled in a palliative and end-of-life nursing elective: A qualitative study. *Nurse Education Today, 35*(6), 777–781. https://doi.org/10.1016/j.nedt.2015.02.011

Karkada, S., Nayak, B. S., & Malathi (2011). Awareness of palliative care among diploma nursing students. *Indian Journal of Palliative Care, 17*(1), 20–23. https://doi.org/10.4103/0973-1075.78445

Khraisat, O. M., Hamdan, M., & Ghazzawwi, M. (2017). Palliative care issues and challenges in Saudi Arabia: Knowledge assessment among nursing students. *Journal of Palliative Care, 32*(3–4), 121–126. https://doi.org/10.1177/0825859717743229

Kirkpatrick, A. J., Cantrell, M. A., & Smeltzer, S. C. (2017). Palliative care simulations in undergraduate nursing education: An integrative review. *Clinical Simulation in Nursing, 13*(9), 414–431. https://doi.org/10.1016/j.ecns.2017.04.009

Kumar, S. P., Jim, A., & Sisodia, V. (2011). Effects of palliative care training program on knowledge, attitudes, beliefs and experiences among student physiotherapists: A preliminary quasi-experimental study. *Indian Journal of Palliative Care, 17*(1), 47–53. https://doi.org/10.4103/0973-1075.78449

Pope, A. (2013). *Palliative care knowledge among bachelors of science nursing students* (Master's thesis). Kennesaw State University, Georgia, USA. Retrieved from https://digitalcommons.kennesaw.edu/cgi/viewcontent.cgi?article=1599&context=etd

Prem, V., Karvannan, H., Kumar, S. P., Karthikbabu, S., Syed, N., Sisodia, V., & Jaykumar, S. (2012). Study of nurses' knowledge about palliative care: A quantitative cross-sectional survey. *Indian Journal of Palliative Care, 18*(2), 122–127. https://doi.org/10.4103/0973-1075.100832

Ross, M. M., McDonald, B., & McGuinness, J. (1996). The palliative care quiz for nursing (PCQN): The development of an instrument to measure nurses' knowledge of palliative care. *Journal of Advanced Nursing, 23*(1), 126–137. https://doi.org/10.1111/j.1365-2648.1996.tb03106.x

Sarhill, N., LeGrand, S., Islambouli, R., Davis, M. P., & Walsh, D. (2001). The terminally ill Muslim: Death and dying from the Muslim perspective. *American Journal of Hospice and Palliative Medicine, 18*(4), 251–255. https://doi.org/10.1177/104990910101800409

Seow, H., & Bainbridge, D. (2018). A review of the essential components of quality palliative care in the home. *Journal of Palliative Medicine, 21*(S1), S37–S44. https://doi.org/10.1089/jpm.2017.0392

Steinberg, S. M. (2011). Cultural and religious aspects of palliative care. *International Journal of Critical Illness and Injury Science, 1*(2), 154–156. https://doi.org/10.4103/2229-5151.84804

Tayeb, M. A., Al-Zamel, E., Fareed, M. M., & Abouellail, H. A. (2010). A "good death": Perspectives of Muslim patients and health care providers. *Annals of Saudi Medicine, 30*(3), 215–221. https://doi.org/10.4103/0256-4947.62836

Usta, E., Aygin, D., & Sağlam, E. (2016). Knowledge and opinions of nursing students on palliative care: A university example. *Journal of Human Sciences, 13*(3), 4405–4415. https://doi.org/10.14687/jhs.v13i3.3917

Williams, A. M., Donovan, R., Stajduhar, K., & Spitzer, D. (2015). Cultural influences on palliative family caregiving: Service recommendations specific to the Vietnamese in Canada. *BMC Research Notes, 8*(1), 280. https://doi.org/10.1186/s13104-015-1252-3

Zeinah, G. F., Al-Kindi, S. G., & Hassan, A. A. (2013). Middle East experience in palliative care. *American Journal of Hospice and Palliative Medicine, 30*(1), 94–99. https://doi.org/10.1177/1049909112439619

22

Exploring the Barriers Faced by Nephrology Nurses in Initiating Patients with Chronic Kidney Disease into Advance Care Planning Using Focus-Group Interviews

Jui-O CHEN[1] • Chiu-Chu LIN[2]*

ABSTRACT

Background: The prevalence of end-stage renal disease in Taiwan is the highest in the world. The rate of signing advance directives in Taiwan is lower than in Western countries, and most of the barriers that have been identified relate to initiating advance care planning (ACP).

Purpose: This study was designed to explore the barriers to discussing ACP with patients with chronic kidney disease faced by nephrology nurses.

Methods: A descriptive qualitative study design was adopted. The Consolidated Criteria for Reporting Qualitative Research was used to report the findings of this study. Data were collected using purposive sampling. A total of 34 nephrology nurses were recruited from hospitals in northern (2 groups, 10 participants), central (1 group, 4 participants), and southern (5 groups, 20 participants) Taiwan. A qualitative content analysis was conducted to analyze the transcripts of the eight focus groups.

Results: Five themes were identified, including (a) lacking the confidence to discuss ACP, (b) difficulty in finding an appropriate opportunity to initiate ACP discussion, (c) personally lacking the characteristics to discuss ACP, (d) conflicting perspectives between doctors and nurses over ACP, and (e) culture and belief-based barriers to discussing ACP.

Conclusions/Implications for Practice: The findings obtained from the interviews revealed that nurses must enhance their ACP-related knowledge and communication skills and foster personal confidence in initiating ACP discussions. Furthermore, nurses must be empowered to work with other healthcare professionals. To implement the initial process of discussing ACP in clinical settings, clinical guidelines should be developed for healthcare professionals on initiating ACP. These measures may facilitate improved collaboration in healthcare settings and further encourage patients and their families to participate in shared decision-making that may help patients complete advance directives and thereby achieve better care quality at the end of life.

KEY WORDS:
advance care planning, advance directives, chronic kidney disease, nephrology nurses.

Introduction

Taiwan has the world's highest prevalence of end-stage renal disease (ESRD; Tsai et al., 2018). Patients with ESRD may depend on hemodialysis for life-sustaining treatment and survival. During hemodialysis, patients may encounter critical conditions and require emergency treatment for which, even after cardiopulmonary resuscitation, the mortality rate is approximately 60% and overall survival averages less than 6 months (Sinclair et al., 2017). Under these circumstances, if they have signed advance directives (ADs), these patients have the latitude not to suffer from resuscitation efforts that are medically futile. In other words, signing an AD in advance is the best way to have a good death, which is defined as dying with a sense of emotional well-being, passing away with dignity, and feeling as though one has completed one's life (Meier et al., 2016). However, only about 740,000 people (around 4%) have signed ADs in Taiwan as of September 2020 (Ministry of Health and Welfare, ROC, 2020). This rate is much lower than in Western countries where the rate ranges from 10% to 20%. In light of the above, identifying the major reasons for the low rate of signing ADs in Taiwan is important.

Advance care planning (ACP) is a means for patients to communicate their wishes, fears, and desires for health decisions that must be made after they lose the ability to consider them (Blackwood et al., 2019). ACP addresses issues including disease prognosis, decision-making in life-sustaining treatment, healthcare proxy appointments, and medical care preferences at the end of life. ADs, as a component of ACP, are legal documents that record patient's treatment and other

[1]PhD, RN, Assistant Professor, Department of Nursing, Tajen University, Pingtung, Taiwan, ROC. • [2]PhD, RN, Professor, School of Nursing; Department of Renal Care, College of Medicine; and Department of Medical Research, Kaohsiung Medical University Hospital, Kaohsiung Medical University, Kaohsiung, Taiwan, ROC.

preferences in the event of incapacity. However, ACP does not always include ADs, such as when a patient does not voice their preferences. How and Koh (2015) indicated that ACP may be as simple as a chat about the patient's end of life wishes with their trusted loved ones and may involve their healthcare providers. These interactions may be documented using available online resources.

Traditionally, the therapeutic relationship between doctors and patients is considered the best platform through which to introduce and initiate the ACP conversation. This is why healthcare professionals are encouraged to initiate patients into ACP and assist them in signing ADs. Detering et al. (2010) noted that clinicians have a responsibility to help patients explore treatment options and formulate their own preferences based on risk–benefit analyses and their personal values to make decisions regarding end of life care. The healthcare provider participating in the ACP discussion does not need to be a clinician. Ideally, that person should be a healthcare provider who is able to work with the medical team and provide information about the prognosis. The existing literature does not indicate the best timing to initiate patients into ACP, and there is currently no related consensus among physicians.

Miller et al. (2019) indicated the incidence of ACP discussions is low and that common barriers to healthcare professionals conducting ACP include perceived lack of time, inadequate training, and lack of experience and confidence. The two important barriers to conducting ACP discussions with patients were insufficient time and lack of knowledge (Beck et al., 2017). Davison (2010) interviewed patients with ESRD and found that they expect their healthcare providers to be capable of initiating ACP with them to help them remain autonomous in making decisions regarding their end of life care. In addition, many felt that ACP should be initiated by the dialysis team at the early stage of the dialysis process. Most desired efficient communication with regard to care plans, prognosis, and ACP. Goff et al. (2015) found that many patients expressed a desire for better education about what to expect from dialysis and more opportunities to participate in medical care decision-making. Likewise, Gjerberg et al. (2015) indicated that a majority of patients with ESRD prefer to be involved in the decision-making process but leave the final decisions to healthcare professionals. Conversations about end of life care issues are emotionally challenging, and few patients discuss these issues with their families. In fact, the reported opinions of relatives regarding a patient's preferences are based primarily on that patient's personal assumptions rather than relatives' statements. However, both patients and their family members expect healthcare providers to raise issues related to ACP (Gjerberg et al., 2015). The purpose of ACP is to help reflect the life values and preferences of patients in their medical care when they are at the end of life. However, the barriers to ACP currently highlighted in the literature reflect mainly the Western perspective. The major reason for the low rate of signing ADs in Taiwan is not clear, and there is scant literature addressing ADs in this country. Therefore, the purpose of this study was to explore the barriers faced by nurses to discussing ACP with patients with chronic kidney disease (CKD).

Methods

Study Design

A descriptive, qualitative design was used in this study, and data were collected from November 2017 to September 2018. The Consolidated Criteria for Reporting Qualitative Research was used to report the findings. Qualitative focus-group interviews were conducted to identify the self-perceived barriers of nephrology nurses to discussing ACP with patients.

Sample and Setting

After receiving institutional review board approval, the researcher contacted the head nurses to explain the purpose of the study and openly recruited nursing staff using purposive sampling. All of the 34 participants enrolled in this study were nephrology nurses who had been working for at least 1 year in the hemodialysis unit or nephrology ward in northern (one hospital with two groups of five participants in each group), central (one hospital with one group of four participants), or southern Taiwan (two hospitals with three and two groups of four participants each). Part-time nurses were excluded. Focus-group interviews were conducted with eight groups of four to five participants each.

Procedures for Data Collection

A 60- to 90-minute interview was conducted with each group by two members of the research team in the meeting room of the hospital where the participants worked. The leader of the group interview sessions was a doctorally prepared nursing teacher who was proficient in group dynamics and qualitative research. Another research team member obtained informed consent from the participants, made the audio recording of the interviews, and took notes. The semistructured interviews asked participants several opening questions regarding ACP. Participant observation also conducted during the interviews was aimed at collecting impressions and rich data regarding how participants interacted in particular situations and contexts. Direct observations brought other insights to the study as well. Once the interviews were finished, the researchers jotted down important messages as a reflection on the interviews. All of the interviews were transcribed in full within 48 hours. The interview guidelines were as follows:

1. Please share your opinions on promoting ACP in your work unit.
2. Have you ever had experience discussing ACP with patients?
   a. If so, could you please talk about how you initiate patients into ACP? Have you encountered any difficulties when discussing ACP with patients? Could you elaborate on your discussions with patients?
   b. If not, could you share the reasons why you have not discussed ACP with your patients?

3. Do you think there are any potential solutions to resolving your problems related to discussing ACP with patients?

Data Analysis

After interviews were transcribed, the data were analyzed in accordance with Colaizzi's (1978) method. The coding of transcripts was conducted by two researchers using the following steps: (a) read and reread all of the verbatim transcripts, (b) identify significant statements, (c) formulate meanings, (d) cluster themes (differences in analyses of key sentences or themes between the two researchers were resolved by inviting qualitative research experts to discuss the data), (e) develop an exhaustive description, (f) generate a fundamental structure, and (g) seek verification of the fundamental structure. In the final step, researchers referred to participants' comments again to validate and clarify the findings. Furthermore, the content of the analysis was reviewed by two participants to validate the original meaning of the data. Based on the principle of theoretical saturation, the focus-group discussion sessions were run until a clear pattern emerged and subsequent groups produced no new information (Krueger & Casey, 2000).

Rigor

Rigor was evaluated using Lincoln and Guba's (1985) criteria to establish analysis rigor. Trustworthiness, dependability, and confirmability were strengthened using an audit trail. To ensure credibility and dependability, the identified themes were reviewed multiple times by the research team. After the interviews, the recordings were transcribed. Transferability indicates the applicability of the results to other groups. In this study, as all of the participants were from CKD-related work units, their experiences and perceptions may be transferable to nephrology nurses in general in Taiwan. To ensure confirmability, the original interview recordings and documents have been preserved and are available for auditing and future study use.

Ethical Considerations

Approval for the study was obtained from Kaohsiung Medical University institutional review board in Taiwan (KMUHIRB-E-(I) 20150279). Before signing informed consent, the participants received full written and verbal explanations of the study. The participants were informed that they could withdraw at any time before the interview began. The data collected for this study were kept confidential and used for this study only. All data and transcripts were anonymized and coded, and personal information was hidden in the data analysis.

Results

Thirty-four female nurses were enrolled as participants. Their ages ranged from 29 to 54 years and averaged 41 years; 94.1% held a bachelor's degree; their working experience ranged from 1 to 25 years (average of 11.2 years); and 12 (35.1%) had experience initiating ACP discussions with patients (N1, N2, N3, N6, N7, N12, N16, N18, N20, N22, N24, and N34). In this study, five major themes were identified, as follows (Table 1).

Theme 1: Lacking the Confidence to Discuss ACP

Lack of ACP-related knowledge and skills, coupled with lack of practical experience, led participants to fear they would not be able to discuss ACP with patients. This theme consists of two subthemes, as follows:

Subtheme 1: Lack of knowledge and communication skills

Participants were consciously unfamiliar with ACP content and the operational process. Furthermore, they feared missing important messages and having insufficient communication skills to open up ACP discussions. One participant said: "Most of the nurses are not familiar with the content and procedures.... Nurses do not know how to register IC cards and may worry that they are not able to answer patients' questions. I feel that I lack relevant knowledge and training experience, so I am not confident about initiating patients into ACP" (excerpt from N1). Another participant said: "I feel that initiating patients into ACP takes lots of time, and I am afraid of missing something important and of not

Table 1

Themes and Subthemes of Barriers to Initiating ACP Discussions Faced by Nephrology Nurses

Theme	Subtheme
1. Lacking the confidence to discuss ACP	• Lack of knowledge and communication skills • Lack of practical experience
2. Difficulty in finding an appropriate opportunity to initiate ACP discussion	• Unpredictability of disease progression • Lack of discussion on clinical guidelines of ACP
3. Personally lacking the characteristics to discuss ACP	• Empathy with high sensitivity
4. Conflicting perspectives between doctors and nurses over ACP	• Cognitive gap related to discussing ACP between physicians and nurses • Initiating ACP is not the responsibility of nurses
5. Culture and belief-based barriers to discussing ACP	• ACP discussion implies misfortune • Reluctance to discuss ACP due to misunderstanding the essence of ACP

Note. ACP = advance care planning.

adequately or accurately elaborating on information. That means that I am not capable of doing this and I think that it is better to have someone more professional initiate the ACP discussion" (excerpt from N9).

Subtheme 2: Lack of practical experience

Participants were conscious that they had no practical experience in discussing ACP and were concerned that they did not have the ability to cope with complex patient problems. Participant N4 said: *"I feel that patients have many other issues. They may shed tears during the discussion. I wonder what I should do when patients get emotional during discussions. How should I comfort them and deal with their emotional issues? These are things I am not certain about."* Participant N2 said: *"You have to have that practical experience to talk to people before you know how to get involved in the process. When you provide the information he wants, he will put his trust in you."*

Theme 2: Difficulty in Finding an Appropriate Opportunity to Initiate Advance Care Planning Discussion

Hemodialysis usually helps patients maintain a good quality of life. Patients often lack disease awareness and cannot understand the significance of discussing ACP. There is a lack of consensus on the appropriate timing to discuss ACP, which makes it hard to determine when to intervene. This theme consists of two subthemes, as follows:

Subtheme 1: Unpredictability of disease progression

The many complications and comorbidities that may occur during hemodialysis make disease trajectories highly unpredictable and make it difficult to determine the appropriate timing for ACP intervention. Participant N14 said: *"There was a patient who was doing well on dialysis but was later diagnosed with lung cancer. He was unaware he had the choice to sign a DNR, and ultimately went on Endo. Prolonging the agony of death was hard on his family."* Participant N17 stated: *"It seems too early to mention ACP, as it is common for young patients to be on dialysis for at least 20 to 30 years. However, we have also come across young patients whose conditions worsened abruptly and unexpectedly, and it was too late for ACP. It is hard to determine the right timing to bring up ACP."* Participant N7 said: *"I think dialysis patients are a high-risk group. There was a patient who collapsed after drinking a sip of water before he was put on the dialysis machine, and CPR did not resuscitate him. Should all new patients be informed of ACP?"*

Subtheme 2: Lack of discussion on clinical guidelines of advance care planning

Nursing staff have expressed the intricacy involved in identifying an appropriate time to introduce ACP to patients without explicit guidelines. For instance, at the initial stages of dialysis, patients usually maintain a good quality of life without much change in lifestyle beyond the need for dialysis. Even at later stages of dialysis, mentioning ACP may cause anxiety in patients and family members who are unprepared to deal with the situation.

Participant N3 said: *"Patients receiving hemodialysis are actually maintaining a good life.... There is no special difference from ordinary persons. If I suddenly initiate them into ACP, they may not be able to understand why. Unless there is a change in patients' condition such as shock or infection, I am not to be able to find a good time to open the conversation about ACP."* Participant N22 said: *"In my opinion, patients may feel that it is not the right time to discuss ACP at the early stage of the disease. But if I initiate a topic of ACP at the critical period of time, the family members may get anxious, and patients may not be ready to face this. I really do not know when the best time to discuss ACP is."* Participant N34 said: *"Sometimes patients think that they are in good condition and wonder why they need to think about ACP.... If receiving hemodialysis improves their quality of life, they do not really have to think ahead on ACP. The most difficult part of conducting ACP is finding a good time to initiate the discussion, as patients' family members may just tell me there is no need to mention this."*

Theme 3: Personally Lacking the Characteristics to Discuss Advance Care Planning

Discussing the complex issue of ACP requires enthusiasm, a caring heart, willingness to listen, and empathy with patients' feelings. This theme consists of one subtheme, as follows:

Subtheme: Empathy with high sensitivity

Nursing staff believe that ACP is unusual in that it involves a wide range of topics and skills such as medical information, emotional states, and the ability to communicate with warmth and convey messages in a way that resonates with patients. Participant N12 stated: *"I think that I need to have the right personality traits to talk about ACP because not all nurses are able to initiate this discussion. Some have knowledge of ACP, but they lack the humanistic characteristics necessary to talk about it.... I feel that hospice nurses are more capable of initiating patients into ACP because they are able to handle patient emotions and know how to reach a patient's heart.... I am not able to do this."* Participant N11 said: *"Having knowledge is not adequate to initiate a discussion on ACP... I think that I need to be aware of the patient's psychological status, I feel I am not able to handle the patient's emotions at any time. I think it is very difficult for me to do so...."* Participant N20 said: *"I think that the one who initiates patients into ACP should have certain personality traits. This means that they have to be able to see people and talk to them with a warm heart. For me, I just feel like I am sharing health education information."*

Theme 4: Conflicting Perspectives Between Doctors and Nurses Over Advance Care Planning

Nursing staff feel frustrated in holding different ideals than physicians regarding the ACP discussion. They believe that physicians should take the lead in initiating and conducting ACP discussions and that these discussions should not be part of the responsibilities of nurses. This theme consists of two subthemes, as follows:

Subtheme 1: Cognitive gap related to discussing advance care planning between physicians and nurses

Nursing personnel believe that when a patient's condition changes, it is time to discuss ACP. But doctors argue that it is good to continue with dialysis treatment, with no need to discuss ACP. The position of physicians completely ignores patients' rights and interests. When medical staff hold conflicting ideals on ACP, nurses are often afraid to initiate discussions with patients out of deference to physician authority. Participant N6 said: *"Once I discussed ACP with a patient at a time when he had experienced hypotension and even shock during hemodialysis. His doctor thought that initiating patients into ACP was not necessary, and I was to blame in this circumstance. I think many doctors give patients lots of hope and rarely mention the risks involved in receiving hemodialysis. I feel that doctors are not supportive, so I feel quite frustrated."* Participant N7 had a similar experience: *"I used to take care of a patient in the ICU, and his condition was not very stable. His family thought of giving up hemodialysis. Before the family meeting regarding this issue, I told the family members that patients could refuse hemodialysis by signing a DNR. As a result, the doctor who was in charge was upset because he preferred to continue treatments for the patient. My point of view is quite different from the doctor and this is the difficult part, as, most likely, doctors differ from nurses with regard to ACP, so I do not know how to deal with this issue."* Participant N16 also said: *"When I occasionally mention DNR, doctors may think that the patient is not in that serious condition and question the necessity of signing a DNR. Doctors think that these patients will just keep receiving hemodialysis until they are unable to do so...I think that doctors are more in control over this."*

Subtheme 2: Initiating advance care planning is not the responsibility of nurses

Explaining the patient's condition and discussing ACP are clinical responsibilities of the physician and not part of the nurse's job. Participant N30 said: *"I think that talking about ACP is the doctor's duty. My primary job should be performing hemodialysis, so I will not take the initiative to talk about it. In addition, discussing ACP is not part of the daily care routine"* (excerpt from N30). Participant N31 also considered it not her job to discuss ACP, and she took a passive role. She said: *"Generally speaking, I do not take the initiative to*

explain patient conditions because it is not my duty. So I am more passive in discussing ACP. Unless patients ask me, I will not answer this type of question." Participant N13 considered the need to train dedicated personnel to perform this duty: *"Healthcare providers focus on their profession, and this type of work should be left to those who are more professional, so the hospital manager should develop a clear flow chart to assist nurses to initiate patients into ACP. Let the professionals do the work instead of any staff nurses."*

Theme 5: Culture and Belief-Based Barriers to Discussing Advance Care Planning

ACP discussions often involve the topic of death, which is a symbol of misfortune and conflict within the Chinese cultural context. Chinese people avoid speaking of death, and discussing ACP is commonly associated with giving up treatment. However, this misinterprets the core values of the ACP discussion. This theme consists of two subthemes, as follows:

Subtheme 1: Advance care planning discussion implies misfortune

Traditional culture takes a conservative point of view toward death, and people regard it as taboo. Participant N18 said: *"Taiwanese do not like to talk about death. Most patients refuse to talk about it when I try to initiate them into ACP, since it is very easy for them to connect ACP with death, which is considered a taboo topic in our culture."* Participant N2 said: *"I used to take care of a patient with diabetic foot. I took the initiative to discuss ACP with her daughter, but she kept refusing to have a conversation about this with me...as she thought that her mom's condition was not near-terminal. So, I stopped talking about this topic with her...I think that family members tend to connect ACP with death. When I am with patients, I am not comfortable talking about death, and patients are also afraid of facing this issue, as this is disallowed in our culture"* (excerpt from N5).

Subtheme 2: Reluctance to discuss advance care planning due to misunderstanding the essence of advance care planning

In Taiwan, people consider having a discussion on ACP is a matter reserved for patients with terminal illness. Patients and their families consider discussing ACP as an abandonment of treatment and a death penalty. They consider ACP as a means to prepare for the end of life. Participant N15 said: *"Once, a patient with hemodialysis asked me if ACP means DNR and if they needed to give up receiving treatment. I think that they do not quite understand the meaning of ACP. They believe that ACP means giving up on life, so half of patients and family members refuse to discuss this issue."* Participant N3 said: *"When I mention ACP, patients and their family think I am cursing them. This is their mindset, so they are unwilling to talk about it, and they wonder why they need ACP at a time when they are in relatively good health. I think that patients and their families are unprepared to make the medical decisions necessary to face end of life in the future."* Participant N24 said: *"I once talked about ACP with a patient, and he asked why I mentioned this as he was doing quite okay.... The hemodialysis center is an open area, so when I mentioned this with this patient, the other patient next to him started to ask questions. The questions may be something like, 'Is that patient going to die?' I think that many patients have no idea about the real meaning of ACP."*

Discussion

In this study, five themes were found related to the barriers faced by nephrology nurses in discussing ACP with patients. Understanding and overcoming these barriers will be necessary to establish ACP as a standard part of a healthcare protocol.

Discussions regarding death and end of life care represent the most challenging aspect of healthcare provider/patient communications (Pfeifer & Head, 2018). Research has identified ACP as a complex and challenging conversation for healthcare professionals to engage in, requiring high-level communication skills, confidence, and emotional and managerial support (Boot & Wilson, 2014). Miller et al. (2019) indicated that, given adequate training and support, nurses are able to initiate and facilitate ACP conversations with patients that result in positive patient outcomes. Increased knowledge is likely to lead to more positive attitudes and greater confidence to undertake these discussions with patients. The findings from previous studies (Boot & Wilson, 2014; Miller et al., 2019; Pfeifer & Head, 2018) support the finding of this study that having professional knowledge and communication skills alone is not adequate for nurses to discuss ACP with patients. These nurses also require specific personality traits such as caring, empathy, and warmth. In other words, even if nurses acquire the requisite knowledge and communication skills related to ACP, they may remain unable to initiate ACP discussions comfortably. In most cases, these nurses have no idea how to discuss ACP and are afraid of causing anxiety in patients.

In addition, the participants in this study expressed uncertainty regarding the best time to initiate patients into ACP. This indicates that nurses are not able to raise the topic of ACP at the "right" moment. If ACP is discussed during the early stage of CKD, patients tend to feel that the issue is abrupt and obtrusive. However, if ACP is discussed at the end of life, patients may be unable to express their medical care preferences and desires, and family members may feel anxious about death. The best timing to initiate patients into ACP has not been indicated in previous studies, and no consensus on this issue exists among physicians. Boot and Wilson (2014) found the decision of nurses to initiate an ACP discussion is influenced by three key factors: patient readiness to discuss the topic, patient physical condition, and the relationship between the nurse and the patient and their family. Therefore, nurses play a key role in promoting and engaging with these discussions based on their close relationship with patients and their families (Blackwood et al., 2019). In addition, some participants considered that the hospice care team or other professionals should be in charge of initiating ACP, as initiating ACP is not part of a nurse's professional responsibilities. This corresponds with Hsieh and Lin (2010), who found that 40% of nurses think that ACP is not part of their responsibility and thus do not take the initiative to discuss this issue. Phillips et al. (2007) indicated that many nurses do not think it is their responsibility to engage in discussions with patients on death because of the lack of related professional training, incompetence, and unclear role boundaries. However, Sinclair et al. (2017) found nurse-led communication facilitates ACP that is acceptable to patients and effective in increasing ACP discussions and further fostering the ACP process. Nurses take care of patients throughout the day and are the ones who best understand the needs of patients and their families. Thus, they play a significant role in initiating patients into ACP (Shepherd et al., 2018). Based on the aforementioned literature, nurse attitudes will likely influence the success of efforts to increase the number of ACP discussions being held.

Omondi et al. (2017) claimed that doctors should take the initiative to discuss ACP with patients, as this is the key element to promote their signing ADs. Tamura and Meier (2013) mentioned that both patients and their family members consider ACP to be part of the daily routine in their healthcare and should be initiated at the early stage of their disease. Howard et al. (2018) indicated that lack of knowledge and lack of support from doctors represented key barriers for nurses. Furthermore, Sellars et al. (2017) noted that some nephrologists continue performing hemodialysis on patients who are unable to communicate and therefore ignore the ACP willingness of these patients. The negligent attitude taken by some doctors toward patient rights with regard to ACP is a point of frustration for nurses and social workers. In Taiwan, physicians hold a still highly respected position of professional authority, and ACP discussions are still predominantly determined and controlled by physicians. The participants mentioned that physicians tend to give patients false hopes and rarely explain the true risks of their disease and treatment. Participants further suggested that physicians should discuss ACP with patients but noted that they appear to be reluctant to do so. This highlights disagreements between nurses and doctors related to initiating patients into ACP. However, if physicians do not take the initiative to discuss ACP with patients, nurses will typically not follow up. This may be a reason for the low signing rate for ADs in Taiwan. This finding echoes Omondi et al. (2017), who identified physicians' involvement and early discussions with patients as key components affecting the signing rate for ADs.

Public attitudes toward death are influenced by culture. In Western societies, respecting the autonomy of terminal patients is of primary importance (Hansdottir et al., 2000). However, in traditional Chinese culture, most family members and medical staff avoid discussions of death with patients who are at end of life because of the fear of death (Yang et al., 2013). In this study, the participants reflected an aversion to discussing death. This aversion creates a barrier to patient healthcare autonomy and limits the ability of healthcare professionals to promote ACP based on the principle of patient autonomy. This echoes Ma et al. (2018), who found that an important reason for the low rate of signing ADs in Taiwan is because death in Chinese culture is considered taboo based on its ominous implications. Therefore, many people do not know how to face death at end of life. The general public in Taiwan is not familiar with the concept of ACP, and they may misunderstand the real meaning behind it. Many are not willing to talk about ACP, as they think ACP implies abandoning treatment (Lee et al., 2015). Other studies have highlighted three important reasons behind the low rate of signing ADs in Taiwan. First, people do not understand their current medical resources. Second, they associate ACP with ominous implications (death), so they do not want to talk about it. Third, they do not understand the meaning and details of ACP or related medical information (Lin et al., 2011). In conclusion, the current results indicate that nurses who are prepared and able to explain the purpose of signing ADs and to clarify patients' misunderstandings should have a significant and positive influence on patient willingness to sign ADs and the ADs signing rate.

Conclusions and Suggestions

Patient-centered care and respect for patient autonomy are core values of ACP. Healthcare professionals who help patients complete ADs often contribute to maintaining a good quality of life in patients who are at end of life. However, in this study, lack of knowledge and communication skills, uncertainties about the best time to initiate ACP discussion, and conflicting perspectives on ACP between doctors and nurses were found to be major barriers to completing ADs. Therefore, nurses must learn the knowledge and skills required to conduct ACP conversations, initiate ACP discussion, and strengthen cooperation with doctors to achieve the goals of ACP.

The participants included nursing personnel in the nephrology departments of medical institutions in northern, central, and southern Taiwan. Manpower and time constraints prevented the researchers from expanding the study to include nursing personnel in other departments to more fully understand the current status of ACP discussions among all relevant nursing personnel in Taiwan. Furthermore, ACP is a person-centered, interdisciplinary, and collaborative approach to patient care. Future studies may further expand recruitment to include other professionals such as physicians, social workers, and psychologists to understand their perspective and barriers in discussing ACP. Only by resolving the barriers faced by various professionals can there be a way to implement a holistic person-centered care.

Implications for Practice

First, nurses must enhance their ACP-related knowledge and skills to facilitate the shared decision-making process. Second, nurses should encourage patients and their families to participate in decision-making to avoid medical futility. Third, nurses must be empowered to initiate ACP and to engage in detailed,

related discussions to improve end of life care. Helping raise awareness of these barriers among nurses and facilitating their working together on this issue are critical to making ACP the norm in healthcare in the near future.

Acknowledgments

This study was funded by the Ministry of Science and Technology, Taiwan, ROC (107-2314-B-037-029-MY3). The authors express their gratitude to all of the participants who shared their valuable experiences.

Author Contributions

Study conception and design: CCL, JOC
Data collection: CCL, JOC
Data analysis and interpretation: CCL, JOC
Drafting of the article: JOC
Critical revision of the article: CCL

References

Beck, E. R., McIlfatrick, S., Hasson, F., & Leavey, G. (2017). Nursing home manager's knowledge, attitudes and beliefs about advance care planning for people with dementia in long-term care settings: A cross-sectional survey. *Journal of Clinical Nursing*, *26*(17–18), 2633–2645. https://doi.org/10.1111/jocn.13690

Blackwood, D. H., Walker, D., Mythen, M. G., Taylor, R. M., & Vindrola-Radros, C. (2019). Barriers to advance care planning with patients as perceived by nurses and other healthcare professionals: A systematic review. *Journal of Clinical Nursing*, *28*(23–24), 4276–4297. https://doi.org/10.1111/jocn.15049

Boot, M., & Wilson, C. (2014). Clinical nurse specialists' perspectives on advance care planning conversations: A qualitative study. *International Journal of Palliative Nursing*, *20*(1), 9–14. https://doi.org/10.12968/ijpn.2014.20.1.9

Colaizzi, P. F. (1978). Psychological research as the phenomenologist views it. In R. S. Valle & M. King (Eds.), *Existential-phenomenological alternatives for psychology* (pp. 48–71). Oxford University Press.

Davison, S. N. (2010). End-of-life care preferences and needs: Perceptions of patients with chronic kidney disease. *Clinical Journal of the American Society of Nephrology*, *5*(2), 195–204. https://doi.org/10.2215/CJN.05960809

Detering, K. M., Hancock, A. D., Reade, M. C., & Silvester, W. (2010). The impact of advance care planning on end of life care in elderly patients: Randomised controlled trial. *BMJ, 340*, Article c1345. https://doi.org/10.1136/bmj.c1345

Gjerberg, E., Lillemoen, L., Førde, R., & Pedersen, R. (2015). End-of-life care communications and shared decision-making in Norwegian nursing homes—Experiences and perspectives of patients and relatives. *BMC Geriatrics, 15*, Article No. 103. https://doi.org/10.1186/s12877-015-0096-y

Goff, S. L., Eneanya, N. D., Feinberg, R., Germain, M. J., Marr, L., Berzoff, J., Cohen, L. M., & Unruh, M. (2015). Advance care planning: A qualitative study of dialysis patients and families. *Clinical Journal of the American Society of Nephrology, 10*(3), 390–400. https://doi.org/10.2215/CJN.07490714

Hansdottir, H., Gruman, C., Curry, L., & Judge, J. O. (2000). Preferences for CPR among the elderly: The influence of attitudes and values. *Connecticut Medicine, 64*(10), 625–630.

How, C. H., & Koh, L. H. (2015). Not that way: Advance care planning. *Singapore Medical Journal, 56*(1), 19–22. https://doi.org/10.11622/smedj.2015005

Howard, M., Bernard, C., Klein, D., Elston, D., Tan, A., Slaven, M., Barwich, D., You, J. J., & Heyland, D. K. (2018). Barriers to and enablers of advance care planning with patients in primary care: Survey of health care providers. *Canadian Family Physician, 64*, e190–e198.

Hsieh, L. Y., & Lin, S. Y. (2010). A pilot study on the perspectives of hemodialysis room nurses on promoting advance directives. *The Journal of Nursing, 57*(4), 59–67. https://doi.org/10.6224/JN.57.4.59 (Original work published in Chinese)

Krueger, R. A., & Casey, M. A. (2000). *Focus groups: A practical guide for applied research* (3rd ed.). Sage.

Lee, H. T. S., Cheng, S. C., Huang, C. F., Wu, Y. M., & Hu, W. Y. (2015). Implementation and barriers for elderly nursing home residents in signing their own advance directives in Taiwan: From culture perspectives of Taoism, Confucianism, and Buddhism. *Taiwan Journal of Hospice Palliative Care, 20*(2), 154–165. https://doi.org/10.6537/TJHPC.2015.20(2).5 (Original work published in Chinese)

Lin, H. M., Yang, C. L., Chen, M. M., Chiu, T. Y., & Hu, W. Y. (2011). Inpatients' willingness on and acceptance of promotion for signing of advance directives. *Taiwan Journal of Hospice Palliative Care, 16*(3), 281–295. https://doi.org/10.6537/TJHPC.2011.16(3).1 (Original work published in Chinese)

Lincoln, Y. S., & Guba, E. G. (1985). *Naturalistic inquiry*. Sage.

Ma, J. C., Yun, C. C., Lin, P. X., Lin, L. S., Hsiao, C. Y., Gu, F. G., & Su, M. I. (2018). Retrospective study of dialysis patients' do-not-resuscitate (DNR) consent in Taiwan. *Formosan Journal of Medicine, 22*(3), 232–241. https://doi.org/10.6320/FJM.201805_22 (3).0002 (Original work published in Chinese)

Meier, E. A., Gallegos, J. V., Thomas, L. P., Depp, C. A., Irwin, S. A., & Jeste, D. V. (2016). Defining a good death (successful dying): Literature review and a call for research and public dialogue. *The American Journal of Geriatric Psychiatry, 24*(4), 261–271. https://doi.org/10.1016/j.jagp.2016.01.135

Miller, H., Tan, J., Clayton, J. M., Meller, A., Hermiz, O., Zwar, N., & Rhee, J. (2019). Patient experiences of nurse-facilitated advance care planning in a general practice setting: A qualitative study. *BMC Palliative Care, 18*(1), Article No. 25. https://doi.org/10.1186/s12904-019-0411-z

Ministry of Health and Welfare, ROC. (2020). *Advance decision, hospice palliative medicine and organ donation willingness information system*. https://hpcod.mohw.gov.tw/HospWeb/index.aspx (Original work published in Chinese)

Omondi, S., Weru, J., Shaikh, A. J., & Yonga, G. (2017). Factors that influence advance directives completion amongst terminally ill patients at a tertiary hospital in Kenya. *BMC Palliative Care, 16*, Article No. 9. https://doi.org/10.1186/s12904-017-0186-z

Pfeifer, M., & Head, B. A. (2018). Which critical communication skills are essential for interdisciplinary end-of-life discussions? *AMA Journal of Ethics, 20*(8), E724–E731. https://doi.org/10.1001/amajethics.2018.724

Phillips, J. L., Davidson, P. M., Ollerton, R., Jackson, D., & Kristjanson, L. (2007). A survey of commitment and compassion among nurses in residential aged care. *International Journal of Palliative Nursing, 13*(6), 282–290. https://doi.org/10.12968/ijpn.2007.13.6.23743

Sellars, M., Tong, A., Luckett, T., Morton, R. L., Pollock, C. A., Spencer, L., Silvester, W., & Clayton, J. M. (2017). Clinicians' perspectives on advance care planning for patients with CKD in Australia: An interview study. *American Journal of Kidney Disease, 70*(3), 315–323. https://doi.org/10.1053/j.ajkd.2016.11.023

Shepherd, J., Waller, A., Sanson-Fisher, R., Clark, K., & Ball, J. (2018). Knowledge of, and participation in, advance care planning: A cross-sectional study of acute and critical care nurses' perceptions. *International Journal of Nursing Studies, 86*, 74–81. https://doi.org/10.1016/j.ijnurstu.2018.06.005

Sinclair, C., Auret, K. A., Evans, S. F., Willimson, F., Dormer, S., Wilkinson, A., Greeve, K., Koay, A., Price, D., & Brims, F. (2017). Advance care planning uptake among patients with severe lung disease: A randomised patient preference trial of a nurse-led, facilitated advance care planning intervention. *BMJ Open, 7*, Article e013415. https://doi.org/10.1136/bmjopen-2016-013415

Tamura, M. K., & Meier, D. E. (2013). Five policies to promote palliative care for patients with ESRD. *Clinical Journal of the American Society of Nephrology, 8*(10), 1783–1790. https://doi.org/10.2215/CJN.02180213

Tsai, M. H., Hsu, C. Y., Lin, M. Y., Yen, M. F., Chen, H. H., Chiu, Y. H., & Hwang, S. J. (2018). Incidence, prevalence, and duration of chronic kidney disease in Taiwan: Results from a community-based screening program of 106,094 individuals. *Nephron, 140*(3), 175–184. https://doi.org/10.1159/000491708

Yang, W. L., Su, Y. L., & Chen, H. N. (2013). Advanced life planning for good death. *Leadership Nursing, 14*(1), 2–9. https://doi.org/10.29494/LN.201303_14(1).0002 (Original work published in Chinese)

23

The Feasibility Study of a Revised Standard Care Procedure on the Capacity of Nasogastric Tube Placement Verification Among Critical Care Nurses

Feng-Huang YANG[1] • Feng-Yu LIN[2,4] • Yueh-Juen HWU[3,4]*

ABSTRACT

Background: Evidence-based studies propose that the aspirate pH test may be easily and reliably conducted to verify the proper placement of nasogastric tubes (NGTs). Nurses rarely implement this procedure because of the lack of related knowledge.

Purpose: The purpose of this study was to explore the feasibility of implementing a revised standard care procedure to enhance nurses' ability to verify placement of the NGT.

Methods: his study used a quasi-experimental, longitudinal research design. Nurses from two intensive care units were randomly assigned to the experimental group ($n = 35$) and the control group ($n = 31$). A revised standard-of-care procedure to confirm the proper placement of an NGT was incorporated into a slideshow presentation, a printed leaflet, and an audit checklist. The experimental group received continuous education and individual teaching on the revised standard-of-care procedure, whereas the control group did not receive additional education and continued to provide conventional care. The study gathered data using scales designed to address knowledge of and attitudes toward verification of NGT placement and the checklist for auditing the NGT care procedure. Scales were implemented before and after the practice program was conducted, in Months 1, 2, and 3, to evaluate the feasibility of the developed improvement measures.

Results: This study found significant improvements in the experimental group in terms of knowledge regarding NGT placement verification and the NGT care auditing procedure. The positive improvement of the intervention on the NGT care auditing procedure remained for at least 3 months after the end of the intervention.

Conclusions: The findings suggest that using an aspirate pH test is a feasible approach to verify NGT placement in critical care units, a crucial aspect of care necessary to promote patient safety and quality of care.

KEY WORDS:
critical care, intervention study, nasogastric tube, placement verification.

Introduction

Patients in intensive care units (ICUs) often experience inability to eat orally and surgery-related dysphagia, improper placement of the endotracheal tube, stroke, and other issues. Some researchers have found that critically ill patients experience delays in enteral feeding initiation and frequently miss meeting nutrition targets (Stewart, Biddle, & Thomas, 2017). Malnutrition, an important issue in the care of the critically ill, is associated with increased costs of care and poor patient outcomes. Inserting a nasogastric tube (NGT) is a measure frequently used to resolve these problems.

Patients of any age may require NGT placement. Thus, the safety of this procedure is worth discussing. NGT placement may increase the risk of resistance and struggle by patients and result in a greater probability of using physical restraints and of unplanned extubations (Lin, Liao, Yu, Chu, & Ho, 2018). The improper placement of NGT may threaten the safety of patients, especially critically ill patients in ICUs (Bourgault et al., 2014). According to a recent literature review (DiBardino & Wunderink, 2015), aspiration pneumonia should be a consideration for critical care patients who are on NGT feeds. Incorrect NGT placement and aspiration place patients at risk. Therefore, NGT placement verification is of great importance in the proper care of ICU patients.

At present, no single, nonradioactive method exists for verifying NGT placement. The current gold standard for NGT placement verification is X-ray. Evidence from numerous research studies has found that the air bolus method and the resultant aspirates are unreliable and cannot correctly determine the placement of NGT. Using multivariate methods to verify NGT placement is thus preferable (Chan et al., 2012; Jiang, Lin, Kao, Lin, & Wu, 2013). Simple and inexpensive detection methods have also been considered clinically, and

[1]MSN, RN, Deputy Director, Department of Nursing at Chung Kang Branch, Cheng Ching Hospital • [2]PhD, Associate Professor, General Education Center, Overseas Chinese University • [3]PhD, RN, Professor, College of Nursing, Central Taiwan University of Science and Technology • [4]Contributed equally.

the aspirate pH test was determined to be the most reliable and economical method for bedside verification of NGT (American Association of Critical-Care Nurses [AACN], 2016).

According to the evidence-based literature, X-rays and aspirate pH tests are most frequently used in the ICU to verify placement of an NGT. In a 3-month study of 100 ICU patients with NGT, all nurses ($N = 42$, 100%) used the aspirate pH test. Only 10 patients received X-ray to verify NGT placement, indicating that it is not feasible even in the ICU (Ke, Lin, Hsieh, Hwu, & Chang, 2014).

To ascertain nurses' knowledge about methods for NGT placement verification and behaviors, this study used a structured questionnaire to survey 200 nurses with direct patient care responsibilities at one regional hospital. One hundred ninety-five valid questionnaires were received and used in subsequent analysis work (response rate: 97.5%). The results revealed that more than half of the participants (50.3%–65.6%) could not answer questions related to the aspirate pH test. Only 4.6% of the participants had used the aspirate pH test to verify NGT placement (Yang, Lin, & Hwu, 2017). This result indicates that many nurses are unfamiliar with the aspirate pH test to confirm NGT placement.

Verifying the correct placement of NGT in critical care settings is imperative and frequently the sole responsibility of nurses. Methods currently in use include obtaining the aspirates (45.6%) and auscultation with insufflation of air (41.5%; Yang et al., 2017); therefore, an additional aspirate pH test to confirm NGT placement is feasible. The incidence of NGT misplacement can easily be significantly reduced when nurses follow revised standard care procedures to confirm NGT placement (Eveleigh, Law, Pullyblank, & Bennett, 2011). Thus, the aim of this quasi-experimental study was to investigate whether a revised standard care procedure could significantly improve NGT placement verification among critical care nurses.

Methods

Study Design and Participants

This study used a quasi-experimental, longitudinal research design and was conducted in two medical–surgical ICUs at one regional teaching hospital in central Taiwan. These two units were similar in terms of the number of beds and personnel. Cluster randomization was used to assign these units as either the experimental group or the control group to avoid cross-contamination. This study was approved by the ethics committee of the participating hospital (HP160043). G-Power Version 3.1.9.2. (Heinrich Heine Universitat, Dusseldorf, Germany; Faul, Erdfelder, Lang, & Buchner, 2007) was used to calculate the sample size. As no prior study had addressed the specific issue taken up in this article, a medium effect size of .5, a significance value (α) of .05, and a statistical power ($1 - \beta$) of .95 were used (Cohen, 1992). On the basis of these measurements, a minimum sample size of 54 participants was determined. The inclusion criteria were nurses who had worked in the ICUs for more than 3 months, had completed the consent

form, and were willing to participate in the study. All of the nurses in the two units met the inclusion criteria and agreed to join in this intervention study. Thirty-five nurses were in the experimental group, and 31 were in the control group.

Intervention

A four-step theoretical domains framework was used to develop the intervention (French et al., 2012). Step 1 identified target behaviors and capabilities related to NGT placement verification. Step 2 chose the theoretical framework most likely to elicit the process of learning effects. Step 3 designed the contents of the NGT practice program. These three steps helped preserve the intellectual integrity of NGT placement verification capabilities. Step 4 used subjective (structured questionnaire to determine nurses' knowledge and attitudes toward the NGT placement verification method) and objective (the checklist for auditing the NGT care procedure) outcomes to evaluate the capacity of NGT placement verification among participants. In addition to relevant knowledge, nurses require practical competence in NGT placement verification (i.e., "know-what" vs. "know-how" knowledge; Schunk, 2007). To gather these data, researchers designed the intervention as follows.

A revised NGT placement verification step was developed based on the literature (AACN, 2016; Metheny & Titler, 2010; Stepter, 2012; Tan, Chang, & Wu, 2012), a quality improvement project (Ke et al., 2014), and the results of a survey (Yang et al., 2017) and was added to the standard care procedure. This intervention was named "You must know the revised standard of care procedure for confirming placement of NGT." The contents of this intervention are described below.

1. Reason for procedural change
   (1) Evidence from many research studies shows that the aspirate obtained and the air bolus methods are unreliable and cannot correctly determine the gastric placement of NGT.
   (2) Although radiographic imaging is the present gold standard for NGT placement verification, it is not feasible for use in critical care settings.
   (3) The most reliable and economical method for verification of NGT at the bedside is the aspirate pH test.

2. Practice recommendations
   (1) Current bedside practice in Taiwan: (a) Aspirate obtained is the primary method, followed by the auscultation of air bolus method. (b) Radiographic imaging is used occasionally.
   (2) AACN recommends that the most reliable and economical method for verifying NGT at the bedside is the aspirate pH test.

3. Key elements of the revised standard care procedure
   (1) An initial X-ray is recommended if unable to confirm NGT placement before administration of a substance via the NGT.

(2) If no substance will be introduced into the NGT (suction or clamped), verify placement via absence of respiratory symptoms and aspiration of gastric contents.

(3) Subsequent verifications of tube placement must be done before each feeding and administration.

(4) Obtain aspirate 0.5–1 ml to check the color.

(5) Test aspirate on pH indicator paper (pH between 1 and 5.5).

(6) Combine one of the other methods as follows:
   · Check whether the tube twines in the mouth.
   · Check tube marking and/or tube length.

(7) Check if the patient is on acid-inhibiting medication.

(8) Nurses must document placement of the NGT every 4 hours and before the administration of any substance.

The amended NGT placement verification procedure was organized as a slideshow presentation, printed on leaflets, and used to develop an audit checklist to promote nurse awareness and application. In addition, two sessions of in-service education were arranged. Written information was distributed to all of the nurses, who were required to read the contents carefully, apply the procedure in a care situation, and propose amendment suggestions in the morning meeting 1 week later. When nurses conduct the aspirate pH test, they may encounter problems such as no aspirate and the need to interpret color change (Boeykens, Steeman, & Duysburgh, 2014). Thus, the head nurse provided instruction at the bedside using the audit checklist for the NGT care procedure to (a) understand the actual problems and difficulties encountered by nurses during implementation of the procedure and (b) provide assistance intended to increase the consistency and correctness of implementation. The NGT placement verification flowchart was posted on the wall in the ICU to remind nurses to verify NGT placement before administration or feeding and to check whether the patient was on acid-inhibiting medication (e.g., H_2 receptor antagonists, proton pump inhibitors; Fan, Tan, & Ang, 2017).

The revised standard care procedure for NGT placement verification was implemented for 2 weeks. After the third posttest, the revised standard care procedure of NGT placement verification continuing education was held for the nurse participants in the control group. These interventions reflect the best learning practices for the clinical setting, which should incorporate reminder, audit, and feedback procedures (French et al., 2012).

Measures

Questionnaires addressing the knowledge and attitudes of nurses toward the nasogastric tube placement verification method

Structured questionnaires were used to ascertain the knowledge and attitudes of the participants toward NGT placement verification. The demographic data collected included age, gender, credentials, years of nursing experience, and the ratio of patients fed via NGTs every day.

Ten items on the questionnaire addressed the knowledge of participants regarding NGT placement verification. Examples included identification of both the best method of NGT placement verification and NGT dislocation. Each correct answer earned a score of 1, and each wrong answer earned a score of 0; the total possible score range was 0–10, with higher scores associated with better knowledge of NGT placement verification. Four items on the questionnaire addressed respondent attitudes, with the aim of discerning opinions on the revised standard care procedure. Scores were based on a 5-point Likert-type scale, with 1 = *strong disagreement* and 5 = *strong agreement*. The total possible score range for this section was 4–20, with higher scores associated with a more positive attitude toward using the revised standard care procedure.

Content validity was verified by a panel of four experts (nursing professor, nursing supervisor, nursing practitioner, and physician). Each item was scored on a scale of 1–5, with 5 indicating highest appropriateness and applicability. Items with a mean panel-wide score of less than 4 were deleted, resulting in a final questionnaire of nine items. The final questionnaire earned a content validity index of .90. Reliability testing was conducted after the questionnaires were collected from the participants. The knowledge-related items, scored dichotomously as either right or wrong, earned a Kuder–Richardson coefficient of .88. The attitude-related items, scored based on a 1- to 5-point scale, showed an internal consistency Cronbach's alpha of .86.

Checklist for auditing the nasogastric tube care procedure

The checklist for auditing the NGT care procedure was developed to evaluate and monitor the integrity of the participants' implementation of the NGT care procedure. The NGT care procedure was divided into six major criteria: (a) implementation of cleaning skills required by the procedure, (b) arranging the patient position during and after administration and feeding, (c) verifying NGT placement, (d) feeding or administering drugs after NGT placement verification, (e) maintaining NGT patency, and (f) recording the observations and assessing and managing patients. Each criterion had its own items (subitems), with 17 subitems in all. The 17 subitems were categorized into "achievement," "failure," and "not applicable." The full score was 17 points, no points were deducted for "not applicable" answers, and 1 point was deducted for the failure of each subitem to evaluate the nurses' NGT care behavior. A pilot study of the checklist for auditing the NGT care procedure was conducted in the ICU of another regional teaching hospital (Wu, Lin, Hwu, Ke, & Chang, 2016). "Nurse informs physician if unable to confirm placement and consider X-ray" was added to this study, resulting in a final audit checklist of 18 items.

The two measurement tools previously discussed were used to evaluate the ability of the participants to verify NGT placement both before and at 1, 2, and 3 months after the intervention. The pretest and posttests were conducted by a nurse who was responsible for quality assurance to maintain the consistency of the evaluation.

Data Collection

Data were collected from November 2016 to May 2017. Before the intervention of the revised standard care procedure, the participants in the experimental and control groups completed the "Structured Questionnaire of Nurses' Knowledge and Attitudes Regarding the NGT Placement Verification Method" and "Checklist for Auditing the NGT Care Procedure." The nurses in the experimental group then received 2 weeks of training on the revised standard of care procedure for confirming placement of NGT, whereas nurses in the control group implemented NGT care procedures according to conventional practice. To explore the sustainable effects of behavioral change, nurses in both groups were given a posttest evaluation of knowledge and attitudes toward NGT placement verification and the checklist for auditing the NGT care procedure at 1, 2, and 3 months after the intervention to compare the immediate and longer-term effects of the intervention (Figure 1).

Data Analysis

Data were analyzed using IBM SPSS Statistics Version 23.0 (IBM, Armonk, NY, USA). Demographic and outcome characteristics were analyzed using descriptive statistics. A chi-square test and independent t tests were used to verify homogeneity between the groups at baseline. To assess the interpretability of the main effects of the intervention between the groups, a separate analysis of covariance (ANCOVA) was conducted by adjusting for baseline on the outcome measures. Finally, to ensure the learning effects of the revised standard care procedure over time, the knowledge and attitudes of participants toward NGT placement verification and NGT care procedure audit responses were compared among the four time points (pretest and three posttests). Between-group differences in the outcomes were analyzed using general linear modeling analysis and a repeated-measures ANCOVA (RANCOVA).

Results

Sample Characteristics

Figure 1 presents the study flowchart. General characteristics such as gender, age, education, years of nursing experience, and ratio of patients requiring NGT feeding showed no significant differences between the two groups, which supported intergroup homogeneity. Moreover, with regard to the three pretest numerical values of the nurses in both groups, although no significant difference in knowledge was found, the results of the attitude and care procedure audit in the control group were superior to those of the experimental group (Table 1).

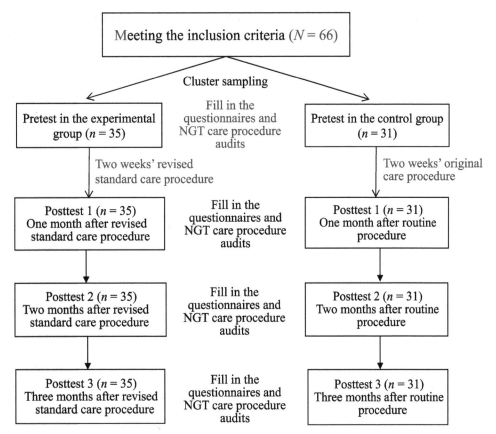

Figure 1. Study flow diagram. NGT = nasogastric tube.

The Immediate and Longer-Term Effects of the Revised Standard Care Procedure on Nasogastric Tube Placement Verification Ability

After using ANCOVA to eliminate the interference of the pretest between both groups (Tu, 2017), the posttest results showed that the experimental group had significantly greater knowledge of NGT placement verification and auditing of NGT care procedure than the control group.

General linear modeling and a sphericity test were used to analyze correlations between changes in outcome variables (knowledge, attitude, and audit levels) over time. RANCOVA with least significance difference was used to examine differences in outcome variables across the four time points.

Knowledge of Nasogastric Tube Placement Verification

The assumption of sphericity was met ($p > .05$). It meant that there were no significant correlations among the four repeated measures. The results from RANCOVA revealed a significant group effect on knowledge of NGT placement verification, $F(1, 33.12) = 6.93, p = .011$, with a higher postintervention mean difference in the experimental group relative to the control group. In terms of time effect, the change in

knowledge of NGT placement verification over time was not significant in either group (Table 2). In addition, there was no significant Group × Time interaction effect on knowledge of NGT placement verification between the groups over time ($p = .496$), as the degree of increased knowledge of NGT placement verification for both groups tended to converge over time (Figure 2).

Attitudes Toward Nasogastric Tube Placement Verification

RANCOVA found no significant main effects of group, time, and Group × Time interaction on attitude. The attitudes toward NGT placement verification in the experimental group rose after the first month and then fell, which was still lower than the pretest after the third month. However, the attitudes in the control group continued to fall until stabilizing after the third month.

Auditing the Nasogastric Tube Care Procedure

The assumption of sphericity was not supported ($p < .05$). A Greenhouse–Geisser correction was conducted because of the significant correlations among the four repeated measures. After a significant repeated-measures result, pairwise comparisons with the least significance difference were used to determine at which points the auditing of NGT care

TABLE 1.
Demographic and Outcome Variables of Participants at Baseline (N = 66)

Variable	Total (N = 66) n	%	Experimental Group (n = 35) n	%	Control Group (n = 31) n	%	χ²	p
Gender							0.49ᵃ	.597
Male	3	4.5	1	2.9	2	6.5		
Female	63	95.5	34	97.1	29	93.5		
Education							1.70	.222
College	29	43.9	18	51.4	11	35.5		
Junior college	37	56.1	17	48.6	20	64.5		
Years of nursing experience							2.17	.538
< 1	12	18.2	7	20.0	5	16.1		
1–5	20	30.3	12	34.3	8	25.8		
> 5	34	51.5	16	45.7	18	58.1		
Ratio of patients requiring NGT feeding (%)							1.76ᵃ	.172
< 50	8	12.1	6	17.1	2	6.5		
≥ 50	58	87.9	29	82.9	29	93.5		
	M	SD	M	SD	M	SD	t	p
Age	28.9	6.3	27.8	6.1	30.1	6.5	−1.48	.144
NGT placement verification knowledge (pretest)	4.6	1.5	4.8	1.4	4.4	1.6	0.97	.338
NGT placement verification attitude (pretest)	16.7	2.4	16.0	2.8	17.4	2.0	−2.17	.034*
NGT care procedure audit (pretest)	11.6	1.6	9.4	1.8	13.8	1.5	−10.86	< .001***

Note. NGT = nasogastric tube.
ᵃFisher's exact test.
*p < .05. ***p < .001.

TABLE 2.
Lasting Effects in Capacity of NGT Placement Verification

Variable Origin	Sphericity Test (p)	Mean Square	Degree of Freedom	F	p	LSD Test
NGT placement verification						
Knowledge	.974					
Group (1, 2, 3, 4)		33.12	1	6.93	.011*	
Time		0.07	3	0.04	.989	
Time × Group		1.43	3	0.80	.496	
Attitude	.999					
Group (1, 2, 3, 4)		28.00	1	2.19	.144	
Time		5.53	3	0.95	.418	
Time × Group		3.65	3	0.63	.598	
Auditing the NGT care procedure	< .001					2 > 3 > 4 > 1
Group (1, 2, 3, 4)		8.88	1	2.99	.088	
Time		231.17	2.39	135.30	< .001***	
Time × Group		173.33	2.39	101.45	< .001***	

Note. NGT = nasogastric tube; LSD = least significant difference; 1 = pretest; 2 = first month; 3 = second month; 4 = third month.
*p < .05. ***p < .001.

procedure differed. RANCOVA adjusted the baseline of the NGT care procedure audit to examine the time effect of the changes in score between groups but did not confirm the significant group effect, $F(1, 8.88) = 2.99$, $p = .088$. In terms of time effect, RANCOVA revealed a statistically significant improvement in the NGT care procedure audit, $F(2.39, 231.17) = 135.30$, $p < .001$. This means that the audit score changed over time. There was also a significant Group × Time interaction effect on the NGT care procedure audit between groups over time, $F(2.39, 173.33) = 101.45$, $p < .001$ (Table 2; Figure 3). Hence, there was an intergroup difference in time effect.

Pairwise comparisons revealed that the pretest for the NGT care procedure audit yielded significantly different scores from those obtained in the 1-, 2-, and 3-month posttests. The frequency of NGT care procedure audits in the experimental group was greater than that in the control group, and differences between the four scores all achieved significance. This indicated that the intervention of the revised standard

procedure achieved a lasting increase in NGT care procedure audits in the experimental group.

Discussion

This article is the first quasi-experimental study to assess the effectiveness of a revised standard care procedure on NGT placement verification in a sample of critical care nurses. The study results show that the scores of NGT placement verification knowledge and NGT care procedure audit in the experimental group were higher than those in the control group. The intergroup differences in NGT care procedure audits persisted across all posttest time points. However, the time effects were not seen in the knowledge of NGT placement verification. The auditing score in the experimental group, lower than that in the control group at pretest (Table 1), significantly improved after the intervention. The main issue addressed in this article was whether the time effects of score changes between the two groups supported

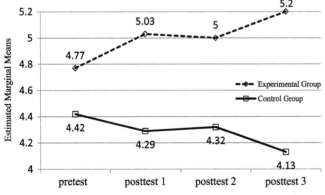

Figure 2. Mean scores for knowledge of NGT placement verification over time.

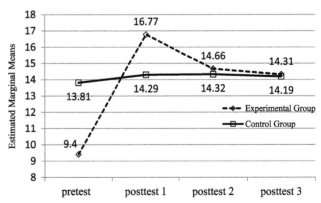

Figure 3. Mean scores for auditing of NGT care procedure.

significant group effects. Therefore, posttests were carried out at 1, 2, and 3 months after completion of the 2-week intervention. Table 2 shows that knowledge and attitudes toward NGT placement verification did not exhibit longitudinal effects and that the NGT care procedure audit did exhibit significant longitudinal effects. This finding suggests that a period of reinforcement is needed to sufficiently internalize the relevant knowledge and attitudes.

Thirteen types of NGT placement verification methods were identified, with X-ray and the aspirate pH test showing the highest verification accuracy (Jiang et al., 2013). Moreover, the pilot programs showed conducting an aspirate pH test before tube feeding and drug administration to be the most reliable method for verifying NGT placement at the bedside (AACN, 2016; Kunis, 2007; Peter & Gill, 2009). Generally speaking, clinical nurses usually observe gastric aspirates to verify NGT placement. Nurses will insufflate air through the NGT for auscultation if no aspirate is found. However, the whooshing sound in the upper abdomen may originate from the tracheobronchial tree or the pleural cavity (Boeykens et al., 2014). Therefore, the aspirate pH test should be conducted to improve the validity of NGT placement verification.

The effects of the revised standard care procedure on participant attitudes toward NGT placement verification were not significantly better than other outcomes, perhaps because the nurses in the experimental group were required to perform an aspirate pH test to verify NGT placement before each administration or feeding. This additional requirement increases nurse workload, which may explain the rise in attitude scores at the first posttest and then the decline thereafter. With increased proficiency, nurses better understood the importance of adding this procedure in terms of ensuring patient safety, leading to a gradual reduction in related complaints.

Several challenges complicate the process of transferring a synthesis of the evidence into clinical application. These include the additional work stress caused by changing care procedures and inadequate support and recognition from supervisors for the implementation efforts of nurses.

This study is affected by three limitations. First, this research was restricted to the ICUs of one teaching hospital in central Taiwan. Thus, the results may not be generalizable to all critical care nurses. In addition, to avoid cross-contamination, a randomized cluster sampling approach was adopted, which may potentially affect the homogeneity of participants. Finally, the effects of the intervention were evaluated at 1, 2, and 3 months after its conclusion. Thus, the longer-term effects of the intervention remain uncertain.

Conclusions

This empirical application of research may encourage practitioners to reexamine and reflect on current NGT care practices. The results of this study highlight the feasibility of applying the aspirate pH test in ICU settings. However, this test may not be applicable in all ICUs.

The recommendations for future related research include increasing the sample size and recruiting participants from different hospitals and geographic areas. We suggest that future researchers consider a crossover or self-comparison design to eliminate preexisting differences between two groups. To assess the longer-term effects of the intervention, the second and third posttest times should be extended to 6 and 12 months, respectively. More research should be published on this issue to promote a sufficiently evidence-based NGT placement verification program.

Acknowledgments

The authors wish to thank all of the critical care nurses who participated in this study. This study was supported by Chung-Kang Branch, Cheng-Ching Hospital Research Fund (Grant No. CH10500199).

References

American Association of Critical-Care Nurses. (2016). AACN practice alert: Initial and ongoing verification of feeding tube placement in adults. *Critical Care Nurse, 36*(2), e8–e13. https://doi.org/10.4037/ccn2016141

Boeykens, K., Steeman, E., & Duysburgh, I. (2014). Reliability of pH measurement and the auscultatory method to confirm the position of a nasogastric tube. *International Journal of Nursing Studies, 51*(11), 1427–1433. https://doi.org/10.1016/j.ijnurstu.2014.03.004

Bourgault, A. M., Heath, J., Hooper, V., Sole, M. L., Waller, J. L., & Nesmith, E. G. (2014). Factors influencing critical care nurses' adoption of the AACN practice alert on verification of feeding tube placement. *American Journal of Critical Care, 23*(2), 134–143. https://doi.org/10.4037/ajcc2014558

Chan, E. Y., Ng, I. H., Tan, S. L., Jabin, K., Lee, L. N., & Ang, C. C. (2012). Nasogastric feeding practices: A survey using clinical scenarios. *International Journal of Nursing Studies, 49*(3), 310–319. https://doi.org/10.1016/j.ijnurstu.2011.09.014

Cohen, J. (1992). A power primer. *Psychological Bulletin, 112*(1), 155–159.

DiBardino, D. M., & Wunderink, R. G. (2015). Aspiration pneumonia: A review of modern trend. *Journal of Critical Care, 30*(1), 40–48. https://doi.org/10.1016/j.jcrc.2014.07.011

Eveleigh, M., Law, R., Pullyblank, A., & Bennett, J. (2011). Nasogastric feeding tube placement: Changing culture. *Nursing Time, 107*(41), 14–16.

Fan, E. M., Tan, S. B., & Ang, S. Y. (2017). Nasogastric tube placement confirmation: Where we are and where we should be heading. *Proceedings of Singapore Healthcare, 26*(3), 189–195. https://doi.org/10.1177/2010105817705141

Faul, F., Erdfelder, E., Lang, A. G., & Buchner, A. (2007). G* power 3: A flexible statistical power analysis program for the social, behavioral, and biomedical sciences. *Behavior Research Methods, 39*(2), 175–191. https://doi.org/10.3758/BF03193146

French, S. D., Green, S. E., O'Connor, D. A., McKenzie, J. E., Francis, J. J., Michie, S., ... Grimshaw, J. M. (2012). Developing theory-informed behaviour change interventions to implement evidence into practice: A systematic approach using the theoretical domains framework. *Implementation Science, 7*, 38–40. https://doi.org/10.1186/1748-5908-7-38

Jiang, Y. X., Lin, F. Y., Kao, M. C., Lin, R. A., & Wu, S. J. (2013). A systematic review of methods for detecting nasogastric tube misplacement after insertion. *The Journal of Long-Term Care, 17*(2), 105–124. (Original work published in Chinese).

Ke, S. C., Lin, F. Y., Hsieh, Y. H., Hwu, Y. J., & Chang, C. N. (2014). Project to increase the nasogastric tube verification practice. *Show Chwan Medical Journal, 13*(3–4), 63–72. https://doi.org/10.3966/156104972014121303002 (Original work published in Chinese)

Kunis, K. (2007). Confirmation of nasogastric tube placement. *American Journal of Critical Care, 16*(1), 19.

Lin, Y. L., Liao, C. C., Yu, W. P., Chu, T. L., & Ho, L. H. (2018). A multidisciplinary program reduces over 24 hours of physical restraint in neurological intensive care unit. *The Journal of Nursing Research, 26*(4), 288–296. https://doi.org/10.1097/jnr.0000000000000251

Metheny, N. A., & Titler, M. G. (2010). Assessing placement of feeding tubes. *The American Journal of Nursing, 101*(5), 36–45. https://doi.org/10.1097/00000446-200105000-00017

Peter, S., & Gill, F. (2009). Development of a clinical practice guideline for testing nasogastric tube placement. *Journal for Specialists in Pediatric Nursing, 14*(1), 3–11. https://doi.org/10.1111/j.1744-6155.2008.00161.x

Schunk, D. H. (2007). *Learning theories: An educational perspective* (5th ed.). Upper Saddle River, NJ: Prentice Hall.

Stepter, C. R. (2012). Maintaining placement of temporary enteral feeding tubes in adults: A critical appraisal of the evidence. *Medsurg Nursing, 21*(2), 61–68.

Stewart, M. L., Biddle, M., & Thomas, T. (2017). Evaluation of current feeding practices in the critically ill: A retrospective chart review. *Intensive and Critical Care Nursing, 38*, 24–30. https://doi.org/10.1016/j.iccn.2016.05.004

Tan, L., Chang, L., & Wu, H. P. (2012). Measuring the pH of gastric aspirate to determine nasogastric tube placement: A systematic review. *Chinese Journal of Practical Nursing, 31*, 57–59. (Original work published in Chinese)

Tu, C. T. (2017). The basic concept of analysis of covariance. In C. T. Tu (Ed.), *Experimental research methods and analysis of covariance* (1st ed., pp. 32–85). Taipei City, Taiwan, ROC: Wu-Nan Book. (Original work published in Chinese)

Wu, S. J., Lin, F. Y., Hwu, Y. J., Ke, S. C., & Chang, C. N. (2016). Evidence utilization of NG tube care in the intensive care units. *Resuscitation & Intensive Care Medicine, 1*(3), 130–141. (Original work published in Chinese)

Yang, F. H., Lin, F. Y., & Hwu, Y. J. (2017). Knowledge, attitude, and behavior of Taiwan nurses toward nasogastric tube placement verification. *Cheng Ching Medical Journal, 13*(1), 55–63. (Original work published in Chinese)

24

Effects of a Case Management Program for Women with Pregnancy-Induced Hypertension

Cheng-Chen CHOU[1] • Jen-Jiuan LIAW[2] • Chuan-Chuan CHEN[3] • Yiing-Mei LIOU[4] • Chi-Jane WANG[5]*

ABSTRACT

Background: Pregnancy-induced hypertension (PIH) is a leading cause of maternal and fetal morbidity and mortality. Although case management programs have been proposed to improve maternal and fetal outcomes in high-risk pregnancies, limited data are available regarding the effect of case management on women with PIH.

Purpose: The aim of this study was to evaluate the effect of an antepartum case management program on stress, anxiety, and pregnancy outcomes in women with PIH.

Methods: A quasi-experimental research design was employed. A convenience sample of women diagnosed with PIH, including preeclampsia, was recruited from outpatient clinics at a medical center in southern Taiwan. Sixty-two women were assigned randomly to either the experimental group ($n = 31$) or the control group ($n = 31$). The experimental group received case management for 8 weeks, and the control group received routine clinical care. Descriptive statistics, independent t or Mann–Whitney U tests, chi-square or Fisher's exact tests, paired t test, and generalized estimating equations were used to analyze the data.

Results: The average age of the participants was 35.1 years ($SD = 4.5$). No significant demographic or clinical differences were found between the control and experimental groups. The results of the generalized estimating equations showed significantly larger decreases in stress and anxiety in the experimental group than in the control group. No significant differences were identified between the two groups with respect to infant birth weeks, infant birth weight, average number of medical visits, or frequency of hospitalization.

Conclusions/Implications for Practice: The nurse-led case management program was shown to have short-term positive effects on the psychosocial outcomes of a population of Taiwanese patients with PIH. These results have important clinical implications for the healthcare administered to pregnant women, particularly in terms of improving the outcomes in those with PIH.

KEY WORDS:
case management, pregnancy-induced hypertension, stress, anxiety.

Introduction

Pregnancy-induced hypertension (PIH) affects 6%–10% of pregnant women worldwide (Kintiraki et al., 2015; Walle & Azagew, 2019) and is a major cause of maternal and fetal death (Wu et al., 2015). This condition involves the development of gestational hypertension and preeclampsia after 20 weeks of pregnancy (Walle & Azagew, 2019). PIH is defined as two occasions of systolic blood pressure (BP) greater than or equal to 140 mmHg or of diastolic BP greater than or equal to 90 mmHg (Muti et al., 2015). The risk factors for PIH include advanced maternal age, primiparity, multiple pregnancy, use of assisted reproduction techniques, being overweight, diabetes mellitus (gestational or otherwise), previous history of PIH, and chronic hypertension (Liu et al., 2018; Zhuang et al., 2019). In Taiwan, PIH is the second leading cause of maternal death (Wu et al., 2015). The incidence of preeclampsia has significantly increased from 0.87% to 1.21%, and the relative risk of developing this complication increases incrementally with age. Hypertensive disorders associated with pregnancy remain a significant challenge for obstetricians in Taiwan because of ongoing changes in society and culture such as the rise in mean maternal age at first birth (Chan et al., 2015).

Women with PIH face increased risks of placental abruption, organ failure, and disseminated intravascular coagulation (Kintiraki et al., 2015). In addition, women with a history of severe preeclampsia may experience headaches, left upper

[1]PhD, RN, Assistant Professor, Institute of Community Health Care, College of Nursing, National Yang Ming Chiao Tung University, Taipei, Taiwan • [2]PhD, RN, Professor, School of Nursing, National Defense Medical Center, Taipei, Taiwan • [3]BSN, RN, Case Manager, Department of Nursing, National Cheng Kung University Hospital, Tainan, Taiwan • [4]PhD, RN, Distinguished Professor, Institute of Community Health Care, College of Nursing, National Yang Ming Chiao Tung University, Taipei, Taiwan • [5]PhD, RN, Associate Professor, Department of Nursing, College of Medicine, National Cheng Kung University, and National Cheng Kung University Hospital, Tainan, Taiwan.

quadrant pain, visual impairment, fatigue, and memory and concentration disturbances after delivery more frequently than women without this history (Brusse et al., 2008). Other long-term risks associated with PIH include atherosclerosis and cardiovascular disease (Watanabe et al., 2015), midlife development of Type 2 diabetes (Timpka et al., 2018), and intracranial hemorrhage (Lin et al., 2016). Furthermore, the fetuses of mothers with PIH face increased risks of intrauterine growth retardation, premature birth, being small for gestational age, and intrauterine death (Kintiraki et al., 2015; Muti et al., 2015). In a study of 17,933 fetal deaths in Norway, 9.2% occurred during the pregnancies of women with hypertensive disorders (Ahmad & Samuelsen, 2012).

Women with PIH also face elevated vulnerability to psychological and physical problems (Abedian et al., 2015; Zhang et al., 2013) that may impact fetal health significantly, even to the point of being life-threatening (Leeners et al., 2008). Evidence has shown that women with PIH experience more stress than healthy pregnant women, and women with preeclampsia often experience higher anxiety and stress levels than pregnant women without preeclampsia (Brusse et al., 2008; Hayase et al., 2014; Thiagayson et al., 2013). The results of previous studies have associated anxiety in early pregnancy with risk of preeclampsia and found that one in four women with preeclampsia experience anxiety problems during their subsequent pregnancy (Habli et al., 2009; Rubertsson et al., 2014). In one study, 67.5% of women with preeclampsia were unaware that they were experiencing this condition before becoming pregnant or being diagnosed, most did not consider it to be a potentially life-threatening condition for mothers, half feared that it threatened the life of their fetuses, and the overwhelming majority (95%) expressed a desire to learn more about it (Frawley et al., 2020).

It has also been reported that women who experience psychological distress during pregnancy may be at increased risks for preterm birth and delivery of low-birth-weight babies. Thus, researchers have emphasized the importance of providing appropriate prenatal mental health support (Glover, 2014; Staneva et al., 2015). Certain relaxation techniques have been shown to be effective in helping pregnant women control anxiety. For example, a randomized, controlled trial involving women in their second trimester found that the experimental group, which participated in a 7-week program involving 90 minutes of relaxation training targeting breathing and muscles, had mean postintervention anxiety and stress levels that were significantly lower than those in the routine-care control group (Bastani et al., 2005). Similarly, Toosi et al. (2017) conducted a study on women receiving in vitro fertilization who participated in a 4-week program of relaxation training that included 10–20 minutes of specific techniques at the end of the course. The training emphasized finding a quiet environment, doing mental preparation, maintaining a passive attitude, remaining comfortable, and relaxing muscles throughout the body, with the experimental group achieving a significant decrease in anxiety at posttest. However, little research has focused on relaxation techniques

that are specifically designed to reduce maternal anxiety or stress in women with PIH (Damodaran, 2015).

Prenatal care during pregnancy is recommended to improve maternal and fetal outcomes, especially during high-risk pregnancies (Till et al., 2012). This care requires case management, which has been defined as "a collaborative process of assessment, planning, facilitation, care coordination, evaluation, and advocacy for options and services to meet an individual's and family's comprehensive health needs through communication and available resources to promote quality, cost-effective outcomes" (Case Management Society of America, 2016). During high-risk pregnancies, case management involves the implementation of systematic, long-term care strategies and includes follow-up consultation to manage risk and reduce morbidity and mortality (Soares & Higarashi, 2019). Maternity case management usually involves screening for diseases and social risks, ongoing contact with case managers, and resource referrals. Curry et al. (2006) conducted a nurse case management study targeting pregnant women at risk for abuse. Women were randomly assigned to the routine-care control group or the experimental group, with members of the latter group provided with videos, telephone access to a nursing case manager, and individualized nursing case management. The findings suggest that nursing case management approaches that assess pregnant women's needs and support their choices may effectively reduce self-perceived stress.

Case management has also proved effective in improving the birth weight of infants and reducing the incidence of preterm births (Slaughter et al., 2013), reducing the frequency at which babies are hospitalized in the neonatal intensive care unit, the healthcare costs associated with pregnancy, and the number of women experiencing high-risk pregnancies (Hutti & Usui, 2004). Moreover, the findings of several studies indicate that case management improves maternal behavior with respect to maintaining and engaging in HIV care at 1-year postpartum (Anderson et al., 2017; Schwartz et al., 2015) and to reducing alcohol consumption and the incidence of fetal alcohol spectrum disorders (de Vries et al., 2015; May et al., 2013). However, as previously noted, little information is available regarding the effectiveness of case management interventions designed to address the needs of women with PIH.

Therefore, the purpose of this study was to evaluate the effect of an antepartum case management program on stress, anxiety, and pregnancy in women in Taiwan with PIH. The primary aim was to assess the impact of an antepartum case management program on the stress and anxiety experienced by pregnant women. The secondary aim was to assess the impact of the program on pregnancy outcomes. Thus, the following research questions were formulated:

- What are the effects of an 8-week antepartum case management program on the stress and anxiety experienced by women with PIH?
- What are the effects of an 8-week antepartum case management program on pregnancy outcomes in women with PIH, including infant birth weeks, infant birth weight, number of medical visits, and frequency of hospitalization?

Methods

Design and Setting

A quasi-experimental approach was used to evaluate the effects of a case management program for women with PIH in terms of stress, anxiety, and pregnancy outcomes. Sixty-two women diagnosed with PIH were recruited from the obstetrics and gynecology clinics at a medical center in southern Taiwan and randomly assigned to either the experimental group or the control group. The experimental group received a case management program, and the control group did not. All of the participants were assessed using the same stress, anxiety, and pregnancy outcome measures. The outcomes were calculated by comparing the differences between measurements taken before the intervention (pretest) and measures taken at 8 weeks after the intervention (posttest).

Participants

Women who met the following criteria were invited to participate: (a) diagnosed by a physician within the previous 20–28 weeks as having PIH (including preeclampsia), (b) $\geq$ 18 years old, (c) free of other major health problems, and (d) able to communicate in Mandarin. Otherwise, qualified individuals with psychiatric conditions or a history of medical–surgical disease, maternal abuse, substance abuse, or multiple pregnancies, as determined via a medical records review, were excluded. In addition, those who had experienced other complications during pregnancy such as bleeding, gestational diabetes, uterine contracture, or rupture of membrane were excluded. Using the F test in G*Power software Version 3.1.6, with the assumptions α = .05, effect size = 0.3, power level = 0.80, and two groups (Chiu, 2007), a minimum sample size of 56 was determined. Using a presumed attrition rate of 10%, a total minimum sample size of 62 was determined for this study. Eighty-three women with PIH met the inclusion criteria for this study, of which 72 were recruited and 62 completed the 8-week program.

Intervention

The case management program for women with PIH was developed after an extensive review of the literature and discussions with experts. The case management program team consisted of physicians, the head nurse, the nursing faculty, and one nurse case manager. Two professors with specialties in maternal nursing and health education were also recruited to serve as the planning committee. The three key components of the case management program were (a) education related to PIH, including its etiology, complications, management, and self-care; (b) instruction in relaxation techniques, including explanations and demonstrations of the various steps; and (c) telephone follow-up evaluations every 2 weeks to identify difficulties faced by the participants, monitor their relaxation practice, and answer questions. A booklet describing case management for PIH, inclusive of all materials

in the health education program, was developed and distributed to the participants for their use as a guide.

The case management process for this study included (a) screening and recruitment by the case manager to identify women meeting the eligibility criteria; (b) assessment and monitoring of the participants' weight, height, BP, blood sugar, urine glucose, proteinuria, bleeding, uterine contracture, and rupture of membrane; (c) implementation of the program, including discussion of the concept of PIH and its etiology, managing symptoms, self-management and monitoring, hospital resources, and relaxation techniques; and (d) evaluation and follow-up consultation by telephone regarding the condition of the pregnant women, weeks of gestation, and the numbers of hospitalizations and visits to clinics or hospitals. Whereas the experimental group participated in the case management program, the control group received the standard care protocol provided by Taiwanese clinics.

Measurements

The measurements included demographic and clinical information, BP, pregnancy outcomes, and self-reported stress and anxiety.

Demographic and clinical information

The demographic data collected from participants included age, education, and marital status. The clinical information that was collected included the participants' pregnancy, childbirth, and PIH histories and any current PIH symptoms such as edema and proteinuria.

Blood pressure

BP was measured 5 minutes before the patients took a rest and 15 minutes afterward using a calibrated, automated, and oscillometric-validated device. All of the measurements were performed by the same researcher at the same time of day at a controlled room temperature.

Pregnancy outcomes

The main concern in this study was to evaluate the pregnancy outcomes of the participants, which included infant birth weeks, infant birth weight, number of hospitalizations, and number of medical visits. Infant birth weeks was defined as the gestational week of birth. Infant birth weight was defined as the weight of the newborn at birth. Number of hospitalizations was defined as the number of participants hospitalized because of PIH. Number of clinic or hospital visits (apart from routine prenatal care) was further subcategorized by reason, including high BP, symptoms related to PIH, and emergency treatment.

Pregnancy stress

The Pregnancy Stress Rating Scale developed by Chen et al. (1983) was used to evaluate prenatal stress. This scale consists of five domains: stress related to concerns about maternal and fetal safety through pregnancy, labor, and childbirth;

newborn care and changes in family relationships; maternal role identification; seeking social support; and physical appearance and changes in function. The participants were asked to rate 30 items keyed to pregnancy-related stressors based on their levels of concern and distress on a Likert scale ranging from 1 (*definitely not concerned or distressed*) to 5 (*very severe concern and distress*). The total possible score was 150, with higher scores correlating with higher levels of prenatal stress. This instrument showed good internal consistency (α = .91) and supporting convergent and discriminate validities (Chen et al., 1983; Chiu, 2007).

Anxiety

Anxiety was measured in this study using one part of the State-Trait Anxiety Inventory (STAI) developed by Spielberger. Twenty items were used to measure state anxiety (STAI-State), which indicated the current feelings of the participants on a 4-point Likert scale ranging from 1 (*not at all*) to 4 (*very much so*); the scores ranged from 20 to 80 for both state anxiety scales, with higher scores correlating with the intensity of the respondents' anxiety. This questionnaire has shown good reliability (Cronbach's α = .830; Delgado et al., 2016).

Procedure

Ethical approval for this study was obtained from the institutional review board of university hospital (B-ER-105-388). The data were collected from January 2017 to January 2018. A nurse with more than 10 years of professional experience served as the case manager and conducted the case management and relaxation course training classes. Eligible participants referred by their physicians were invited to participate. Written informed consent was obtained from the participants after explaining the study thoroughly. The participants were randomly assigned to either the experimental group or the control group. Those assigned to the experimental group were instructed to fill out the pretest measure, which included demographic and clinical information, information related to pregnancy stress, and the state anxiety questionnaires, which took about 20 minutes to complete. Next, these participants received one-on-one health education related to PIH for about 30 minutes and spent 20 minutes on the relaxation techniques. The intervention was conducted for an 8-week period, and every participant received a copy of the aforementioned PIH case management booklet. The posttest, administered after the intervention, gathered data on pregnancy stress, state anxiety, number of medical visits, and number of hospitalizations. By contrast, the participants who were assigned to the control group received routine care and completed both the pretest and posttest measures. Information on infant birth weeks and infant birth weight was obtained from the participants' medical records. All of the data collected were treated confidentially, and the participants were informed that they were free to withdraw from the study at any time and for any reason without affecting their treatment or care.

Ethical Considerations

The confidential information associated with this study was stored on a password-protected computer in a locked cabinet. The researchers explained the purpose, process, and method of the study to the participants along with their related rights and interests. Signed, informed consent was obtained from all of the participants before data collection. To maintain the principle of equality, the members of the control group had access to routine hospital care during their pregnancies. To further ensure the confidentiality and privacy of participants, all data were anonymously encoded and not publicly disclosed.

Data Analysis

The data were analyzed using SPSS for Windows software Version 25.0 (IBM Inc., Armonk, NY, USA). Descriptive statistical analysis served to describe the study variables and the demographic and clinical characteristics of the participants. Independent t tests or Mann–Whitney U tests were used for the continuous variables, and chi-square tests or Fisher exact tests were used for the categorical variables to examine the homogeneity between the experimental and control groups. In addition, paired-sample t tests were used to compare intragroup differences in the outcome variables between T1 and T2, and generalized estimation equations were used to evaluate the differences in the changes between the groups (p < .05) between pretest and posttest.

Results

Seventy-two qualified individuals consented to participate in the study, with 10 lost to follow-up for reasons including transfer to another hospital, inability to complete the intervention, or being moved away from the area. Thus, data for 62 participants were available for analysis, including 31 in the experimental group and 31 in the control group. No significant intergroup differences were identified in terms of either demographics (Table 1) or clinical-related information.

Levels of stress and anxiety did not differ significantly between the two groups at either pretest or posttest (Table 2). In the experimental group, the mean score for stress during pregnancy decreased significantly, from 62.3 (SD = 15.8) at pretest to 52.5 (SD = 8.8; p < .001) at posttest, and the mean score for anxiety status declined significantly from 40.0 (SD = 12.8) at pretest to 36.9 (SD = 10.0) at posttest (p = .003). In the control group, no significant improvement was observed for either stress or anxiety status. In terms of intergroup comparisons, the posttest mean anxiety score was significantly lower in the experimental group than in the control group (p = .03). In terms of posttest pregnancy outcomes, no significant differences were found between the two groups with respect to infant birth weeks, infant birth weight, number of medical visits, or number of hospitalizations.

The interactions between the groups and time were analyzed using a generalized estimation equation analysis of the changes in stress and anxiety after the case management intervention (Table 3). The results showed that posttest stress (Pregnancy Stress Rating Scale) scores were significantly lower in the

Table 1

Demographic and Clinical Information, by Group (N = 62)

Variable	Total (N = 62)		Experimental Group (n = 31)		Control Group (n = 31)		p
	n	%	n	%	n	%	
Age (years; M and SD)	35.1	4.5	34.8	4.9	35.4	4.1	.639
Marital status							1.000
Married	58	93.5	29	93.5	29	93.5	
Not married	4	6.5	2	6.5	2	6.5	
Educational level							.155
High school or less	17	27.4	11	35.5	6	19.4	
Post-high school	45	72.6	20	64.5	25	80.6	
Religious							.189
Yes	23	37.1	14	45.2	9	29.0	
No	39	62.9	17	54.8	22	71.0	
Employed (n = 60)							.142
Yes	38	63.0	15	52.0	23	74.0	
No	22	37.0	14	48.0	8	26.0	
Health insurance (n = 60)							.416
Yes	54	90.0	25	86.0	29	94.0	
No	6	10.0	4	14.0	2	6.0	
Gestational weeks (M and SD)	24.4	2.5	24.3	2.3	24.5	2.7	.835
Hypertensive disorder subtype							.309
Gestational hypertension	30	48.0	13	42.0	17	54.0	
Mild or severe preeclampsia	32	52.0	18	58.0	14	46.0	
Previous deliveries							.611
0	32	51.6	17	54.8	15	48.4	
≥ 1	30	48.4	14	45.2	16	51.6	
Previous preterm deliveries							1.000
0	55	88.7	28	90.3	27	87.1	
1	7	11.3	3	9.7	4	12.9	
Previous PIH experience							.562
Yes	16	25.8	9	29.0	7	22.6	
No	46	74.2	22	71.0	24	77.4	
SBP (mmHg; M and SD)	146.6	8.8	147.3	10.6	145.8	6.7	.488
DBP (mmHg; M and SD)	88.6	9.1	88.7	9.1	88.6	9.3	.989
Edema							.297
Yes	24	38.7	14	45.2	10	32.3	
No	28	61.3	17	54.8	21	67.7	
Proteinuria							.544
Yes	14	22.6	8	25.8	6	19.4	
No	48	77.4	23	74.2	25	80.6	

Note. PIH = pregnancy-induced hypertension; SBP = systolic blood pressure; DBP = diastolic blood pressure.

experimental group ($B = -8.92$, $p = .013$) than in the control group. Moreover, group and time interaction effects were observed on the anxiety (STAI-State) score ($B = -4.69$, $p = .031$).

Discussion

This study was the first to explore the effect of case management on stress, anxiety, and pregnancy outcomes in women with PIH. The stress and anxiety scores of the participants

who undertook the 8-week intervention decreased significantly more than their control group peers. These results indicate that the case management program used in this research may have positive effects on the psychological outcomes of pregnant women with hypertension in Taiwan.

Previous research has found inconsistent results from case management programs that target pregnancy-related stress (Churchill et al., 2018; Curry et al., 2006). In this study, the significantly stronger improvement in stress scores seen

Table 2

Stress, Anxiety, and Pregnancy Outcomes, by Group (N = 62)

Variable	Experimental Group (n = 31)		Control Group (n = 31)		p
	M	SD	M	SD	
Pregnancy Stress Rating Scale					
Pretest	62.3	15.8	59.5	13.5	.457
Posttest	52.5	8.8	56.6	15.0	.238
p Value	< .001		.317		
State Trait Anxiety Inventory-State					
Pretest	40.0	12.8	41.5	10.8	.610
Posttest	36.9	10.0	42.6	10.3	.030
p Value	.003		.550		
Pregnancy outcomes					
Infant birth weeks	36.3	2.38	37.4	2.2	.082
Infant birth weight (grams)	2639.1	660.1	2857.0	622.6	.190
Number of medical visits	5.2	1.9	5.1	1.3	.646
Frequency of hospitalization	0.4	0.6	0.3	0.4	.353

in the experimental group versus the control group supports the effectiveness of the developed intervention protocol. This finding has significance for clinical practice because psychosocial stress during pregnancy is a risk factor for preterm birth (Staneva et al., 2015). This correlation may be attributable to the stimulation, in response to stress, of adrenaline production and the sympathetic nerves, which accelerates respiratory and heart rates. The relaxation techniques taught to members of the experimental group in this study were based on established stress-management strategies (Mohammadi & Parandin, 2019). The effectiveness of the case management program in this study may also be attributable in part to its implementation by a nursing case manager in the form of one-on-one consultation and education, which, in the experimental

group, raised awareness of the disease, suggested ways to manage stress and PIH symptoms, and provided psychological support. Further study is needed to determine the long-term effectiveness of this case management approach to managing stress and to compare the specific effects of the individual elements of this case management program such as relaxation techniques, educational booklets, and consultations.

In this study, the case management approach significantly reduced the anxiety perceived by women with PIH. This finding is consistent with previous studies on the efficacy of using case management to treat anxiety in various populations (Hsu & Tai, 2014; Wang et al., 2016). In clinical settings, pregnant women with hypertension may experience various symptoms over time, including high BP, dizziness, headaches, proteinuria,

Table 3

Generalized Estimating Equation Analysis of Changes in PSRS and STAI-S From Baseline (T1) to 8 Weeks (T2)

Variable	PSRS				STAI-S			
	B	95% Wald CI Low	High	p	B	95% Wald CI Low	High	p
(Intercept)	33.80	9.80	57.80	.006	28.49	11.03	45.95	.001
Time								
8 weeks (T2) vs. baseline (T1)	−1.48	−6.88	3.91	.590	1.29	−2.60	5.18	.510
Group								
Experimental vs. control	3.97	−2.54	10.49	.230	−1.74	−7.25	3.75	.530
Group × Time								
Experimental vs. control with 8 weeks (T2) vs. baseline (T1)	−8.92	−16.01	−1.84	.013	−4.69	−8.97	−0.42	.031

Note. Controlled variables included age, education, past pregnancy-induced hypertension experience, systolic blood pressure, diastolic blood pressure, edema, and proteinuria. PSRS = Pregnancy Stress Rating Scale; STAI-S = State Trait Anxiety Inventory-State; CI = confidence interval.

and edema in the lower limbs. Effective nurse case managers are knowledgeable about PIH, capable of identifying related symptoms, and able to make decisions regarding the best treatment. Case management may also be effective in terms of limiting the fragmentation and discontinuity of care associated with referrals and arrangements (Soares & Higarashi, 2019), which may subsequently reduce the anxiety felt by pregnant women who are at a high risk for complications associated with this condition. The positive psychological effects of case management make this a promising approach for patients dealing with PIH-related issues.

The lack of significant differences in infant birth weeks and infant birth weights between the experimental and control groups was unexpected. This finding may be attributable to dosage issues associated with case management. An earlier study found that women who received more than 6 hours of antenatal coordination services were less likely to have poor neonatal outcomes than those who received fewer than 6 hours of these services (Van Dijk et al., 2011). Another study found that women who received case management characterized by frequent and long-duration contacts beginning in the first or second trimester were less likely to have low-birth-weight or preterm deliveries than those who received less extensive case management (Slaughter & Issel, 2012). However, as most of the participants in this study were in their second trimester, the intervention period of 8 weeks was chosen in light of the manner in which PIH develops (i.e., after 20 weeks of pregnancy). Future research is needed to examine the effects of the initiation, duration, and intensity of nursing case management on maternal and neonatal outcomes.

In addition, no significant differences were found between the experimental and control groups with respect to numbers of medical visits or hospitalizations. One possible explanation for this is the effective dissemination of information online by most hospitals in Taiwan. As pregnant women with hypertension are able to access information through the internet that can help alleviate their complications or symptoms, they are less likely to seek hospitalization or outpatient services. Another reason for this may reflect inaccurate reporting, as medical visit and hospitalization numbers were self-reported by the participants. Researchers conducting similar future studies may consider using medical records of other pregnancy outcomes such as the number of babies hospitalized in the neonatal intensive care unit or number of mothers with high-risk conditions to assess the effect of the case management approach on pregnant women (Hutti & Usui, 2004).

This study was subject to several limitations. As the data were collected while the participants were pregnant, the results are not generalizable to the postpartum period. Further study is needed to shed light on the longer-term case management of women with PIH. A further limitation was the use of subjective questionnaires to measure stress and anxiety. Future studies may employ more-objective measures of psychological change.

Conclusions

The results of this study support the effectiveness of the case management approach in improving psychological outcomes

in women with PIH. Specifically, the participants in the experimental group had significantly lower levels of stress and anxiety after the conclusion of the case management intervention than their counterparts who received routine care only. Prenatal case management services should be further evaluated using a larger sample to validate and identify the program characteristics of intervention programs that improve psychological and birth outcomes for women with PIH.

Acknowledgments

This work was supported by a grant from the Taiwan Nurses Association (TWNA-1062010).

Author Contributions

Study conception and design: CC Chou, CJW
Data collection: CC Chen
Data analysis and interpretation: CC Chou, JJL, YML, CJW
Drafting of the article: CC Chou, CJW
Critical revision of the article: JJL, YML, CJW

References

Abedian, Z., Soltani, N., Mokhber, N., & Esmaily, H. (2015). Depression and anxiety in pregnancy and postpartum in women with mild and severe preeclampsia. *Iranian Journal of Nursing and Midwifery Research, 20*(4), 454–459. https://doi.org/10.4103/1735-9066.161013

Ahmad, A. S., & Samuelsen, S. O. (2012). Hypertensive disorders in pregnancy and fetal death at different gestational lengths: A population study of 2 121 371 pregnancies. *British Journal of Obstetrics and Gynaecology, 119*(12), 1521–1528. https://doi.org/10.1111/j.1471-0528.2012.03460.x

Anderson, E. A., Momplaisir, F. M., Corson, C., & Brady, K. A. (2017). Assessing the impact of perinatal HIV case management on outcomes along the HIV care continuum for pregnant and postpartum women living with HIV, Philadelphia 2005–2013. *AIDS and Behavior, 21*(9), 2670–2681. https://doi.org/10.1007/s10461-017-1714-9

Bastani, F., Hidarnia, A., Kazemnejad, A., Vafaei, M., & Kashanian, M. (2005). A randomized controlled trial of the effects of applied relaxation training on reducing anxiety and perceived stress in pregnant women. *Journal of Midwifery & Women's Health, 50*(4), e36–e40. https://doi.org/10.1016/j.jmwh.2004.11.008

Brusse, I., Duvekot, J., Jongerling, J., Steegers, E., & De Koning, I. (2008). Impaired maternal cognitive functioning after pregnancies complicated by severe pre-eclampsia: A pilot case-control study. *Acta Obstetricia et Gynecologica Scandinavica, 87*(4), 408–412. https://doi.org/10.1080/00016340801915127

Case Management Society of America. (2016). *Standards of practice for case management*. Little Rock.

Chan, T.-F., Tung, Y.-C., Wang, S.-H., Lee, C.-H., Lin, C.-L., & Lu, P.-Y. (2015). Trends in the incidence of pre-eclampsia and eclampsia in Taiwan between 1998 and 2010. *Taiwanese Journal of Obstetrics & Gynecology, 54*(3), 270–274. https://doi.org/10.1016/j.tjog.2013.06.021

Chen, C.-H., Yu, Y.-M., & Hwang, K.-K. (1983). Psychological stressors perceived by pregnant women during their third trimester. *Formosan Journal of Public Health, 10*(1), 88–98. (Original work published in Chinese)

Chiu, W. H. (2007). *The effectiveness of case management style for the twin pregnancy women*, [Unpublished master's thesis]. National Taipei University of Nursing and Health Sciences, Taipei. (Original work published in Chinese)

Churchill, S. S., Leo, M. C., Brennan, E. M., Sellmaier, C., Kendall, J., & Houck, G. M. (2018). Longitudinal impact of a randomized clinical trial to improve family function, reduce maternal stress and improve child outcomes in families of children with ADHD. *Maternal and Child Health Journal, 22*(8), 1172–1182. https://doi.org/10.1007/s10995-018-2502-5

Curry, M. A., Durham, L., Bullock, L., Bloom, T., & Davis, J. (2006). Nurse case management for pregnant women experiencing or at risk for abuse. *Journal of Obstetric, Gynecologic, & Neonatal Nursing, 35*(2), 181–192. https://doi.org/10.1111/j.1552-6909.2006.00027.x

Damodaran, D. (2015). Effect of progressive muscle relaxation technique in terms oi anxiety and physiological parameters of antenatal mothers with pregnancy-induced hypertension. *The Nursing Journal of India, 106*(6), 254–257.

de Vries, M. M., Joubert, B., Cloete, M., Roux, S., Baca, B. A., Hasken, J. M., Barnard, R., Buckley, D., Kalberg, W. O., Snell, C. L., Marais, A. S., Seedat, S., Parry, C. D. H., & May, P. A. (2015). Indicated prevention of fetal alcohol spectrum disorders in South Africa: Effectiveness of case management. *International Journal of Environmental Research and Public Health, 13*(1), Article 13010076. https://doi.org/10.3390/ijerph13010076

Delgado, A. M., Freire, A. D., Wanderley, E. L., & Lemos, A. (2016). Analysis of the construct validity and internal consistency of the State-Trait Anxiety Inventory (STAI) State-Anxiety (S-Anxiety) Scale for pregnant women during labor. *Revista Brasileira de Ginecologia e Obstetrícia, 38*(11), 531–537. https://doi.org/10.1055/s-0036-1593894

Frawley, N., East, C., & Brennecke, S. (2020). Women's experiences of preeclampsia: A prospective survey of preeclamptic women at a single tertiary centre. *Journal of Obstetrics and Gynaecology, 40*(1), 65–69. https://doi.org/10.1080/01443615.2019.1615040

Glover, V. (2014). Maternal depression, anxiety and stress during pregnancy and child outcome; what needs to be done. *Best Practice & Research Clinical Obstetrics & Gynaecology, 28*(1), 25–35. https://doi.org/10.1016/j.bpobgyn.2013.08.017

Habli, M., Eftekhari, N., Wiebracht, E., Bombrys, A., Khabbaz, M., How, H., & Sibai, B. (2009). Long-term maternal and subsequent pregnancy outcomes 5 years after hemolysis, elevated liver enzymes, and low platelets (HELLP) syndrome. *American Journal of Obstetrics and Gynecology, 201*(4), 385.e1–385.e5. https://doi.org/10.1016/j.ajog.2009.06.033

Hayase, M., Shimada, M., & Seki, H. (2014). Sleep quality and stress in women with pregnancy-induced hypertension and gestational diabetes mellitus. *Women and Birth, 27*(3), 190–195. https://doi.org/10.1016/j.wombi.2014.04.002

Hsu, C. C., & Tai, T. Y. (2014). Long-term glycemic control by a diabetes case-management program and the challenges of diabetes care in Taiwan. *Diabetes Research and Clinical Practice, 106*(Suppl. 2), S328–S332. https://doi.org/10.1016/S0168-8227(14)70738-7

Hutti, M. H., & Usui, W. M. (2004). Nursing telephonic case management and pregnancy outcomes of mothers and infants. *Lippincott's Case Management, 9*(6), 287–299. https://doi.org/10.1097/00129234-200411000-00008

Kintiraki, E., Papakatsika, S., Kotronis, G., Goulis, D. G., & Kotsis, V. (2015). Pregnancy-induced hypertension. *Hormones (Athens, Greece), 14*(2), 211–223. https://doi.org/10.14310/horm.2002.1582

Leeners, B., Stiller, R., Neumaier-Wagner, P., Kuse, S., Schmitt, A., & Rath, W. (2008). Psychosocial distress associated with treatment of hypertensive diseases in pregnancy. *Psychosomatics, 49*(5), 413–419. https://doi.org/10.1176/appi.psy.49.5.413

Lin, L. T., Tsui, K. H., Cheng, J. T., Cheng, J. S., Huang, W. C., Liou, W. S., & Tang, P. L. (2016). Increased risk of intracranial hemorrhage in patients with pregnancy-induced hypertension: A nationwide population-based retrospective cohort study. *Medicine (Baltimore), 95*(20), e3732. https://doi.org/10.1097/md.0000000000003732

Liu, Q., Wang, X. X., Zhang, Y. K., Li, J. H., & Wang, L. (2018). Correlation between pregnancy-induced hypertension and age in pregnant women from Hebei province, 2016. *Zhonghua Liu Xing Bing Xue Za Zhi, 39*(9), 1270–1273. https://doi.org/10.3760/cma.j.issn.0254-6450.2018.09.024 (Original work published in Chinese)

May, P. A., Marais, A. S., Gossage, J. P., Barnard, R., Joubert, B., Cloete, M., Hendricks, N., Roux, S., Blom, A., Steenekamp, J., Alexander, T., Andreas, R., Human, S., Snell, C., Seedat, S., Parry, C. C., Kalberg, W. O., Buckley, D., & Blankenship, J. (2013). Case management reduces drinking during pregnancy among high risk women. *International Journal of Alcohol and Drug Research, 2*(3), 61–70. https://doi.org/10.7895/ijadr.v2i3.79

Mohammadi, M. M., & Parandin, S. (2019). Effect of the combination of Benson's relaxation technique and brief psychoeducational intervention on multidimensional pain and negative psychological symptoms of pregnant women: A randomized controlled trial. *Journal of Education and Health Promotion, 8*, 91. https://doi.org/10.4103/jehp.jehp_286_18

Muti, M., Tshimanga, M., Notion, G. T., Bangure, D., & Chonzi, P. (2015). Prevalence of pregnancy induced hypertension and pregnancy outcomes among women seeking maternity services in Harare, Zimbabwe. *BMC Cardiovascular Disorders, 15*, Article No. 111. https://doi.org/10.1186/s12872-015-0110-5

Rubertsson, C., Hellström, J., Cross, M., & Sydsjö, G. (2014). Anxiety in early pregnancy: Prevalence and contributing factors. *Archives of Women's Mental Health, 17*(3), 221–228. https://doi.org/10.1007/s00737-013-0409-0

Schwartz, S. R., Clouse, K., Yende, N., Van Rie, A., Bassett, J., Ratshefola, M., & Pettifor, A. (2015). Acceptability and feasibility of a mobile phone-based case management intervention to retain mothers and infants from an option B+ program in postpartum HIV care. *Maternal and Child Health Journal, 19*(9), 2029–2037. https://doi.org/10.1007/s10995-015-1715-0

Slaughter, J. C., & Issel, L. M. (2012). Developing a measure of prenatal case management dosage. *Maternal and Child Health Journal, 16*(5), 1120–1130. https://doi.org/10.1007/s10995-011-0840-7

Slaughter, J. C., Issel, L. M., Handler, A. S., Rosenberg, D., Kane, D. J., & Stayner, L. T. (2013). Measuring dosage: A key factor when assessing the relationship between prenatal case management and birth outcomes. *Maternal and Child Health Journal, 17*(8), 1414–1423. https://doi.org/10.1007/s10995-012-1143-3

Soares, L. G., & Higarashi, I. H. (2019). Case management as a high-risk prenatal care strategy. *Revista Brasileira de Enfermagem, 72*(3), 692–699. https://doi.org/10.1590/0034-7167-2018-0483

Staneva, A., Bogossian, F., Pritchard, M., & Wittkowski, A. (2015). The effects of maternal depression, anxiety, and perceived stress during pregnancy on preterm birth: A systematic review. *Women and Birth, 28*(3), 179–193. https://doi.org/10.1016/j.wombi.2015.02.003

Thiagayson, P., Krishnaswamy, G., Lim, M. L., Sung, S. C., Haley, C. L., Fung, D. S., Allen, J. C., & Chen, H. (2013). Depression and anxiety in Singaporean high-risk pregnancies—Prevalence and screening. *General Hospital Psychiatry, 35*(2), 112–116. https://doi.org/10.1016/j.genhosppsych.2012.11.006

Till, S. R., Everetts, D., Haas, D. M., & Cochrane Pregnancy and Childbirth Group. (2012). Incentives for increasing prenatal care use by women in order to improve maternal and neonatal outcomes. *Cochrane Database of Systematic Reviews, 12*, Article CD009916. https://doi.org/10.1002/14651858.CD009916.pub2

Timpka, S., Markovitz, A., Schyman, T., Mogren, I., Fraser, A., Franks, P. W., & Rich-Edwards, J. W. (2018). Midlife development of type 2 diabetes and hypertension in women by history of hypertensive disorders of pregnancy. *Cardiovascular Diabetology, 17*(1), Article No. 124. https://doi.org/10.1186/s12933-018-0764-2

Toosi, M., Akbarzadeh, M., & Ghaemi, Z. (2017). The effect of relaxation on mother's anxiety and maternal–fetal attachment in primiparous IVF mothers. *Journal of the National Medical Association, 109*(3), 164–171. https://doi.org/10.1016/j.jnma.2017.03.002

Van Dijk, J. W., Anderko, L., & Stetzer, F. (2011). The impact of prenatal care coordination on birth outcomes. *Journal of Obstetric,* *Gynecologic, and Neonatal Nursing, 40*(1), 98–108. https://doi.org/10.1111/j.1552-6909.2010.01206.x

Walle, T. A., & Azagew, A. W. (2019). Hypertensive disorder of pregnancy prevalence and associated factors among pregnant women attending ante natal care at Gondar town health Institutions, North West Ethiopia 2017. *Pregnancy Hypertension, 16*, 79–84. https://doi.org/10.1016/j.preghy.2019.03.007

Wang, Y. C., Hsieh, L. Y., Wang, M. Y., Chou, C. H., Huang, M. W., & Ko, H. C. (2016). Coping card usage can further reduce suicide reattempt in suicide attempter case management within 3-month intervention. *Suicide & Life-Threatening Behavior, 46*(1), 106–120. https://doi.org/10.1111/sltb.12177

Watanabe, K., Kimura, C., Iwasaki, A., Mori, T., Matsushita, H., Shinohara, K., Wakatsuki, A., Gosho, M., & Miyano, I. (2015). Pregnancy-induced hypertension is associated with an increase in the prevalence of cardiovascular disease risk factors in Japanese women. *Menopause, 22*(6), 656–659. https://doi.org/10.1097/gme.0000000000000361

Wu, T. P., Huang, Y. L., Liang, F. W., & Lu, T. H. (2015). Underreporting of maternal mortality in Taiwan: A data linkage study. *Taiwanese Journal of Obstetrics & Gynecology, 54*(6), 705–708. https://doi.org/10.1016/j.tjog.2015.10.002

Zhang, S., Ding, Z., Liu, H., Chen, Z., Wu, J., Zhang, Y., & Yu, Y. (2013). Association between mental stress and gestational hypertension/preeclampsia: A meta-analysis. *Obstetrical & Gynecological Survey, 68*(12), 825–834. https://doi.org/10.1097/ogx.0000000000000001

Zhuang, C., Gao, J., Liu, J., Wang, X., He, J., Sun, J., Liu, X., & Liao, S. (2019). Risk factors and potential protective factors of pregnancy-induced hypertension in China: A cross-sectional study. *The Journal of Clinical Hypertension, 21*(5), 618–623. https://doi.org/10.1111/jch.13541

25

Relationships Between Job Satisfaction and Job Demand, Job Control, Social Support and Depression in Iranian Nurses

Majid BAGHERI HOSSEIN ABADI[1] • Ebrahim TABAN[2] • Narges KHANJANI[3] • Zahra NAGHAVI KONJIN[4] • Farahnaz KHAJEHNASIRI[5] • Seyed Ehsan SAMAEI[4]*

ABSTRACT

Background: Nurses often experience a wide variety of stressful situations. Excessive work stress influences the physical and mental health of nurses and decreases their life quality and professional efficacy. In addition, high levels of psychological stress may cause job dissatisfaction and job strain.

Purpose: The objective of this study was to explore the relationship between several work-related risk factors and job satisfaction in Iranian nurses.

Methods: A cross-sectional study was conducted on 730 nurses from four public hospitals in, respectively, northern, southern, eastern, and western Iran. Variables in the job demand–control–support (JDCS) model were measured using the Job Content Questionnaire, and job satisfaction was measured using the Minnesota Satisfaction Questionnaire.

Results: The mean score for job satisfaction was 62.94 ± 14.24, which is considered moderate. Nurses with a low level of job satisfaction had significantly higher psychological and physical job demands ($p < .05$). Significant relationships were found between job satisfaction and several dimensions of the JDCS model, including psychological job demands ($\beta = -0.11$, $p < .001$), physical job demands ($\beta = -0.86$, $p = .004$), skill discretion ($\beta = 0.48$, $p = .033$), decision authority ($\beta = 0.43$, $p = .028$), and supervisor support ($\beta = 1.85$, $p = .004$). The sociodemographic and JDCS model variables used in this study explained 42% of the variation in job satisfaction ($R^2 = .42$).

Conclusions/Implications for Practice: Enhancing the job satisfaction of nurses is possible by creating a balance between job demands, job control, and social support.

KEY WORDS:
Job Content Questionnaire, job demand–control–support model, Minnesota Satisfaction Questionnaire, nurses.

Introduction

Job satisfaction impacts significantly on productivity and work absenteeism in nurses. Previous studies have shown that increasing job satisfaction in nurses results in higher quality medical services and leads to better healthcare outcomes and higher patient satisfaction (Janicijevic et al., 2013; Negahban et al., 2017). Job satisfaction is a complicated subject, with low levels of job satisfaction associated with increased intention to leave the nursing profession (De Simone & Planta, 2017). Researchers are currently assessing the critical factors that affect job satisfaction to establish and improve evidence-based job satisfaction theories and management interventions for nurses. Demographic, occupational characteristic, and organizational factors are known to affect job satisfaction (Al Maqbali, 2015; Lu et al., 2016; Schwendimann et al., 2016).

Numerous studies have reported on a strong negative relationship between occupational stress and job satisfaction, suggesting that occupational stress in nurses may lead to intention to leave and reduce nursing quality (Bagheri Hosseinabadi et al., 2018; Gadirzadeh et al., 2017; Sveinsdóttir et al., 2006). Occupational stress has been described as negative emotional and physical reactions that occur when job demands (psychological or physical) do not match a worker's capabilities (Rao & Chandraiah, 2012).

Job demand is a factor that plays a key role in increasing occupational stress. Nursing is a job known for its high psychological and physical demands (Chen et al., 2015). A study by Hülsheger and Schewe (2011) showed that high psychological demand often causes low self-monitoring, which has negative effects on employees' general well-being. Several studies have been conducted to identify the risk factors of occupational stress. These studies have developed models of job/occupational stress such as the job demand–control–

[1]MS, School of Public Health, Shahroud University of Medical Science, Shahroud, Iran • [2]PhD, Assistant Professor, Social Determinants of Health Research Center, Department of Occupational Health Engineering, Mashhad University of Medical Sciences, Mashhad, Iran • [3]PhD, Professor, Neurology Research Center, Kerman University of Medical Sciences, Kerman, Iran • [4]PhD, Assistant Professor, Health Sciences Research Center, Addiction Institute, Mazandaran University of Medical Sciences, Sari, Iran • [5]PhD, Associate Professor, Department of Community Medicine, Faculty of Medicine, Tehran University of Medical Sciences, Tehran, Iran.

support (JDCS) model and highlighted the harmful effects of occupational stress on worker health (Negussie & Kaur, 2016; Rhee, 2010; Sharma et al., 2014). On the basis of the JDCS model, high job demand and low job control in addition to increasing physical and psychological stress may cause cardiovascular diseases and mental health problems (Nieuwenhuijsen et al., 2010).

Karasek has defined high job demand as high workload. Using the JDCS model, job demand and social support (including supervisor and coworkers support) were shown to influence job satisfaction in Ethiopian nurses (Negussie & Kaur, 2016). Furthermore, studies have shown that job satisfaction and social support in nurses may be affected by burnout (Hamaideh, 2011). Job control, defined as the extent of a person's independence to make decisions and control actions during their occupational tasks, is negatively correlated with job dissatisfaction (Clumeck et al., 2009).

Demographic variables such as age, gender, and marital status are known to influence job satisfaction (Tabatabaei et al., 2013), and many efforts have been made to illustrate the relationship between job satisfaction and job-related stress (Bagheri et al., 2017; Lee et al., 2019). However, further investigation of these factors is needed, as there is wide variability among nursing work conditions, particularly in developing countries, that may exacerbate or alleviate perceived job stress (Bagheri Hosseinabadi et al., 2018; Khamisa et al., 2017).

Several studies have examined the effective factors of job satisfaction among nurses in developed countries. Because of differences between developed and developing countries in terms of healthcare systems and nurses' job structure, more research in developing countries is desperately needed to identify occupational factors that affect job satisfaction to help health services managers improve organizational culture and nurses' job satisfaction (Bagheri Hosseinabadi et al., 2018; Khamisa et al., 2017; San Park & Hyun Kim, 2009). Creating an appropriate organizational culture is a well-known first step to creating good working conditions (Banaszak-Holl et al., 2015). Therefore, this study was conducted to evaluate the relationship between job satisfaction and, respectively, job demand, job control, and social support among Iranian nurses.

Methods

Design and Sample

This cross-sectional study was conducted to evaluate the respective effects of physical and psychological work demands, social and coworker support, and job control on job satisfaction in nurses. Data were collected from March 2016 to February 2017.

The participants were nurses who were currently working in one of four public hospitals in, respectively, northern, southern, eastern, and western Iran (in the respective cities of Babol, Kerman, Mashhad, and Hamedan). The inclusion criteria were being a full-time nurse with more than 1-year clinical experience in the current ward. The exclusion criteria

included having a second job or currently under treatment by a psychiatrist. The total number of nurses working in these hospitals was 1,687. Thus, a target sample size of 694 was calculated using the table suggested by Krejcie and Morgan (1970) to obtain a 95% confidence level and 3.5% margin of error. Nurses were selected randomly from all of the wards in the target hospitals. The questionnaires were delivered to 730 nurses, but only 701 were returned, and an additional seven questionnaires were excluded because of incompleteness.

Data Collection

Sociodemographic variables

The demographic questionnaire contained questions about age, gender, educational level, employment status, ward, clinical experience, and work status (fixed and rotating shifts).

The job demand–control–support model

In this study, components of the JDCS model were measured using the Job Content Questionnaire (JCQ). This questionnaire is a self-assessment tool that was designed to measure the psychological and social characteristics of occupations (Karasek et al., 1998). This questionnaire is available in several languages, including Persian, and was approved by the JCQ Center (Choobineh et al., 2011). The three dimensions of the 27-item JCQ respectively measure job demand, job control (decision latitude), and social support.

Job demand covers the physical and psychological aspects of a job that impose an ongoing physical or psychological burden on cognition and perception. Karasek described a high level of job demand as "work overload." The amount of workload is continuously used in JDC studies to show the level of job demand for employees. In this study, job demand was measured using two scales measuring, respectively, psychological job demands and physical job demands. These scales include 10 items, including working fast, working hard, no excessive work, enough time, conflicting demands, too much physical effort, lifting heavy loads, rapid physical activity, awkward body position, and awkward arm positions. The final job demand score was obtained by summing the respective scores of these two scales.

Job control is the extent to which a person is able to make decisions and control his or her actions independently during occupational tasks. In this study, job control was measured using the two scales of skill discretion and decision authority, which included nine items, including learning new things, repetitive work, requiring creativity, high skills level, variety, developing abilities, allowing to make own decisions, little decision freedom, and lots of say. The job control score was obtained by summing the respective scores of the two scales.

Social support incorporates the concepts of perceived support in the workplace and organizational trust. In this study, social support was measured using the two scales of coworker support and supervisor support, which included eight items, including supervisor concern, supervisor attention, supervisor helpfulness, supervisor being a good organizer, the coworker component, coworker interest, coworkers friendliness, and coworker helpfulness. The social support score was obtained by summing the respective scores of the two scales.

Each of item was scored using a Likert scale ranging from 1 (*strongly disagree*) to 4 (*strongly agree*). Scoring and calculations for each dimension were done in accordance with the JCQ user's guide (Choobineh et al., 2011).

Job satisfaction

The aspect of job satisfaction was measured using the short Minnesota Satisfaction Questionnaire (MSQ). The MSQ is an extensively used tool for evaluating satisfaction in different occupations. This questionnaire contains 20 items that measure three facets of job satisfaction, including intrinsic satisfaction (12 items), extrinsic satisfaction (six items), and general satisfaction (two items). Intrinsic satisfaction relates to working conditions and perceptions regarding specific features of occupational tasks. Extrinsic satisfaction relates to environmental conditions and perceptions regarding job characteristics outside the workplace. The participants answered this questionnaire using a 5-point Likert scale ranging from "highly dissatisfied" to "highly satisfied" (Abugre, 2014). The Persian-version short MSQ is as valid and reliable tool that has been used extensively by Iranian researchers (Hadizadeh Talasaz et al., 2014). The overall job satisfaction score is obtained by summing the intrinsic satisfaction, extrinsic satisfaction, and general satisfaction scale scores.

Statistical Analyses

Descriptive statistics for all of the variables were reported. The Kolmogorov–Smirnov and Levene's tests were used to investigate the normality of quantitative data and equality of variances, respectively. Pearson correlation coefficients were used to estimate the relationship between the scales and subscales of JCQ and job satisfaction. In addition, backward, multiple linear regression was used to determine the variables with the most significant impact on job satisfaction. For regression analysis, all categorical variables were converted into dummy variables. All statistical tests were set at a significance level of $p < .05$. All analysis work was done on SPSS Version 18 (IBM, Inc., Armonk, NY, USA).

Ethical Considerations

This study was approved by the Ethics Committee of Kerman University of Medical Science (Approval No. IRB-1392.644). After gaining permission from the hospitals, the researchers visited each department in the target hospitals. The study aim was explained to the people in charge of each ward, and written permission was obtained from the authorities. After obtaining oral consent from the nurses, the purpose of the study as well as instructions regarding how the questionnaires should be completed were explained to the participants. The researchers assured the participants that the collected data would not be used for any purpose other than the study objectives and that their information would be de-identified. The participants were informed that they could leave the study at any time.

Results

Most of the participants were female and married. Over half had work experience of less than 10 years (Table 1). Most held a bachelor of science degree, over two thirds did shift work, and 71% worked more than 30 shifts per month.

Psychological and physical job demands earned the highest mean scores. The correlation results between job satisfaction and job demands, job control, and social support are shown in Table 2. In this study, job satisfaction was shown to be inversely related to psychological demand and physical demand, and direct relationships were found between job satisfaction and skill discretion, decision authority, supervisor support, and coworker support.

The correlations between JDCS model variables and job satisfaction showed job satisfaction as related inversely to job demands and related directly to social support (Table 3).

The effective predictors of job satisfaction in the participants, according to backward multiple linear regression models ($R^2 = .42$), are shown in Table 4. On the basis of these results, job satisfaction decreased with increased age. In addition, higher education was shown to be significantly associated with poorer job satisfaction; psychological and physical demands were both shown to be inversely and significantly related to job satisfaction; and higher levels of skill discretion, decision authority, and supervisor support were each shown to be significantly and directly related to job satisfaction.

Discussion

Studies have shown that job satisfaction in healthcare workers, especially nurses, is related to intention to leave, job burnout, and medical care quality. Identifying the factors that relate to job satisfaction in healthcare workers, including nurses, is a high priority for health service managers. Perceived occupational stress from job demands, control, and social support may influence job satisfaction. In this study, the relationships between the psychological aspects of workplaces and job satisfaction were assessed using a sample of nurses working at four general hospitals in northern, southern, eastern, and western Iran.

In this study, the mean score for job satisfaction was 3.14 (*SD* = 0.71), with the participants reporting a higher mean level of job satisfaction than Chinese nurses (2.95, *SD* = 0.75) and a lower mean level of job satisfaction than Turkish nursing managers (3.63, *SD* = 0.64; Kantek & Kaya, 2017; Yang et al., 2014).

These different results may be because of cultural differences in terms of how individuals in different countries perceive questions about job satisfaction (Kristensen & Johansson, 2008), which may make job satisfaction difficult to compare and interpret across cultures.

Table 1

Demographic Characteristics of the Participants (N = 694)

Variable	n	%	M	SD	p
Gender					.451[a]
Female	593	85.4	62.61	14.33	
Male	101	14.6	65.09	14.09	
Age (years)					.067[b]
20–29	191	27.5	67.18	13.83	
30–39	321	46.3	62.77	14.63	
≥ 40	182	26.2	60.51	13.92	
Marital status					.712[a]
Married	517	74.5	62.67	13.88	
Unmarried	177	25.5	63.64	15.07	
Employment status					.911[a]
Permanent	153	22.0	63.13	14.12	
Contract	541	78.0	62.72	14.95	
Educational level					.007[b]
LPN	144	20.7	70.1	10.72	
BSN	474	68.3	62.91	16.09	
MSN/PhD	76	11.0	60.78	14.28	
Clinical experience (years)					.491[b]
≤ 10	416	59.9	63.53	14.58	
11–20	187	27.0	60.74	14.24	
≥ 21	91	13.1	64.66	12.72	
Job position					.224[b]
Nurse	459	66.1	61.55	15.22	
Head nurse	125	18.0	66.66	11.53	
Supervisor	110	15.9	67.92	12.07	
Number of shifts per month					.234[a]
≤ 30	201	29.0	65.23	15.21	
> 30	493	71.0	62.13	13.82	
Ward					.543[b]
General ward	364	52.4	61.82	14.51	
Operating room	234	33.7	63.93	14.49	
Critical care unit	96	13.9	65.17	12.77	
Shift work					.974[a]
Fixed	244	35.2	63.19	15.73	
Rotating	450	64.8	62.89	3.64	

Note. LPN = licensed practical nurse; BSN = bachelor of science in nursing; MSN = master of science in nursing; PhD = doctor of philosophy.
[a]Independent *t* test. [b]One-way analysis of variance.

In this study, the job demand dimensions (psychological and physical job demands) earned the highest mean scores of the JCQ dimensions, which is in line with other studies of nurses in Iran (Bagheri et al., 2017; Barzideh et al., 2014). Canadian nurses have reported the highest scores for job control (Morgan et al., 2002), which reflect social and cultural differences between developed and developing countries. However, Morgan et al.'s study was conducted on 110 nurses only, which is significantly lower than two other studies.

In this study, an inverse correlation was found between age and job satisfaction, with job satisfaction decreasing with increasing age. However, Guglielmi et al. (2013) did not find a similar relationship between age and job satisfaction in emergency nurses. Moreover, job satisfaction was not significantly correlated with age in Semachew et al. (2017) study, in which almost half (49.6%) of the participants were male and nearly two thirds (62.3%) were diploma holders. In this study, only around 15% and 20% of the participants were male and licensed practitioners, respectively. The inverse relationship between age and job satisfaction found in this study may be related to decreased physical abilities and higher occupational stress in older nurses as well as to higher workload because of being more experienced.

In addition, an inverse relation was found between level of education and job satisfaction. Han et al. reported that nurses with more education had less job satisfaction (*OR* = 1.61, 95% CI [1.06, 2.44]; Han et al., 2015). Furthermore, Lu et al. (2016) found that healthcare workers in China with more education reported lower levels of job satisfaction. This is possibly because nurses with more education expect to have fewer work-related demands, greater control, and more social support.

The results of regression model showed a significant, inverse correlation between physical and psychological job demand and satisfaction, and decreasing job satisfaction related to increases in this demand. Bagheri et al. and Han et al. found that Iranian and American nurses, respectively, who scored higher for physical and psychological demand reported lower levels of job satisfaction (Bagheri et al., 2017; Han et al., 2015). On the basis of these results, higher psychological demands (such as workload and time restraints) and physical demand (such as patient handling and repositioning of patients) are stress factors that may lead to job dissatisfaction.

In this study, a direct relationship was found between job satisfaction with, respectively, skill discretion and decision authority, with job satisfaction increasing as these components increased. A similar result was found among Italian nurses (Karanikola et al., 2014). Moreover, in a systematic review by Cicolini et al. (2014), 12 studies from different countries, including Italy, Canada, Malaysia, and China, were reviewed, with results showing psychological empowerment (e.g., decision authority) and structural empowerment (e.g., leadership, guidance, and feedback received from supervisors and colleagues) to be significantly associated with job satisfaction. Elliott et al. (2017) reported higher job satisfaction as associated with greater job control and lower depression in their study of 173 aged care nurses. Similarly, in this study, job satisfaction was found to correlate significantly with job control (skill discretion and decision authority). However, the job control dimension was found to have only a marginally significant correlation with job satisfaction. Moreover, in this study, the effect of job control on decision making was related to treatment and patient care practices, with higher levels of job control improving nursing care performance and patient conditions (Skår, 2010). In addition,

Table 2

Correlations Between the Subscales of Job Content Questionnaire and Job Satisfaction (N = 695)

Item	Score Range	M	SD	1	2	3	4	5	6
Job content questionnaire									
1. Job demand									
Psychological	12–48	38.00	6.29	–					
Physical	5–20	17.21	2.51	.17*	–				
2. Job control									
Skill discretion	12–48	32.91	5.60	.24**	.21**	–			
Decision authority	12–48	28.13	6.41	−.18*	.06	.20*	–		
3. Social support									
Supervisor support	4–16	12.14	2.60	−.17*	−.17*	.17*	.18*	–	
Coworker support	4–16	12.21	2.33	−.17*	.03	.19*	.20*	.57**	–
Job satisfaction	1–5	3.14	0.71	−.43**	−.26**	.16*	.29**	.40**	.35**

*p < .05. **p < .01.

job control, making decisions, and independence all increase self-efficiency, confidence, and sense of success in nurses, which may increase job satisfaction (Elliott et al., 2017). Increased job control has been found to have a consistent and positive impact on self-reported health (Bambra et al., 2009) and is considered an important variable in nurses' mental health (Elliott et al., 2017).

In this study, a direct relationship was found between supervisor support and job satisfaction. However, Elliott et al. reported no association between supervisor support and job satisfaction (Elliott et al., 2017). The participants in the Elliott et al. study were aged care nurses, which may result in different working conditions than those experienced by the nurses in this study and thus may lead to different results. Some studies have reported a significant relationship between job satisfaction and supervisor support (Bagheri Hosseinabadi et al., 2019; Fila et al.,

2014), suggesting that supervisors giving nursing teams positive perceptions of emotional support may help promote a common sense of satisfaction in the work environment. Therefore, providing acknowledgment, trust, and empathy may be an important strategy for supervisors to enhance the quality of interpersonal relationships and job satisfaction (Gok et al., 2015).

Limitations and Strengths

The studied population included participants from northern, southern, eastern, and western Iran and was thus relatively representative of nurses working in Iran. In addition, this study attempted to assess job factors related to job satisfaction, which had not been considered in previous research in Iran.

A limitation of this study was that the collected information was subjective, which may either overestimate or

Table 3

The Correlation Between the Dimensions of JDCS Model and Job Satisfaction

Item	Score Range	M	SD	Score of 100	Item		
					1	2	3
1. Job demand (PsyJD and PhyJD)	17–68	55.33	7.09	81.36	–		
2. Job control (SD and DA)	24–96	60.93	9.27	63.46	.07 (p = .541)	–	
3. Social support (SupSupp and CoSupp)	8–32	24.29	4.28	75.90	−.22 (p = .035)	.27 (p = .002)	–
Job satisfaction	1–5	3.14	0.71	62.80	−.47 (p < .001)	.19 (p = .061)	.42 (p < .001)

Note. JDCS = Job Demand–Control–Support; PsyJD = psychological job demands; PhyJD = physical job demands; SD = skill discretion; DA = decision authority; SupSupp = supervisor support; CoSupp = coworker support.

Table 4

Results of Multivariate Linear Regression Analysis of Job Satisfaction (N = 694)

Predictor	Adjusted B	t	95% CI		p
			Lower	Upper	
Age (years)					
31–40 vs. ≤ 30	−8.74	2.49	−15.71	−1.77	.015
≥ 41 vs. ≤ 30	−8.41	2.01	−16.71	−0.11	.047
Educational level					
BSN vs. LPN	−1.74	−1.81	−2.37	−0.12	.043
MSN/PhD vs. LPN	−8.99	−2.37	−16.52	−1.46	.021
Psychological job demands	−0.11	−4.13	−0.16	−0.06	< .001
Physical job demands	−0.86	−3.16	−1.42	−0.31	.004
Skill discretion	0.48	2.18	0.04	0.93	.033
Decision authority	0.43	1.88	0.05	0.83	.028
Supervisor support	1.85	2.95	0.61	3.10	.004

Note. BSN = bachelor of science in nursing; LPN = licensed practical nurse; MSN = master of science in nursing; PhD = doctor of philosophy.

underestimate level of job satisfaction, psychological demand, and physical demand variables. Another limitation of this study was the shift-work classification used. We classified regular shifts as fixed shifts and irregular shift as rotating shifts, but we did not take into account the effect of different shift working times (i.e., morning, evening, and night shifts) on job satisfaction. Furthermore, this was a cross-sectional study and thus was not designed to show changes in job satisfaction over time. Finally, as all variables were assessed simultaneously, the causal direction among job satisfaction, job demands, job control, and support could not be assessed.

Conclusions

The job satisfaction of nurses is affected by multiple factors. The findings of this study indicate that nurses with lower levels of psychological and physical demand, greater skill discretion, greater decision authority, and more social support tend to be more satisfied with their job. Nurse managers may enhance the job satisfaction of nurses by improving work-related factors and decreasing work-related stress. For example, managers may decrease dissatisfaction by giving more autonomy to nurses in terms of making decisions related to patient care. Furthermore, maintaining an appropriate nurse-to-patient ratio may help reduce workload and physical demands and enhance job satisfaction. Finally, paying greater attention to nurses who are older and more educated may also help raise overall job satisfaction.

Acknowledgments

We thank the anonymous reviewers for their detailed and helpful comments on this article and express appreciation to those who helped us conduct this research project, particularly head nurses and nursing staffs in the participating hospitals.

Author Contributions

Study conception and design: MBHA, SES
Data collection: ET, SES
Data analysis and interpretation: NK, ZNK
Drafting of the article: SES, MBHA
Critical revision of the article: SES, FK

References

Abugre, J. B. (2014). Job satisfaction of public sector employees in sub-Saharan Africa: Testing the Minnesota Satisfaction Questionnaire in Ghana. *International Journal of Public Administration, 37*(10), 655–665. https://doi.org/10.1080/01900692.2014.903268

Al Maqbali, M. A. (2015). Job satisfaction of nurses in a regional hospital in Oman: A cross-sectional survey. *The Journal of Nursing Research, 23*(3), 206–216. https://doi.org/10.1097/jnr.0000000000000081

Bagheri Hosseinabadi, M., Ebrahimi, M. H., Khanjani, N., Biganeh, J., Mohammadi, S., & Abdolahfard, M. (2019). The effects of amplitude and stability of circadian rhythm and occupational stress on burnout syndrome and job dissatisfaction among irregular shift working nurses. *Journal of Clinical Nursing, 28*(9–10), 1868–1878. https://doi.org/10.1111/jocn.14778

Bagheri Hosseinabadi, M., Etemadinezhad, S., Khanjani, N., Ahmadi, O., Gholinia, H., Galeshi, M., & Samaei, S. E. (2018). Evaluating the relationship between job stress and job satisfaction among female hospital nurses in Babol: An application of structural equation modeling. *Health Promotion Perspectives*, *8*(2), 102–108. https://doi.org/10.15171/hpp.2018.13

Bagheri, M., Taban, E., Khanjani, N., Galeshi, M., & Etemadinezhad, S. (2017). The effect of psychological stress on job satisfaction among intensive care nurses. *International Journal of Hospital Research*, *6*(3), 24–34. http://ijhr.iums.ac.ir/article_76952.html

Bambra, C., Gibson, M., Sowden, A. J., Wright, K., Whitehead, M., & Petticrew, M. (2009). Working for health? Evidence from systematic reviews on the effects on health and health inequalities of organisational changes to the psychosocial work environment. *Preventive Medicine*, *48*(5), 454–461. https://doi.org/10.1016/j.ypmed.2008.12.018

Banaszak-Holl, J., Castle, N. G., Lin, M. K., Shrivastwa, N., & Spreitzer, G. (2015). The role of organizational culture in retaining nursing workforce. *The Gerontologist*, *55*(3), 462–471. https://doi.org/10.1093/geront/gnt129

Barzideh, M., Choobineh, A., & Tabatabaee, H. (2014). Comparison of job stress dimensions in Iranian nurses with those from other countries based on the demand–control–support model. *Journal of Health Sciences and Surveillance System*, *2*(2), 66–71.

Chen, I. H., Brown, R., Bowers, B. J., & Chang, W. Y. (2015). Job demand and job satisfaction in latent groups of turnover intention among licensed nurses in Taiwan nursing homes. *Research in Nursing Health*, *38*(5), 342–356. https://doi.org/10.1002/nur.21667

Choobineh, A., Ghaem, H., & Ahmedinejad, P. (2011). Validity and reliability of the Persian (Farsi) version of the Job Content Questionnaire: A study among hospital nurses. *Eastern Mediterranean Health Journal*, *17*(4), 335–341.

Cicolini, G., Comparcini, D., & Simonetti, V. (2014). Workplace empowerment and nurses' job satisfaction: A systematic literature review. *Journal of Nursing Management*, *22*(7), 855–871. https://doi.org/10.1111/jonm.12028

Clumeck, N., Kempenaers, C., Godin, I., Dramaix, M., Kornitzer, M., Linkowski, P., & Kittel, F. (2009). Working conditions predict incidence of long-term spells of sick leave due to depression: Results from the Belstress I prospective study. *Journal of Epidemiology & Community Health*, *63*(4), 286–292. https://doi.org/10.1136/jech.2008.079384

De Simone, S., & Planta, A. (2017). The intention to leave among nurses: The role of job satisfaction, self-efficacy and work engagement. *Work, Environment and Health (La Medicina del Lavoro; in Italiano)*, *108*(2), 87–97. https://doi.org/10.23749/mdl.v108i2.6074

Elliott, K. E. J., Rodwell, J., & Martin, A. J. (2017). Aged care nurses' job control influence satisfaction and mental health. *Journal of Nursing Management*, *25*(7), 558–568. https://doi.org/10.1111/jonm.12493

Fila, M. J., Paik, L. S., Griffeth, R. W., & Allen, D. (2014). Disaggregating job satisfaction: Effects of perceived demands, control, and support. *Journal of Business and Psychology*, *29*(4), 639–649. https://doi.org/10.1007/s10869-014-9358-5

Gadirzadeh, Z., Adib-Hajbaghery, M., & Matin Abadi, M. J. A. (2017). Job stress, job satisfaction, and related factors in a sample of Iranian nurses. *Nursing and Midwifery Studies*, *6*(3), 125–131. https://doi.org/10.4103/nms.nms_26_17

Gok, S., Karatuna, I., & Karaca, P. O. (2015). The role of perceived supervisor support and organizational identification in job satisfaction. *Procedia-Social and Behavioral Sciences*, *177*, 38–42. https://doi.org/10.1016/j.sbspro.2015.02.328

Guglielmi, D., Simbula, S., Mazzetti, G., Tabanelli, M. C., & Bonfiglioli, R. (2013). When the job is boring: The role of boredom in organizational contexts. *Work*, *45*(3), 311–322. https://doi.org/10.3233/WOR-121528

Hadizadeh Talasaz, Z., Nourani Saadoldin, S., & Taghi Shakeri, M. (2014). The relationship between job satisfaction and job performance among midwives working in healthcare centers of Mashhad, Iran. *Journal of Midwifery and Reproductive Health*, *2*(3), 157–164. https://doi.org/10.22038/jmrh.2014.2623

Hamaideh, S. H. (2011). Burnout, social support, and job satisfaction among Jordanian mental health nurses. *Issues in Mental Health Nursing*, *32*(4), 234–242. https://doi.org/10.3109/01612840.2010.546494

Han, K., Trinkoff, A. M., & Gurses, A. P. (2015). Work-related factors, job satisfaction and intent to leave the current job among United States nurses. *Journal of Clinical Nursing*, *24*(21–22), 3224–3232. https://doi.org/10.1111/jocn.12987

Hülsheger, U. R., & Schewe, A. F. (2011). On the costs and benefits of emotional labor: A meta-analysis of three decades of research. *Journal of Occupational Health Psychology*, *16*(3), 361–389. https://doi.org/10.1037/a0022876

Janicijevic, I., Seke, K., Djokovic, A., & Filipovic, T. (2013). Healthcare workers satisfaction and patient satisfaction—Where is the linkage? *Hippokratia*, *17*(2), 157–162.

Kantek, F., & Kaya, A. (2017). Professional values, job satisfaction, and intent to leave among nursing managers. *The Journal of Nursing Research*, *25*(4), 319–325. https://doi.org/10.1097/jnr.0000000000000164

Karanikola, M. N. K., Albarran, J. W., Drigo, E., Giannakopoulou, M., Kalafati, M., Mpouzika, M., Tsiaousis, G. Z., & Papathanassoglou, E. D. E. (2014). Moral distress, autonomy and nurse–physician collaboration among intensive care unit nurses in Italy. *Journal of Nursing Management*, *22*(4), 472–484. https://doi.org/10.1111/jonm.12046

Karasek, R., Brisson, C., Kawakami, N., Houtman, I., Bongers, P., & Amick, B. (1998). The Job Content Questionnaire (JCQ): An instrument for internationally comparative assessments of psychosocial job characteristics. *Journal of Occupational Health Psychology*, *3*(4), 322–355. https://doi.org/10.1037/1076-8998.3.4.322

Khamisa, N., Peltzer, K., Ilic, D., & Oldenburg, B. (2017). Effect of personal and work stress on burnout, job satisfaction and general health of hospital nurses in South Africa. *Health SA Gesondheid*, *22*, 252–258. https://doi.org/10.1016/j.hsag.2016.10.001

Krejcie, R. V., & Morgan, D. W. (1970). Determining sample size for research activities. *Educational and Psychological Measurement*, *30*(3), 607–610. https://doi.org/10.1177/001316447003000308

Kristensen, N., & Johansson, E. (2008). New evidence on cross-country differences in job satisfaction using anchoring vignettes. *Labour Economics*, *15*(1), 96–117. https://doi.org/10.1016/j.labeco.2006.11.001

Lee, J. H., Hwang, J., & Lee, K. S. (2019). Job satisfaction and job-related stress among nurses: The moderating effect of mindfulness. *Work*, *62*(1), 87–95. https://doi.org/10.3233/wor-182843

Lu, Y., Hu, X.-M., Huang, X.-L., Zhuang, X.-D., Guo, P., Feng, L.-F., Hu, W., Chen, L., & Hao, Y.-T. (2016). Job satisfaction and associated factors among healthcare staff: A cross-sectional study in Guangdong Province, China. *BMJ Open, 6*(7), Article e011388. https://doi.org/10.1136/bmjopen-2016-011388

Morgan, D. G., Semchuk, K. M., Stewart, N. J., & D'Arcy, C. (2002). Job strain among staff of rural nursing homes. A comparison of nurses, aides, and activity workers. *The Journal of Nursing Administration, 32*(3), 152–161.

Negahban, T., Ansari Jaberi, A., & Manssouri, H. (2017). Nurses' job satisfaction and their perceived organizational justice in Kerman University of Medical Sciences: An evaluation for the Iranian health system transformation plan. *Journal of Occupational Health and Epidemiology, 6*(1), 47–55. https://doi.org/10.18869/acadpub.johe.6.1.47

Negussie, N., & Kaur, G. (2016). The effect of job demand–control–social support model on nurses' job satisfaction in specialized teaching hospitals, Ethiopia. *Ethiopian Journal of Health Sciences, 26*(4), 311–320. https://doi.org/10.4314/ejhs.v26i4.3

Nieuwenhuijsen, K., Bruinvels, D., & Frings-Dresen, M. (2010). Psychosocial work environment and stress-related disorders, a systematic review. *Occupational Medicine, 60*(4), 277–286. https://doi.org/10.1093/occmed/kqq081

Rao, J. V., & Chandraiah, K. (2012). Occupational stress, mental health and coping among information technology professionals. *Indian Journal of Occupational and Environmental Medicine, 16*(1), 22–26. https://doi.org/10.4103/0019-5278.99686

Rhee, K. Y. (2010). Different effects of workers' trust on work stress, perceived stress, stress reaction, and job satisfaction between Korean and Japanese workers. *Safety and Health at Work, 1*(1), 87–97. https://doi.org/10.5491/SHAW.2010.1.1.87

San Park, J., & Hyun Kim, T. (2009). Do types of organizational culture matter in nurse job satisfaction and turnover intention? *Leadership in Health Services, 22*(1), 20–38. https://doi.org/10.1108/17511870910928001

Schwendimann, R., Dhaini, S., Ausserhofer, D., Engberg, S., & Zúñiga, F. (2016). Factors associated with high job satisfaction among care workers in Swiss nursing homes—A cross sectional survey study. *BMC Nursing, 15*, Article No. 37. https://doi.org/10.1186/s12912-016-0160-8

Semachew, A., Belachew, T., Tesfaye, T., & Adinew, Y. M. (2017). Predictors of job satisfaction among nurses working in Ethiopian public hospitals, 2014: Institution-based cross-sectional study. *Human Resources for Health, 15*(1), Article No. 31. https://doi.org/10.1186/s12960-017-0204-5

Sharma, P., Davey, A., Davey, S., Shukla, A., Shrivastava, K., & Bansal, R. (2014). Occupational stress among staff nurses: Controlling the risk to health. *Indian Journal of Occupational & Environmental Medicine, 18*(2), 52–56. https://doi.org/10.4103/0019-5278.146890

Skår, R. (2010). The meaning of autonomy in nursing practice. *Journal of Clinical Nursing, 19*(15–16), 2226–2234. https://doi.org/10.1111/j.1365-2702.2009.02804.x

Sveinsdóttir, H., Biering, P., & Ramel, A. (2006). Occupational stress, job satisfaction, and working environment among Icelandic nurses: A cross-sectional questionnaire survey. *International Journal of Nursing Studies, 43*(7), 875–889. https://doi.org/10.1016/j.ijnurstu.2005.11.002

Tabatabaei, S., Ghaneh, S., Mohaddes, H., & Khansari, M. M. (2013). Relationship of job satisfaction and demographic variables in Pars Ceram factory employees in Iran. *Procedia - Social and Behavioral Sciences, 84*, 1795–1800. https://doi.org/10.1016/j.sbspro.2013.07.036

Yang, J., Liu, Y., Chen, Y., & Pan, X. (2014). The effect of structural empowerment and organizational commitment on Chinese nurses' job satisfaction. *Applied Nursing Research, 27*(3), 186–191. https://doi.org/10.1016/j.apnr.2013.12.001

26

Impact of Training Based on Orem's Theory on Self-Care Agency and Quality of Life in Patients with Coronary Artery Disease

Fatma TOK YILDIZ[1*] • Mağfiret KAŞIKÇI[2]

ABSTRACT

Background: Coronary artery disease (CAD) is a primary cause of death worldwide. CAD negatively affects individuals because it reduces their functional skills and self-care abilities and disrupts quality of life.

Purpose: This study was designed to assess the impact of a training program based on Orem's self-care deficit nursing theory (SCDNT) on self-care abilities and quality of life in patients with CAD.

Methods: This study was conducted using a randomized, controlled, pretest/posttest experimental design. One hundred two patients with CAD were divided evenly into either the intervention or control group, with sample randomization based on gender, age, low-density lipoprotein cholesterol level, and Self-Care Agency Scale scores. For both groups, interviews were conducted in two sessions held, respectively, at the hospital and at home. Study data were collected using the patient information form, Self-Care Agency Scale, MacNew Heart Disease Health-Related Quality of Life Questionnaire (MacNew), Quality of Life Questionnaire (15D), and training booklet.

Results: A highly significant difference was found between the two groups in terms of the average posttest scores on the Self-Care Agency Scale, MacNew, and 15D. For the intervention group, the posttest scores on the Self-Care Agency Scale, MacNew, and 15D were significantly higher than the pretest scores, whereas average pretest and posttest scores on these measures were similar for the control group.

Conclusions: The training program developed in this study based on Orem's SCDNT improved self-care agency as well as disease-specific and overall quality of life in patients with CAD. Nurses should pay attention to the CAD-related educational level of patients when teaching them how to live with their disease. Moreover, nurses should use Orem's SCDNT to strengthen the self-care agency of these patients to increase quality of life and the effectiveness of related education efforts. Finally, medical institutions and governments should develop appropriate education policies for patients at risk of CAD and for those with CAD.

KEY WORDS:

training, coronary artery disease, Orem's self-care deficit nursing theory, self-care agency, quality of life.

Introduction

According to the global implementation plan of the World Health Organization (WHO) on preventable and controllable noncommunicable diseases, cardiovascular disease, cancer, chronic respiratory tract diseases, and diabetes are the primary causes of deaths worldwide, with incidences of 48%, 21%, 12%, and 3.5%, respectively (WHO, 2019). Cardiovascular disease is the leading cause of morbidity and mortality in Turkey. According to the 2009 Cardiac Diseases and Risk Factors in Turkish Adults report, coronary artery disease (CAD) is the largest cause of death in Turkey (Onat, 2009).

CAD negatively affects an individual's course of life, maintenance of health, and progression of disease owing to its accompanying physical, psychological, social, and economic problems (Hassani et al., 2010; Sevinç & Akyol, 2010). In addition, this disease reduces functional skills and self-care abilities (Hassani et al., 2010), prevents completion of self-care responsibilities, and disrupts quality of life (Dilek et al., 2010; Durmaz et al., 2009; Norris et al., 2009). Studies on CAD have identified a high prevalence of modifiable risk factors and determined that effective risk factor management may substantially reduce the pace of morbidity and mortality and, eventually, improve health and quality of life (Durmaz et al., 2009; Saffi et al., 2014; Sevinç & Akyol, 2010).

Education is crucial to increasing awareness to protect and help individuals maintain health and make necessary changes in lifestyle (Hall, 2013; Taylor et al., 2011). Previous studies have revealed that providing education to patients with CAD improves self-care agency (Hassani et al., 2010), quality of life (Küçükberber et al., 2011), and self-care information as well as motivation and skill levels (Mohammadpour et al., 2015).

[1]PhD, RN, Assistant Professor, Program of Anaesthesia, Department of Medical Services and Techniques, Vocational School of Health Services, Sivas Cumhuriyet University, Sivas, Turkey • [2]PhD, RN, Professor, Faculty of Nursing, Atatürk University, Erzurum, Turkey.

In nursing practice, the use of theory helps systematize care planning, organizes professional knowledge into a conceptual framework, and guides nurses on how and why certain steps must be taken, thereby increasing the effectiveness of services by providing cost-effective care (Johnson, 2015). A crucial issue in improving quality of life in patients with chronic illness is ensuring patient participation in their treatment and care (Johnson, 2015). In this context, a basic principle of self-care is patient participation and assumption of responsibility (Hassani et al., 2010). Self-care, defined as performing individual duties to protect life, health, and well-being, develops gradually through communication, culture, education, and interaction (Berbiglia & Banfield, 2014; Fawcett & DeSanto-Madeya, 2013; Johnson, 2015). Orem's self-care deficit nursing theory (SCDNT) considers each individual as a self-care agent with the necessary ability to perform self-care activities individually (Berbiglia & Banfield, 2014; Fawcett & DeSanto-Madeya, 2013; Johnson, 2015).

In promoting the health status of patients with CAD, it is critical to effectively combat interchangeable risk factors, increase awareness, and improve self-care agency and quality of life (Butcher & Castelluci, 2011; Hassani et al., 2010). Therefore, training that is based on Orem's SCDNT has been hypothesized as an effective approach to preventing disease progression, reducing recurrent hospitalizations, minimizing financial expenses, improving self-care agency and quality of life, encouraging patient education, protecting health, and providing behavioral change by raising awareness toward development and teaching home care methods. This study was designed to determine the impact of a training program based on Orem's SCDNT on self-care agency and quality of life in patients with CAD.

Methods

This randomized, controlled, pretest/posttest experimental study was conducted between January 2015 and February 2017. The study population comprised patients with CAD from a cardiology clinic of a university and public hospital. One hundred two patients, 51 of whom were assigned to the intervention group and 51 of whom were assigned to the control group, were randomized according to gender, age (unmodifiable risk factors that increase the risk of CAD), low-density lipoprotein (LDL) cholesterol level ($\geq$ 70 mg/dl; modifiable risk factors that increase the risk of CAD), and Self-Care Agency Scale score ($\geq$ 120 points; Figure 1). The

Figure 1

Flow diagram

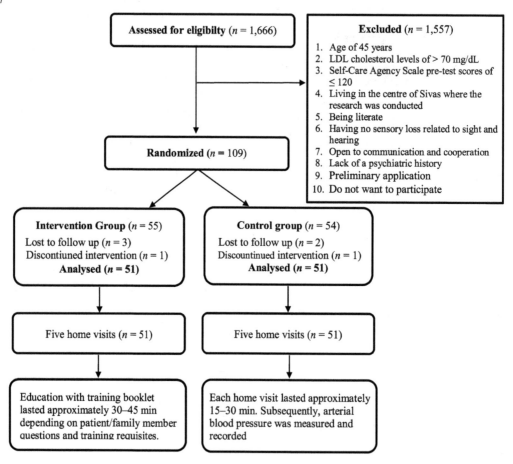

sampling criteria were as follows: (a) age of ≥ 45 years, (b) LDL cholesterol levels of > 70 mg/dl, (c) Self-Care Agency Scale pretest scores of ≤ 120, (d) living in the center of Sivas where the research was conducted, (e) being literate, (f) having no sensory loss related to sight or hearing, (g) being open to communication and cooperation, and (h) lack of a psychiatric history.

The study data were collected using the patient information form, Self-Care Agency Scale, MacNew Heart Disease Health-Related Quality of Life Questionnaire (MacNew), and Quality of Life Questionnaire (15D) during the second and third interviews, which were conducted, respectively, before hospital discharge and during the outpatient visit conducted 5–6 months after discharge.

Patient Information Form

This form comprised 26 questions, including concomitant diseases, medications used, and general information, which were used to determine the risk factors for CAD (Butcher & Castelluci, 2011; Durmaz et al., 2009; Lukkarinen & Hentinen, 2006).

Self-Care Agency Scale

The Self-Care Agency Scale, developed by Kearney and Fleischer (1979), with its validity and reliability in Turkish reported by Nahcivan (1993) in healthy young individuals and by Pınar (1995) in chronic diseases, has been adapted for use in Turkish settings. In this study, the version of the scale adapted by Pınar was used (Pınar, 1995). Validity and reliability study of the scale for use on patients with chronic diseases revealed a test–retest reliability of .80 and an internal consistency of .89 (Pınar, 1995). Furthermore, the pretest and posttest values of Cronbach's alpha reliability coefficient were determined to be .89 and .93, respectively. The Self-Care Agency Scale has been used to determine the self-care abilities of individuals, with high total scores indicating a high level of independence and abilities in achieving self-care. There are 35 items in the Turkish form, with each item evaluated using a score ranging from 0 to 4: 0 = *does not describe me at all*; 1 = *does not describe me very well*, 2 = *no idea*, 3 = *describes me a little*, and 4 = *describes me very well*. Eight of the scale items (3, 6, 9, 13, 19, 22, 26, and 31) are negatively stated, so the scoring method is reversed. The evaluation is based on 140 points, with a score below 82 points considered low, 82–120 points considered medium, and above 120 points considered high (Pınar, 1995).

MacNew

MacNew, developed by the MacNew Group (MacNew, 2014), was tested for validity and reliability in Turkish and adapted to Turkish society by Daskapan et al. (2008). MacNew was designed to measure heart-disease-specific quality of life (MacNew, 2014). MacNew is a valid and easily applicable scale for patients with myocardial infarction, angina pectoris, or heart failure. There are strong correlations between MacNew

and other quality-of-life scales, suggesting that MacNew is a valid and reliable quality-of-life measurement tool for patients with CAD (MacNew, 2014). In Daskapan et al., the Cronbach's alpha reliability coefficient of the questionnaire was determined to be .89. In this study, the pretest and posttest values of the Cronbach's alpha reliability coefficient for MacNew were .95 and .96, respectively. MacNew includes 27 items, each of which is scored using a 7-point Likert-type response, that are grouped into three subdimensions (emotional, physical, and social) as well as assessed as a total score. After assessing subdimensions, the averages of the items in each dimension are used. Therefore, the average scores vary from 1 to 7, with lower scores indicating worse quality of life and higher scores indicating better quality of life (MacNew, 2014). Only the total score for MacNew was used in this study.

Quality of Life Questionnaire (15D)

15D, developed by Sintonen (2009) and tested for validity and reliability in Turkish by Akinci et al. (2005), has been adapted to Turkish settings to measure overall quality of life. The Cronbach's alpha reliability coefficient of 15D was found to be .99 in Akinci et al. (2005), and the pretest and posttest values were determined to be .62 and .83, respectively, in this study. 15D items are designed to assess movement, vision, hearing, breathing, sleeping, eating, speaking, excretion, normal activities, mental function, discomfort, depression, distress, vitality, and sexual activity. Each item offers five choices and is scored as 1 point. In 15D, individuals select one option, and scores are calculated. The first choice indicates the highest level, whereas the fifth choice indicates the lowest level. The obtained score is converted to a total score between 1 and 0, which indicates quality of life in terms of subjective health (1 = *quality of life with best health*, 0 = *quality of life with worst health*; Lukkarinen & Hentinen, 2006; Sintonen, 2009).

Training Booklet

CAD-specific information was integrated into a training booklet in accordance with Orem's SCDNT by conducting a literature review and canvassing the opinions of related experts. Information on CAD was structured into three parts in the training booklet, covering the requisites of universal self-care, developmental self-care, and health deviation self-care. Universal self-care requisites include information on CAD such as maintaining adequate respiration, sustaining adequate fluid intake, maintaining adequate nutrient intake, maintaining adequate excretion, maintaining exercise–rest balance, maintaining balance between loneliness and the social environment, having protection from dangers that affect life and well-being, and being able to perform normal functions. Developmental self-care requisites include information on identifying and managing high-risk individuals. Finally, health deviation self-care requisites address the following topics: What is the responsibility of the heart? What is CAD? What are the risk factors for CAD? Which are the unmodifiable risk factors? Which are the modifiable risk factors? What should be done to achieve quality life with CAD? How can serum lipid level, hypertension, obesity, diabetes mellitus, stress, behavior patterns, and homocysteine level be controlled? How can one make lifestyle changes related to physical inactivity? What should be considered in drug treatment?

Interviews were conducted after completion of the 6-month postdischarge monitoring of behavioral changes and support provision. The participants were informed that they could use the training booklet as a guide but that they should not use the booklet as a substitute for referral/treatment by a physician. Furthermore, the participants were advised that they could call the researcher if they had any questions or concerns.

Ethical Consideration

Before implementing this study, approval from the Faculty of Health Science Clinical Studies Ethics Committee of Erzurum Atatürk University (resolution number: 10/12/2014) was obtained and written permission from Sivas Cumhuriyet University, Healthcare Research Hospital, and Sivas Public Hospital was received. Written informed consent was obtained from each patient who met the inclusion criteria. The patients were informed that their participation in this study was their choice, that their names would be written on data-gathering forms, and that all personal information would be kept confidential. No intervention was included in the routine treatment of the two groups.

Nursing Practice

All of the interviews were performed by the researcher F. T. Y. The research data from the preliminary practice were collected via face-to-face interviews from the patients who agreed to participate.

In the intervention group, data were collected during two sessions: at the hospital before discharge and at home after discharge. On average, 8–10 phone calls were made by the researcher to each of the participants or their relatives to plan home visits or to address questions/concerns.

Interview 1 was conducted at the cardiology clinic when hemodynamic indicators were normal on the first or second day after discharge from the intensive care unit. The participant was informed about the study, and verbal and written informed consents were obtained.

Interview 2 was conducted a day after the first interview at the cardiology clinic. The Self-Care Agency Scale was implemented, and LDL cholesterol level was recorded. The patients were randomized into an intervention group and a control group using the simple random sampling method based on age, gender, Self-Care Agency Scale score, and LDL cholesterol level.

Interview 3 was held a day after the second interview at the cardiology clinic. The pretest measurements (patient information form, MacNew, and 15D) were filled out by the researcher, and the participants' routine triglyceride–total cholesterol–HDL

(high-density lipoprotein) cholesterol levels and arterial blood pressure were recorded at the hospital. The training was held in a quiet and calm private room with normal lighting and temperature to ensure comfort. Before the training, the patients were informed about the aim and goal of the training, including that the training would last approximately 40–50 minutes, that it would be interrupted and paused if necessary, and that questions could be asked whenever desired. The training booklet prepared to support learning with written and visual materials was given to participants, and the training content was projected on a projection screen.

Interview 4 was conducted at home after hospital discharge. At the first home visit, arterial blood pressure was measured and recorded.

Interview 5 was held at home within 3 days after the outpatient checkup in the first month. At the second home visit, arterial blood pressure was measured and recorded.

Interview 6 was held at home 4 weeks after the fifth interview. At the third home visit, arterial blood pressure was measured and recorded.

Interview 7 was held at home 3 days after the outpatient checkup in the third month. At the fourth home visit, arterial blood pressure, body mass index (BMI), and waist circumference were measured. The patients' triglyceride, total cholesterol, HDL cholesterol, and LDL cholesterol levels, which were routinely measured at the hospital, were recorded. The initial levels of modifiable risk factors were compared with the present levels. Changes that positively or negatively affected CAD were determined.

Interview 8 was conducted at home within 3 days after the outpatient checkup in the sixth month. At the fifth home visit, the patients' posttest measurements such as arterial blood pressure, BMI, and waist circumference were measured, and triglyceride–total cholesterol–HDL cholesterol–LDL cholesterol levels, which were routinely measured at the hospital during the outpatient visit in the sixth month, were recorded. The Self-Care Agency Scale, MacNew, and 15D were then filled out by F. T. Y.

In the intervention group, each home visit, conducted after hospital discharge, lasted approximately 30–45 minutes depending on each patient's questions and training requirements. The researcher asked each participant 12 questions that were prepared based on the content of the training, and behavioral changes were investigated. If deemed necessary, training was again provided to the participant during the interview.

In the control group, data were collected from two sessions, including that conducted before hospital discharge (Interview 1, Interview 2, and Interview 3) and after discharge. The pretest measurements, including the patient information form, MacNew, and 15D, were filled out by F. T. Y., and the participants' routine triglyceride–total cholesterol–HDL cholesterol levels and arterial blood pressure were recorded at the hospital during Interview 3. Each home visit after discharge (Interview 4, Interview 5, Interview 6, Interview 7, and Interview 8) lasted approximately 15–30 minutes.

Subsequently, arterial blood pressure was measured and recorded. Counseling sessions on CAD for patients or their relatives were provided when deemed necessary. In addition, 8–10 phone calls were made to plan home visits and/or provide counseling to each patient or his or her relatives. In Interview 8, the patients' posttest measurements, including arterial blood pressure, BMI, and waist circumference, were measured and recorded. Triglyceride–total cholesterol–HDL cholesterol–LDL cholesterol levels, which were routinely measured at the hospital during the outpatient visit in the sixth month, were recorded, and the Self-Care Agency Scale, MacNew, and 15D were filled out by F. T. Y. Training was conducted, and the training booklet was provided to the control group patients at the end of the interviews (Interview 8).

Evaluation of Data

Analyses of the study data were performed using IBM SPSS Statistics Version 20.0 (IBM, Inc., Armonk, NY, USA), and tables were created. Statistical results were presented as frequency and percentage based on the distribution of group characteristics related to the descriptive characteristics and CAD risk factors of the study groups. Chi-square analysis was performed to evaluate the characteristic distribution of the patients in the study groups with respect to descriptive characteristics and CAD risk factors and percentage distributions. Chi-square analysis was used for the homogeneity test, the Kolmogorov–Smirnov test was used to determine whether the pretest data were suitable for normal distribution to select the appropriate statistical analyses, and the Levene's test was used to determine the homogeneity of variances. Nonparametric tests were applied in all analyses because the normality analysis and the homogeneity of variance test did not show normal distribution. The Mann–Whitney U test was used for intergroup comparisons of the pretest and posttest values of triglyceride, total cholesterol, HDL cholesterol, LDL cholesterol, arterial blood pressure, BMI, waist circumference, and Self-Care Agency Scale, MacNew, and 15D scores. A Wilcoxon's signed-rank test was used for intragroup comparisons. Correlation analysis was used to determine the relationship between the average pretest and posttest scores on the Self-Care Agency Scale, MacNew, and 15D measures. Correlation coefficients of .00–.30 were considered low, .30–.70 were considered medium, and .70–1 were considered high (Büyüköztürk, 2010).

Results

The distribution and comparison of the descriptive characteristics of the patients with CAD who participated in this study are summarized in Table 1. No significant difference was observed between the groups in terms of descriptive characteristics, and the groups were homogeneous in terms of the study variables ($p > .05$).

Regarding hereditary CAD, serum lipid level, BMI, waist circumference, hypertension, diabetes, smoking, alcohol,

Table 1

Distribution and Comparison of Patients by Descriptive Characteristics

Characteristic	Intervention Group ($n = 51$)		Control Group ($n = 51$)		χ^2	p
	n	%	n	%		
Age (years; M and SD)	59.98	7.42	56.74	7.55	5.76	.21
45–49	4	7.8	6	11.8		
50–54	9	17.7	18	35.3		
55–59	12	23.5	10	19.6		
60–64	16	31.4	9	17.6		
65 and above	10	19.6	8	15.7		
Gender					0.92	.33
Female	42	82.4	38	74.5		
Male	9	17.6	13	25.5		
Marital status					1.38	.24
Single	5	9.8	2	3.9		
Married	46	90.2	49	96.1		
Educational level					7.74	.17
Literate	3	5.9	2	3.9		
Primary	31	60.8	33	64.7		
Secondary	2	3.9	5	9.8		
High school	9	17.6	11	21.6		
University	5	9.8	–	–		
Master/doctorate	1	2.0	–	–		
Occupation					4.94	.29
Retired	32	62.7	29	56.9		
Housewife	7	13.7	13	25.5		
Civil servant	7	13.7	3	5.9		
Other	5	9.9	6	11.8		
Income level					0.67	.71
Lower than expenses	46	90.2	13	25.5		
Balanced	–	–	35	68.6		
Higher than expenses	5	9.8	3	5.9		
Lifestyle					2.53	.86
Single	2	3.9	2	3.9		
With spouse	12	23.5	10	19.6		
With spouse and children	34	66.7	35	68.6		
Other	3	5.9	4	7.9		
Diagnosis					0.40	.52
Angina pectoris	15	29.4	18	35.3		
Myocardial infarction	36	70.6	33	64.7		
Chronic disease					0.40	.52
Yes	33	64.7	36	70.6		
No	18	35.3	15	29.4		

sedentary lifestyle, and stressors related to CAD risk factors, no significant difference was identified between the two groups ($p > .05$). In addition, the groups had similar characteristics in terms of the study variables related to CAD risk factors. In both groups, the pretest values for LDL cholesterol level, total cholesterol level, triglyceride level, and waist circumference were high. Furthermore, the posttest LDL cholesterol and total cholesterol levels of the two groups showed lower intragroup average scores, with a highly significant intergroup difference ($p < .01$; Table 2).

When the average pretest and posttest scores on the Self-Care Agency Scale were compared, the average intragroup scores of the intervention group were found to be significantly higher than those of the control group ($p < .01$). In addition, there was a significantly greater increase in the last average score of the control group than that of the intervention group ($p > .05$). However, the average posttest scores on the Self-Care Agency Scale were significantly higher in the intervention group than in the control group ($p < .01$; Table 3).

Table 3 shows a comparison of the average pretest and posttest scores on MacNew. According to the pretest intragroup scores on this measure, the average posttest scores were significantly higher in the intervention group than in the control group ($p < .01$), which recorded a decline in average posttest scores ($p > .05$). In addition, the average intergroup posttest scores on MacNew were significantly higher in the intervention group than in the control group ($p < .01$).

With regard to the average pretest and posttest scores on 15D (Table 3), the intervention group showed an increase in average scores ($p < .01$), and in the intergroup analysis, the average posttest score was significantly higher in the intervention group than in the control group ($p < .01$).

A statistically significant correlation was found at the low–medium level on the positive side, ranging from .288 to .587 between the average pretest and posttest scores on the Self-Care Agency Scale and MacNew in both groups. Moreover, a statistically significant correlation was found at the low–medium level on the positive side, ranging from .369 to .482 between the average pretest and posttest scores on the Self-Care Agency Scale and 15D in both groups. Furthermore, a statistically significant correlation was noted at the medium–high level on the positive side, ranging from .677 to .852 on MacNew and 15D in both groups.

Discussion

When the distribution according to CAD risk factors was examined, it was found that both groups widely shared family histories of CAD and lived a sedentary lifestyle and stressful lives. The posttest LDL cholesterol level was found to be higher than the pretest level in both groups. Similarly, previous studies have found that individuals with CAD tend to have a family history of the disease (Herman et al., 2014; Kang & Yang, 2013; Saffi et al., 2014), to live a sedentary lifestyle (Saffi et al., 2014; Tokgözoğlu et al., 2010), and to have stressful lives (Herman et al., 2014). In this study, the two groups were distributed homogeneously based on CAD risk factors, with results consistent with results previously reported in the literature. Steps toward identifying effective risk factors in CAD formation, providing primary protection to the population

Table 2

Distribution and Comparison of Patients by CAD Risk Factors

Distribution	Intervention Group (n = 51)		Control Group (n = 51)		χ²	p
	n	%	n	%		
Hereditary					0.20	.65
Yes	37	72.5	39	76.5		
No	14	27.5	12	25.5		
Serum lipids: LDL cholesterol (mg/dl; posttest)[a]					0.63	.42
≤ 70	7	13.7	10	19.6		
> 70	44	86.3	41	80.4		
Total cholesterol (mg/dl; pretest)					0.99	.31
≤ 200	31	60.8	26	51.0		
> 200	20	39.2	25	49.0		
Total cholesterol (mg/dl; posttest)					0.82	.36
≤ 200	36	70.6	40	78.4		
> 200	15	29.4	11	21.6		
Triglyceride (mg/dl; pretest)					0.98	.32
≤ 150	23	45.1	28	54.9		
> 150	28	54.9	23	45.1		
Triglyceride (mg/dl; posttest)					0.35	.55
≤ 150	30	58.8	27	52.9		
> 150	21	41.2	24	47.1		
HDL cholesterol (mg/dl; pretest)					0.36	.54
≥ 40	23	45.1	20	39.2		
< 40	28	54.9	31	60.8		
HDL cholesterol (mg/dl; posttest)					0.62	.42
≥ 40	23	45.1	27	52.9		
< 40	28	54.9	24	47.1		
BMI (kg/m²; pretest)					0.36	.54
≤ 30	32	62.7	29	56.9		
> 30	19	37.3	22	43.1		
BMI (kg/m²; posttest)					1.02	.31
≤ 30	33	64.7	28	54.9		
> 30	18	35.3	23	45.1		
Waist circumference (cm; pretest)					0.05	.81
♀: ≤ 88, ♂: ≤ 95	12	23.5	13	25.5		
♀: ≥ 88, ♂: ≥ 95	39	76.5	38	74.5		
Waist circumference (cm; posttest)					0.92	.33
♀: ≤ 88, ♂: ≤ 95	13	25.5	9	17.6		
♀: ≥ 88, ♂: ≥ 95	38	74.5	42	82.4		
Hypertension[b]					2.54	.11
Yes	26	78.8	22	61.1		
No	7	21.2	14	38.9		
Diabetes[b]					0.16	.68
Yes	14	42.4	17	47.2		
No	19	57.6	19	52.8		
Cigarette					1.32	.51
Smoking	21	41.2	24	47.1		
No smoking	15	29.4	17	33.3		
Quit smoking	15	29.4	10	19.6		

(continues)

Table 2

Distribution and Comparison of Patients by CAD Risk Factors, Continued

Distribution	Intervention Group (n = 51)		Control Group (n = 51)		χ^2	p
	n	%	n	%		
Alcohol					0.37	.82
Drinking	1	2.0	2	3.9		
No drinking	38	74.5	38	74.5		
Quit drinking	12	23.5	11	21.6		
Sedentary lifestyle					2.13	.14
Yes	14	27.5	21	41.2		
No	37	72.5	30	58.8		
Stressors					0.56	.81
Yes	40	78.4	39	76.5		
No	11	21.6	12	23.5		

Note. CAD = coronary artery disease; BMI = body mass index; HDL = high-density lipoprotein; LDL = low-density lipoprotein.

[a]LDL cholesterol pretest measurement of >70 mg/dl is the sampling criterion and so is not included in the table.

[b]Numbers of patients with chronic diseases: intervention group, n = 33; control group, n = 36.

and to high-risk individuals, providing secondary protection through the identification of the current risk factors for CAD, and improving quality of life and tertiary protection, including morbidity and mortality rate reduction and rehabilitation implementation, have gained in importance (Onat, 2009; WHO, 2019). In this respect, the fact that the risk factors of CAD were identified in this study as well as in the control group

patients is considered to be an indicator that the patient sample was properly selected.

In both groups, only the average posttest LDL cholesterol and total cholesterol levels were low, and the intragroup difference was statistically significant. Studies have reported a decrease in intergroup levels of LDL cholesterol (Jiang et al., 2007; Saffi et al., 2014; Wood et al., 2008), triglyceride (Jiang et al., 2007), and total cholesterol (Jiang et al., 2007; Wood et al., 2008), whereas intergroup differences have been found to be highly significant only in these studies (Jiang et al., 2007; Wood et al., 2008). The training provided by a researcher on cholesterol-lowering drug therapy and dietary and lifestyle changes may account for the decrease in the LDL cholesterol and total cholesterol levels in the intervention group. The decrease in LDL cholesterol and total cholesterol levels in the control group may be associated with the recommendations of cardiologists and nurses regarding cholesterol-lowering drug treatments and dietary and lifestyle changes given before discharge and during outpatient clinic visits, as no statistically significant differences were observed between the average intergroup pretest and posttest scores for serum lipid levels, arterial blood pressure, and waist circumference.

The average intragroup and intergroup posttest scores for the intervention group on the Self-Care Agency Scale were found to be significantly higher than those for the control group (Table 3). In a prior study conducted to determine self-care agency in patients with CAD, self-care agency (59.13 ± 12.62) was found to be low (Hassani et al., 2010). In this study, the higher average self-care agency score and better self-care agency in the intervention group than in the control group are consistent with the findings previously reported in the literature. Therefore, the training program

Table 3

Comparison of Pretest and Posttest Mean Scores of Self-Care Agency Scale, MacNew, and 15D

Scale	Intervention Group			Control Group			U	p
	M	SD	Median	M	SD	Median		
Self-Care Agency Scale								
Pretest	93.09	18.30	96.00	87.68	23.44	87.00	1110.0	.20
Posttest	119.96	12.27	121.00	91.23	21.04	92.00	287.5	< .001
	z = −5.923, p < .001			z = −1.275, p = .20				
MacNew								
Pretest	5.09	1.36	5.40	5.03	1.38	5.07	1270.5	.84
Posttest	6.40	0.61	6.59	5.01	1.10	5.25	271.0	< .001
	z = −5.672, p < .001			z = −0.145, p = .88				
15D								
Pretest	0.85	0.06	0.84	0.85	0.07	0.85	1279.0	.88
Posttest	0.95	0.05	0.96	0.86	0.08	0.85	455.0	< .001
	z = −5.952, p < .001			z = −0.994, p = .32				

Note. MacNew = MacNew Heart Disease Health-Related Quality of Life Questionnaire; U = Mann–Whitney U test; z = Wilcoxon sign test; 15D = Quality of Life Questionnaire.

based on Orem's SCDNT increased the level of CAD-related awareness and improved lifestyle habits and disease risk factors. Furthermore, the intervention was effective in improving self-care agency by increasing awareness of, ability to utilize, and ability to further enhance their self-care agency.

In addition, the average posttest scores on MacNew for the intervention group were significantly higher than those for the control group (Table 3). In studies using MacNew to assess quality of life in patients with cardiac disease (Daskapan et al., 2008; Höfer et al., 2012; Sevinç & Akyol, 2010), good results have been reported. In comparing the results of this study with those in the literature (Daskapan et al., 2008; Höfer et al., 2012; Sevinç & Akyol, 2010), the average quality-of-life score related to CAD was found to be higher in the intervention group than in the control group. This result suggests that the training based on Orem's SCDNT resulted in positive behavioral changes in the intervention group that allowed participants to better manage their disease.

Table 3 shows the comparison between average pretest and posttest scores on 15D. In the intervention group, the difference between the average intragroup and intergroup posttest scores on 15D was significantly larger than that in the control group. In previous studies that used 15D (Heiskanen et al., 2016; Sintonen, 2009), patients were found to have a good quality of life (mean score: 0.82–0.95). The overall quality of life of the intervention group in this study seems to be better than that of patients in other studies (Heiskanen et al., 2016; Sintonen, 2009). This result may relate to the fact that the training based on Orem's SCDNT improved self-care agency and cardiac-disease-specific quality of life by effectively promoting lifestyle changes. The nursing initiative that was employed to improve self-care skills in the intervention group may also have improved self-care abilities and disease-related adjustments, while also boosting overall quality of life by improving functional abilities and promoting the effective management of disease progression.

To the best of our knowledge, no previous study has evaluated the correlation among the Self-Care Agency Scale, MacNew, and 15D in patients with CAD. However, several studies have evaluated the correlation between various scales such as the Self-Care Agency Scale, the Short Form-36, EuroQoL-5 dimension, 15D, and MacNew in chronic diseases such as CAD, chronic obstructive pulmonary disease, and diabetes (Heiskanen et al., 2016; Höfer et al., 2008). In these studies, self-care agency and disease-specific and overall quality of life were found to affect each other at low (Heiskanen et al., 2016), middle (Höfer et al., 2008), and high (Akinci et al., 2005) levels. Therefore, determining self-care agency and the disease-specific and overall quality of life of patients with CAD positively contributes to current scholarly knowledge on this subject.

This study is affected by several limitations. Although CAD is among the most frequently observed diseases and a common cause of death worldwide, the number of patients included in this study was limited (102). In addition, conducting the last follow-up during the autumn–winter season limited this study to home environments and ended the measurement of physiological parameters (BMI and waist circumference) in early autumn.

In conclusion, the Orem's SCDNT-based training program used in this study significantly increased self-care agency and disease-specific and overall quality of life in the intervention group. The use of theory in nursing practice systematizes care planning and organizes professional knowledge into a conceptual framework, providing an effective guide to nurses in terms of what to do and why actions should be taken. In addition, nurses should pay closer attention to the CAD-related educational level of their patients with CAD to best teach them how to live with their disease. Therefore, it is suggested that Orem's SCDNT be used as a guide to strengthen self-care and increase quality of life in patients with CAD from the time of hospital admission and discharge through the postdischarge period. Furthermore, medical institutions and governments should develop educational policies for patients at risk of CAD and for those with CAD.

Acknowledgments

This study was supported by the Scientific and Technological Research Council of Turkey (TUBİTAK). We thank Associate Professor Ahmet Altun for his help in data analysis. We also thank all of the patients and their families for their participation.

Author Contributions

Study conception and design: FTY, MK
Data collection: FTY
Data analysis and interpretation: FTY, MK
Drafting of the article: FTY, MK
Critical revision of the article: FTY, MK

References

Akinci, F., Yildirim, A., Ogutman, B., Ates, M., Gozu, H., Deyneli, O., Aydar, S., Isci, E., Balcioglu, L., & Sayhan, O. Z. (2005). Translation, cultural adaptation, initial reliability, and validation of Turkish 15D's version: A generic health-related quality of life (HRQoL) instrument. *Evaluation & Health Professions*, *28*(1), 53–66. https://doi.org/10.1177/0163278704273078

Berbiglia, V. A., & Banfield, B. (2014). Self-care deficit theory of nursing. In M. R., Alligood (Ed.), *Nursing theorists and their work* (8th ed., pp. 240–257). Elsevier.

Butcher, L., & Castelluci, D. (2011). Nursing management: Coronary artery disease and acute coronary syndrome. In S. L., Lewis, S. R., Dirksen, M. M., Heitkemper, L., Bucher, & I. M., Camera (Eds.), *Medical-surgical nursing: Assessment and management of clinical problems* (8th ed., pp. 760–796). Elsevier Mosby.

Büyüköztürk, Ş. (2010). *Data analysis handbook for social sciences* (12th ed., pp. 31–37). Pegem Academy.

Daskapan, A., Höfer, S., Oldridge, N., Alkan, N., Muderrisoglu, H., & Tuzun, E. H. (2008). The validity and reliability of the Turkish version of the MacNew Heart Disease Questionnaire in patients with angina. *Journal of Evaluation in Clinical Practice, 14*(2), 209–213. https://doi.org/10.1111/j.1365-2753.2007.00834.x

Dilek, F., Ünsar, S., & Süt, N. (2010). Assessment quality of life in patients with coronary artery disease. *Fırat Sağlık Hizmetleri Dergisi (Fırat Health Services Journal), 5*(13), 29–44. (Original work published in Turkish)

Durmaz, T., Özdemir, Ö., Özdemir, B. A., Keleş, T., Bayram, N. A., & Bozkurt, E. (2009). Factor affecting quality of life in patients with coronary heart disease. *Turkish Journal of Medical Sciences, 39*(3), 343–351. https://doi.org/10.3906/sag-0901-26

Fawcett, J., & DeSanto-Madeya, S. (2013). *Contemprorary nursing knowledge: Analysis and evuluation of nursing models and theories* (3rd ed.). F. A. Davis Company.

Hall, A. M. (2013). Patient education. In P. A., Potter, A. G., Perry, P., Stockert, & A., Hall (Eds.), *Fundamentals of nursing* (8th ed., pp. 328–348). Mosby.

Hassani, M., Farahani, B., Zohour, A. R., & Azar, P. (2010). Self-care ability based on Orem's theory in individuals with coronary artery disease. *Iranian Journal of Critical Care Nursing, 3*(2), 87–91.

Heiskanen, J., Tolppanen, A.-M., Roine, R. P., Hartikainen, J., Hippeläinen, M., Miettinen, H., & Martikainen, J. (2016). Comparison of EQ-5D and 15D instruments for assessing the health-related quality of life in cardiac surgery patients. *European Heart Journal: Quality of Care & Clinical Outcomes, 2*(3), 193–200. https://doi.org/10.1093/ehjqcco/qcw002

Herman, R., Liebergall, M., & Rott, D. (2014). Correlation between participation in a cardiac rehabilitation program and quality of life of patients with coronary artery disease. *Rehabilitation Nursing, 39*(4), 192–197. https://doi.org/10.1002/rnj.118

Höfer, S., Saleem, A., Stone, J., Thomas, R., Tulloch, H., & Oldridge, N. (2012). The MacNew Heart Disease Health-Related Quality of Life Questionnaire in patients with angina and patients with ischemic heart failure. *Value in Health, 15*(1), 143–150. https://doi.org/10.1016/j.jval.2011.07.003

Höfer, S., Schmid, J. P., Frick, M., Benzer, W., Laimer, H., Oldridge, N., & Saner, H. (2008). Psychometric properties of the MacNew heart disease health-related quality of life instrument in patients with heart failure. *Journal of Evaluation Clinical Practice, 14*(4), 500–506. https://doi.org/10.1111/j.1365-2753.2007.00905.x

Jiang, X., Sit, J. W., & Wong, T. K. (2007). A nurse-led cardiac rehabilitation programme improves health behaviours and cardiac physiological risk parameters: Evidence from Chengdu, China. *Journal of Clinical Nursing, 16*(10), 1886–1897. https://doi.org/10.1111/j.1365-2702.2006.01838.x

Johnson, B. M. (2015). Nursing theory. In B. M., Johnsson & P. B., Webber (Eds.), *An introduction to theory and reasoning in nursing* (pp. 158–161). Wolters Kluwer Health.

Kang, Y., & Yang, I. S. (2013). Cardiac self-efficacy and its predictors in patients with coronary artery diseases. *Journal of Clinical Nursing, 22*(17–18), 2465–2473. https://doi.org/10.1111/jocn.12142

Kearney, B. Y., & Fleischer, B. J. (1979). Development of an instrument to measure exercise of self-care agency. *Research in Nursing & Health, 2*(1), 25–34. https://doi.org/10.1002/nur.4770020105

Küçükberber, N., Ozdilli, K., & Yorulmaz, H. (2011). Evaluation of factors affecting healthy life style behaviors and quality of life in patients with heart disease. *The Anatolian Journal of Cardiology, 11*(7), 619–626. https://doi.org/10.5152/akd.2011.166 (Original work published in Turkish)

Lukkarinen, H., & Hentinen, M. (2006). Treatments of coronary artery disease improve quality of life in the long term. *Nursing Research, 55*(1), 26–33.

MacNew, G. (2014). *Measuring outcome in heart disease: MacNew heart disease health-related quality of life instrument.* http://www.macnew.org/wp

Mohammadpour, A., Rahmati Sharghi, N., Khosravan, S., Alami, A., & Akhond, M. (2015). The effect of a supportive educational intervention developed based on the Orem's self-care theory on the self-care ability of patients with myocardial infarction: A randomised controlled trial. *Journal of Clinical Nursing, 24*(11–12), 1686–1692. https://doi.org/10.1111/jocn.12775

Nahcivan, N. (1993). *Effect of domestic environments and self-care on healthy young people* [Unpublished doctoral dissertation]. Istanbul University, Turkey. (Original work published in Turkish)

Norris, C. M., Patterson, L., Galbraith, D., & Hegadoren, K. M. (2009). All you have to do is call; a pilot study to improve the outcomes of patients with coronary artery disease. *Applied Nursing Research, 22*(2), 133–137. https://doi.org/10.1016/j.apnr.2007.06.003

Onat, A. (2009). *Prevalence of heart disease in our adults, new coronary events and prevalence of death from heart.* https://file.tkd.org.tr/PDFs/TEKHARF-2017.pdf (Original work published in Turkish)

Pınar, R. (1995). *Investigation of factors affecting quality of life and quality of life of patients with diabetes mellitus* [Unpublished doctoral dissertation]. Istanbul University, Turkey. (Original work published in Turkish)

Saffi, M. A., Polanczyk, C. A., & Rabelo-Silva, E. R. (2014). Lifestyle interventions reduce cardiovascular risk in patients with coronary artery disease: A randomized clinical trial. *European Journal of Cardiovascular Nursing, 13*(5), 436–443. https://doi.org/10.1177/1474515113505396

Sevinç, S., & Akyol, A. D. (2010). Cardiac risk factors and quality of life in patients with coronary artery disease. *Journal of Clinical Nursing, 19*(9–10), 1315–1325. https://doi.org/10.1111/j.1365-2702.2010.03220.x

Sintonen, H. (2009). The 15D instrument of health-related quality of life: Properties and applications. *Annals of Medicine, 33*(5), 328–336. https://doi.org/10.3109/07853890109002086

Taylor, C. R., Lillis, C., Lemone, P., & Lynn, P. (2011). *Fundamentals of nursing the art and science of nursing care* (7th ed.). Lippincott Williams & Wilkins.

Tokgözoğlu, L., Kaya, E. B., Erol, Ç., Ergene, O., & EUROASPIRE III Turkey Study Group. (2010). EUROASPIRE III: A comparison between Turkey and Europe. *Archives Turkish Society of Cardiology, 38*(3), 167–172. (Original work published in Turkish)

Wood, D. A., Kotseva, K., Connolly, S., Jennings, C., Mead, A., Jones, J., Holden, A., De Bacquer, D., Collier, T., De Backer, G., Faergeman, O., & EUROACTION Study Group. (2008). Nurse-coordinated multidisciplinary, family-based cardiovascular disease prevention programme (EUROACTION) for patients with coronary heart disease and asymptomatic individuals at high risk of cardiovascular disease: A paired, cluster-randomised controlled trial. *The Lancet, 371*(9629), 1999–2012. https://doi.org/10.1016/s0140-6736(08)60868-5

World Health Organization. (2019). *Global action plan for the prevention and control of NCDs 2013–2020.* http://www.who.int/nmh/publications/ncd-action-plan/en/

Permissions

All chapters in this book were first published by Wolters Kluwer; hereby published with permission under the Creative Commons Attribution License or equivalent. Every chapter published in this book has been scrutinized by our experts. Their significance has been extensively debated. The topics covered herein carry significant findings which will fuel the growth of the discipline. They may even be implemented as practical applications or may be referred to as a beginning point for another development.

The contributors of this book come from diverse backgrounds, making this book a truly international effort. This book will bring forth new frontiers with its revolutionizing research information and detailed analysis of the nascent developments around the world.

We would like to thank all the contributing authors for lending their expertise to make the book truly unique. They have played a crucial role in the development of this book. Without their invaluable contributions this book wouldn't have been possible. They have made vital efforts to compile up to date information on the varied aspects of this subject to make this book a valuable addition to the collection of many professionals and students.

This book was conceptualized with the vision of imparting up-to-date information and advanced data in this field. To ensure the same, a matchless editorial board was set up. Every individual on the board went through rigorous rounds of assessment to prove their worth. After which they invested a large part of their time researching and compiling the most relevant data for our readers.

The editorial board has been involved in producing this book since its inception. They have spent rigorous hours researching and exploring the diverse topics which have resulted in the successful publishing of this book. They have passed on their knowledge of decades through this book. To expedite this challenging task, the publisher supported the team at every step. A small team of assistant editors was also appointed to further simplify the editing procedure and attain best results for the readers.

Apart from the editorial board, the designing team has also invested a significant amount of their time in understanding the subject and creating the most relevant covers. They scrutinized every image to scout for the most suitable representation of the subject and create an appropriate cover for the book.

The publishing team has been an ardent support to the editorial, designing and production team. Their endless efforts to recruit the best for this project, has resulted in the accomplishment of this book. They are a veteran in the field of academics and their pool of knowledge is as vast as their experience in printing. Their expertise and guidance has proved useful at every step. Their uncompromising quality standards have made this book an exceptional effort. Their encouragement from time to time has been an inspiration for everyone.

The publisher and the editorial board hope that this book will prove to be a valuable piece of knowledge for researchers, students, practitioners and scholars across the globe.

List of Contributors

Knar Sagherian
College of Nursing, The University of Tennessee Knoxville, USA

Linsey M. Steege
School of Nursing, University of Wisconsin-Madison, USA

Jeanne Geiger-Brown
School of Nursing, George Washington University, USA

Donna Harrington
School of Social Work, University of Maryland, Baltimore, USA

Shing-Chia Chen
School of Nursing, College of Medicine, National Taiwan University and Supervisor, Department of Nursing, National Taiwan University Hospital

Shih-Kai Lee
Department of Nursing, Tsaotun Psychiatric Center, Ministry of Health and Welfare

Jiin-Ru Rong
School of Nursing, National Taipei University of Nursing and Health Sciences

Chien-Chang Wu
Department and Graduate Institute of Medical Education and Bioethics, College of Medicine, National Taiwan University

Wen-I Liu
School of Nursing, National Taipei University of Nursing and Health Sciences

Su Jung LEE and Mi So KIM
Korea University College of Nursing, Seoul, Republic of Korea

You Jin JUNG
National Evidence-Based Healthcare Collaborating Agency, Seoul, Republic of Korea

Leili BORIMNEJAD
Center for Nursing Care Research, Iran University of Medical Sciences, Tehran, Iran

Marjan MARDANI-HAMOOLEH
Iran University of Medical Sciences, Tehran, Iran

Naimeh SEYEDFATEMI
Center for Nursing Care Research, Iran University of Medical Sciences, Tehran, Iran

Mamak TAHMASEBI
Cancer Institute, Tehran University of Medical Sciences, Tehran, Iran

Mi So KIM, Su Jung LEE and Min Sun PARK
College of Nursing, Korea University, Seoul

Gyu-Tae KIM
School of Electrical Engineering, Korea University, Seoul

Eun-hye JEONG
College of Nursing, Korea University, Seoul

Sung Ok CHANG
College of Nursing, Korea University, Seoul
College of Nursing, Korea University, ROK
Korea University College of Nursing, Seoul, Republic of Korea

Sun-Young LIM
College of Nursing, Baekseok Culture University, ROK

Wei-Fang WANG
Nursing Department and Education Center, National Cheng Kung University Hospital, College of Medicine, National Cheng Kung University and Doctoral Candidate, School of Nursing, Kaohsiung Medical University, Taiwan, ROC

Chich-Hsiu HUNG
School of Nursing, Kaohsiung Medical University and Adjunct Research Professor, Department of Medical Research, Kaohsiung Medical University Hospital, Taiwan, ROC

Chung-Yi LI
Department of Public Health, College of Medicine, National Cheng Kung University, Taiwan, ROC

Seher ÜNVER
Faculty of Health Sciences, Department of Surgical Nursing, Trakya University, Edirne, Turkey

Remziye SEMERCI
Faculty of Health Sciences, Department of Child Health and Disease Nursing, Trakya University, Edirne, Turkey

Zeynep Kızılcık ÖZKAN
Faculty of Health Sciences, Department of Surgical Nursing, Trakya University, Edirne, Turkey

İlker AVCIBAŞI
Faculty of Health Sciences, Department of Public Health Nursing, Trakya University, Edirne, Turkey

Hyangjin PARK
Department of Prevention and Public Relations & Research and Development Team, Korea Center on Gambling Problems, Seoul, Republic of Korea

Haeryun CHO
Department of Nursing, Wonk wang University, Iksan, Republic of Korea

Emmanuel Zamokwakhe HLUNGWANE and Benedict Raphael OAMEN
Department of Nursing Science, Nelson Mandela University, Port Elizabeth, South Africa

Wilma TEN HAM-BALOYI
Faculty of Health Sciences, Nelson Mandela University, Port Elizabeth, South Africa

Portia JORDAN
Faculty of Medicine and Health Sciences, Department of Nursing and Midwifery, Stellenbosch University, South Africa

Mihyun PARK
College of Nursing, The Catholic University of Korea, Seoul, ROK

Eun-Jun PARK
Department of Nursing, Konkuk University, ROK

Ahmad RAYAN
Psychiatric and Mental Health Nursing, Zarqa University, Jordan

Mo'men SISAN
BSN, RN, Oncology Specialist Nurse, King Abdullah Medical City, Mecca, Saudi Arabia

Omar BAKER
College of Nursing, King Saud University, Riyadh, Saudi Arabia

Zhen LI
Gynaecology and Obstetrics Division, the Affiliated Hospital of Putian University, Putian, People's Republic of China

Fei-Fei HUANG
School of Nursing, Fujian Medical University, Fuzhou, People's Republic of China

Shiah-Lian CHEN
Department of Nursing, National Taichung University of Science and Technology, Taichung, Taiwan, Republic of China

Anni WANG
School of Nursing, Fudan University, Shanghai, People's Republic of China

Yufang GUO
School of Nursing, Shandong University, People's Republic of China

Hatice KARABULAK
MSN, RN, Ministry of Health, Turkey

Fadime KAYA
Faculty of Health Sciences, Department of Mental Health and Psychiatric Nursing, Kafkas University, Kars, Turkey

Fatemeh SHIRAZI
Department of Nursing, School of Nursing and Midwifery, Shiraz University of Medical Sciences, Shiraz, Iran

Shiva HEIDARI
Department of Nursing, Urmia Branch, Islamic Azad University, Urmia, Iran

Yi-Ya CHANG
Department of Nursing and Clinical Competency Center, Chang Gung University of Science and Technology and Assistant Research Fellow, Chang Gung Medical Foundation, Taiwan, ROC

Miao-Chuan CHEN
Department of Nursing, Chang Gung University of Science and Technology, Taiwan, ROC

Ru-Wen LIAO
Department of Nursing, Taipei Tzu Chi Hospital, Buddhist Tzu Chi Medical Foundation

Mei-Ling YEH
School of Nursing, National Taipei University of Nursing and Health Sciences

Kuan-Chia LIN
Institute of Hospital and Health Care Administration, National Yang-Ming University

Kwua-Yun WANG
Rui Guang Health care Group and Jointly Appointed Professor, School of Nursing, National Defense Medical Center

Kyung Eun Lee
Department of Nursing, Keimyung College University, Daegu, South Korea

Ying-Ying KO
MSN, RN,NP, Department of Nursing, Kaohsiung Medical University Hospital, Kaohsiung Medical University, Taiwan, ROC

Yi LIU
School of Nursing, Kaohsiung Medical University, Taiwan, ROC

Hsing-Mei CHEN
Department of Nursing, College of Medicine, National Cheng Kung University, Taiwan, ROC

Hsiu-Yun LIAO
School of Nursing, Kaohsiung Medical University, Taiwan, ROC

Yu-Mei LIAO
Department of Nursing, Kaohsiung Medical University Hospital, Kaohsiung Medical University, Taiwan, ROC

Hsiao-Ying HUNG and Yu-Wen WANG, Jui-Ying FENG and Esther Ching-Lan LIN
Department of Nursing, College of Medicine, National Cheng Kung University

Ying-Ju CHANG
Institution of Allied Health Sciences and Department of Nursing, College of Medicine, National Cheng Kung University and Director, Department of Nursing, National Cheng Kung University Hospital, College of Medicine, National Cheng Kung University

Ahmad E. ABOSHAIQAH
College of Nursing, King Saud University, Saudi Arabia

Jui-O CHEN
Department of Nursing, Tajen University, Pingtung, Taiwan, ROC

Chiu-Chu LIN
School of Nursing; Department of Renal Care, College of Medicine; and Department of Medical Research, Kaohsiung Medical University Hospital, Kaohsiung Medical University, Kaohsiung, Taiwan, ROC

Feng-Huang YANG
Department of Nursing at Chung Kang Branch, Cheng Ching Hospital

Feng-Yu LIN
General Education Center, Overseas Chinese University

Yueh-Juen HWU
College of Nursing, Central Taiwan University of Science and Technology

Cheng-Chen CHOU
Institute of Community Health Care, College of Nursing, National Yang Ming Chiao Tung University, Taipei, Taiwan

Jen-Jiuan LIAW
School of Nursing, National Defense Medical Center, Taipei, Taiwan

Chuan - Chuan CHEN
Department of Nursing, National Cheng Kung University Hospital, Tainan, Taiwan

Yiing-Mei LIOU
Institute of Community Health Care, College of Nursing, National Yang Ming Chiao Tung University, Taipei, Taiwan

Chi-Jane WANG
Department of Nursing, College of Medicine, National Cheng Kung University and National Cheng Kung University Hospital, Tainan, Taiwan
Department of Nursing, College of Medicine, National Cheng Kung University, Taiwan, ROC
Department of Nursing, College of Medicine, National Cheng Kung University

Majid BAGHERI HOSSEIN ABADI
MS, School of Public Health, Shahroud University of Medical Science, Shahroud, Iran

Ebrahim TABAN
Social Determinants of Health Research Center, Department of Occupational Health Engineering, Mashhad University of Medical Sciences, Mashhad, Iran

Narges KHANJANI
Neurology Research Center, Kerman University of Medical Sciences, Kerman, Iran

Zahra NAGHAVI KONJIN and Seyed Ehsan SAMAEI
Health Sciences Research Center, Addiction Institute, Mazandaran University Medical Sciences, Sari, Iran

Farahnaz KHAJEHNASIRI
Department of Community Medicine, Faculty of Medicine, Tehran University of Medical Sciences, Tehran, Iran

Fatma TOK YILDIZ
Program of Anaesthesia, Department of Medical Services and Techniques, Vocational School of Health Services, Sivas Cumhuriyet University, Sivas, Turkey

Mağfiret KAŞIKÇI
Faculty of Nursing, Atatürk University, Erzurum, Turkey

Index

Printed in the USA
CPSIA information can be obtained
at www.ICGtesting.com
JSHW051406091023
49903JS00006B/296